~The~
Qur'anic
Prescription

~

Unlocking the Secrets to Optimal Health

MADIHA M. SAEED, MD

KUBE
PUBLISHING

The Qur'anic Prescription: Unlocking the Secrets to Optimal Health

First published in England by
Kube Publishing Ltd,
Markfield Conference Centre,
Ratby Lane, Markfield,
Leicestershire, LE67 9SY,
United Kingdom Tel: +44 (0) 1530 249230

Website: www.kubepublishing.com
Email: info@kubepublishing.com

Cataloguing-in-Publication Data is available from the British Library

ISBN Paperback: 978-1-84774-161-5
ISBN Ebook: 978-1-84774-162-2

Cover design and Arabic calligraphy: Jannah Haque
Internal Design and Typesetting: LiteBook Prepress Services
Printed by Elma Basim, Turkey

"And We send down of the Qur'an that which is healing and mercy for the believers, but it does not increase the wrongdoers except in loss."

(Qur'an 17:82)

Dedication

In memory of Zaina Batal Seede
Can't thank Allah enough for bringing you into my life!
A friendship started in heaven
She enhanced the world of everyone she met
Radiating love and gratitude
May Allah place her in the highest Jannah
May her children, Noah and Isaac continue to exemplify all she taught them

Acknowledgements

I Can't Thank Allah Enough!

And [remember] when your Lord proclaimed, 'If you are grateful, I will surely increase you [in favour].... (Qur'an 14:7)

Allah is the Ar-Rahman, Ar-Raheem. I can't thank Allah enough for opening my eyes and heart to this mission. Can't thank Allah enough for all the blessings in my life, most of all— my parents, my family. My parents sacrificed everything, literally everything for me and my siblings to be where we are today. They sacrificed and sold our home, left loved ones, family and friends, moved multiple times and so much more—only because my parents wanted us to live our lives without debt, a life without interest, live our lives according to our dīn. My parents sacrificed everything in the name of Allah, putting full tawakkul (trust in Allah), opening my heart to the power of unconditional love, gratitude and what it truly means to trust Allah, when the world is telling you different.

I can't thank Allah enough for my husband, Omer, my siblings, Athar, Fasiha, Sophi and Atif and in-laws, who supported me through every hurdle, took on my "crazy" ideas and respected me and loved me through everything I learned. I've had to change my entire lifestyle, change foods, change dietary habits, and my family tolerated and supported me. Finding new restaurants, changed foods at large family events, attending my talks, watching and spoiling my children, spoiling me, letting me take a break and shower—I have been truly blessed. I can't thank Allah enough for gifting me with the most loving and supportive family. Love you all so much!

I can't thank Allah enough for friends and family who support me, edit my books, listen to my ideas on educating the world and encouraging me every step of the way. Can't thank Allah enough for Zaina Batal Seede. We met at Whole Foods talking to each other across the aisles, living blocks away with our children in the same classes--we were so much alike! I've never met someone so positive, loving, friendly, packed with optimism and energy. She taught me so much, exemplifying

vi

what it means to have faith. Cheering me on every step of the way. Dropping off halal and tayyib treats at my doorstep, reading all my books, implementing all she learned, we were in this together. She edited every book I wrote multiple times, including this one two weeks before she passed away. When this mission seemed too big, she would tell me, "Middo, Allah put you on this planet for his purpose, don't let anyone tell you otherwise." Zaina, I love you so much, your support, love and friendship has meant more to me than you will ever know. Can't thank Allah and her parents for bringing her into this world and into my life, when I needed her most. May Allah protect her children, Noah and Isaac, to exemplify all she taught them to be righteous human beings.

I can't thank Allah enough for adopted parents, Uncle Fahim, Aunty Naseem, Sr Jill and Dr Ahmad who blessed me with their wisdom and support. Thank you, Jazak Allah Khair for opening my eyes to, deepening my love for the Qur'an and Sunnah, helping me to understand the Qur'an in a whole different light. Can't thank Allah enough for Aunty Ayesha, Dr Uthman and Susan Cavallo that opened my eyes to the wonders of integrative, holistic and functional medicine.

I can't thank Allah enough for Kube Publishing, helping me make my dreams a reality. I can't thank Allah for all the leaders in functional, integrative and holistic medicine, that have educated and opened my eyes to real whole system healing, and the importance of a healthy lifestyle and helping me understand tayyib in more detail.

Most importantly, my children, Abdullah, Zain, Emaad, Qasim—my gifts from Allah. While writing this book one day, while they fold laundry, I asked them, "Why did Allah bless me with such amazing children?" They replied, "Mama, Allah made a deal with you. If He gave you good children, you would have to work for Allah, teaching people how to take care of the blessings Allah gave us. You start it and we can work with you!"

May Allah continue to bless each step we all take. May every word I speak, and even letter I write, continue to shower those that blessed my life with Allah's infinite blessings. The power of unconditional love and sacrifice, completely for the sake of Allah, can open doors that one could have never even imagined.

My Lord, enable me to be grateful for Your favor which You have bestowed upon me and upon my parents and to work righteousness of which You will approve and make righteous for me my offspring. Indeed, I have repented to You, and indeed, I am of the Muslims.

(Qur'an 46:15)

Contents

ix

Disclaimer

This book represents reference material only. It is not intended as a medical manual, and the data presented here are meant to assist the reader in making informed choices regarding wellness. This book is not a replacement for treatment that the reader's personal physician may have suggested. If the reader believes he or she is experiencing a medical issue, professional medical help is recommended. Mention of particular products, companies, or authorities in this book does not entail endorsement by the publisher or author.

Foreword

I'll never forget the night I went to bed with an itchy red thumb on 5 December 2017. I shrugged it off as a mild allergic reaction to something I must have touched while visiting my parents in Florida. Little did I know that that tiny itch would be the beginning of something much more serious. The next morning, I woke up to a bright red, swollen face, hands and feet. Within two weeks, I was diagnosed with Pityriasis Rubra Pilaris (PRP). I was prescribed a few intense medications by my dermatologist and was left wondering how the days ahead would unfold. Over the next several days, the palms of my hands and the soles of my feet became thicker than normal; with the skin constantly peeling and feeling thick, like plastic. It was painful and difficult to grip with my hands and it hurt to walk on my feet. I couldn't even get out of bed without first filling the deep cracks in the soles of my feet with mounds of Aquaphor, then putting on my socks and shoes just to make walking bearable, both in and outside the house.

I felt ugly. I wore gloves to hide my hands. The hair on my eyebrows and head were noticeably thinning. My face and scalp were scaling and peeling. The rest of my body was intensely burning, turning purple, and shedding. No one had ever heard of my ultra-rare autoimmune disease, and it felt as if no one knew what I was going through. My nails turned yellow, thickened and became disfigured. Even though my body burned and itched, I also felt cold all the time. On top of that, I had insomnia, which made it difficult since all I could do was lie awake in utter pain and discomfort. One night, I remember waking up cold, with every pore on my body on fire, and it was then I thought to myself, 'Now I know what suffering feels like.' But the physical aspect of the disease was not the only difficulty. The disgusted looks, remarks, the subconscious pulling away when I drew near, and the discomfort people exhibited when my skin fell on their clothes or furniture was painful and heartbreaking. I remember feeling very connected to Prophet Ayūb (peace upon him) and his trial with his health.

Fast forward three weeks to the end of December 2017. I had been invited to speak at the MAS-ICNA Convention in Chicago months before I got sick. Now I had two options before me – stay home and be miserable, or travel with a peeling and burning body. It was Allah's ultimate mercy and guidance that inspired me to go. And what a blessing it was to go, since a miracle would take place and change my life forever.

During the convention, I gave a lecture, where I made a passing reference to my autoimmune disease. The next day, I prayed Maghrib along with thousands of others in the prayer hall. After finishing, I shook hands with the sister on my right and then with the sister to the right of her. That woman held on to my hand and yelled, 'Oh my God! Sister Lobna? I prayed to Allah I would meet you!' I was taken aback by her enthusiastic energy. So who was this person? She was none other than Dr. Madiha Saeed! Madiha told me that she was at my lecture just the day before and after hearing that I had an autoimmune disease, she tuned out everything else I said during the lecture while she tried to figure out how she could meet me. There in the prayer hall, Madiha handed me her then newly published book, *Holistic Rx*, and the rest is history.

How amazing is it that just a few hours earlier in the hotel room I had to give myself an injection, feeling deflated, as the expensive medicine spilled out of the needle instead of going into my skin and, later, out of hundreds of attendees sitting in the lecture hall, Dr. Madiha would be there to make *du'a* for me. And how amazing is it that when my dermatologist first told me about PRP, she told me, 'We don't know what triggers this disease and there is no cure,' yet when I met Dr. Madiha in the middle of the bustling prayer hall she said, 'We know what causes PRP and we know the cure!' And, finally, how amazing is it that I would get sick in Florida, go back home to Los Angeles to get diagnosed, and then fly to Chicago to find my cure, all within a span of three weeks. Truly Allah is the best of planners!

After returning home, I called Madiha, and so began my journey to healing. But first I was to take another journey. 'I need to leave,' I remember telling my husband. He knew it was for the best and so I booked a ticket to Florida to be with my parents for a week. That one-week visit turned into a one-month healing intensive. I left my husband, my four kids, missed my son getting his driver's license and endured the pleas of my younger children as they urged me to come home. I even missed my daughter speaking in front of 2,000 people at her county-level Academic Decathlon competition. I so badly wanted to go home, but we all knew it would delay my healing. During that time, I was grateful to my whole family, including my in-laws, who supported me greatly during this entire journey.

Based on the extensive lab work requested, Madiha recommended the Gut and Psychology Syndrome (GAPS) diet, homeopathic medications, supplements, daily salt baths and other lifestyle changes. I had been sick for two excruciating months, yet the *very* day I started the GAPS diet (with the dedicated and loving help of my mother), the intense burning lessened dramatically. All I ate, day and night, for a whole month, was boiled meat and vegetables in bone broth. No coffee, no salad, no fruit, *nada!* At one point, I was ready to go off all conventional medications. I not only received much hesitation from some of my family but also from my dermatologist who even wanted me to try an even more intensive drug. With full confidence in Madiha's conventional medical background (she is an MD after all), her success in curing her own multiple autoimmune diseases, her knowledge as a certified holistic, functional and integrative doctor, as well as her success with hundreds of patients, I stopped taking all conventional medication (after consulting with Dr. Madiha of course).

After a month, I went home excited to see my family. Yet my homecoming was bittersweet. Problems that were already brewing at home, came to a head. One of my children was struggling greatly and on top of it all, my marriage suffered immensely. We went to counseling, I made lots of supplication, cried and called Madiha several times. One key piece of advice from Madiha was crucial to maintaining my health during this crisis: gratitude – mindful and intentional gratitude. *If you are grateful, verily I will increase you in favour.* (14: 7) She reminded me of this verse in the noble Qur'an again and again. And even with so much going on, my body was healing, slowly and steadily. *Alhamdulillah* during this time, Allah not only healed me, but my family and my marriage as well.

Many of those who have my disease suffer for months and years on end; yet, thankfully, after only four months, I was completely cured! And not only that, I lost over thirty pounds as a side effect of clean living and eating. *Allāhu akbar!* Thinking back to that time, I now know that before I was diagnosed with PRP, I was already suffering from three other autoimmune diseases, all of which I dismissed as annoying symptoms that I just had to deal with. Yet, following the principles of Dr. Madiha's book, I was cured not only of PRP, but of three other diseases as well!

Looking at a year in review is quite revealing. Who knew that back in September of 2017, when I registered to participate in the Los Angeles Marathon, that not only would I be unable to run, but by the spring of 2018, I would barely be able to walk? And who knew that just one year after my diagnosis, I would go on a three-day, 33-mile backpacking trip, carrying thirty-five pounds on my back (and still sticking to my diet)?

"Verily with difficulty, comes ease. Verily with difficulty, comes ease." (Qur'an 94:5–6)

I am a firsthand witness and beneficiary to the success of Madiha's methodology. I now feel so strongly about this way of living that I want to share it with the world. I have dramatically changed the way my entire household eats so that it is "halal and *ṭayyib*", and everyone has benefitted. I gradually cleared out my pantry, throwing away toxic food and donating the rest. I changed out all household products, from hand soap, to detergents, to lotions. There was a lot of resistance, crying and complaining, but we got through it.

Dear reader, I must forewarn you: one big obstacle lies ahead of you – your thoughts. 'I don't have the discipline to change my diet,' will stop you from even trying. If I can do it, so can you. As a carbohydrate lover, former diet soda addict, and former processed and fast food fan, I was able to overcome my intense cravings. Learning about the science behind inflammation and understanding Allah's calling upon humanity to *eat that which is lawful and pure*, will hopefully give you the motivation you need to move forward in this journey, as it did for me. Another obstacle lies ahead of you as well: your well-meaning family, friends, and even co-workers. 'That's so hard!' 'Just a little cheating won't hurt.' 'You're not going to eat what I made?!' Just smile and say, 'I'm following Allah's orders and my doctor's, too.' So how do you start? – one thought and one meal at a time. May Allah grant you success in all your endeavors, *āmīn*.

Sincerely,

Lobna Mulla
Creator, YouTube Channel, Double Shot Mocha
Member, Yaqeen Institute, Board of Directors
Chaplain at UCLA, Institute of Knowledge

A Note from Renowned Islamic Scholars

"A wonderful book about how to care for ourselves in a way that allows us to improve not just the quality of our lives, but our worship as well." – **Imam Dr. Omar Suleiman**

"Dr. Madiha Saeed has written some important works given that, unfortunately, very few of our highly qualified physicians are paying attention to the importance of integral medicine and recognizing the many effective health modalities that are not limited to the allopathic tradition. Dr. Saeed is a board certified family physician and has studied holistic medicine from other traditions. She gives excellent advice in her books on how to have a more holistic approach to health. Health is partly a choice, and we all have a choice to actually maintain our health. Too many people neglect the maintenance of their health, and when they fall ill, they pray for a miraculous recovery. God, however, has given us everything we need. He's given us a phenomenal immune system and gifted us extraordinary foods that nourish and sustain. The Prophet Muhammad, peace and blessings be upon him, has warned us on lifestyle choices that can harm us both physically and spiritually. When the Muslims first came to Egypt, one of the great physicians, when he heard the verse from the Qur'an, "Eat and drink but not to excess," said, "Your Prophet hasn't left anything for the physicians."" – **Shaykh Hamza Yusuf**

"Dr. Madiha Saeed has performed a great service to the Muslim Ummah with her book, "The Qur'anic Prescription." Plunging into the deep and rich waters of the Qur'an and Sunnah, she brings forth priceless pearls of life enhancing wisdom. More than just a medical text, "The Qur'anic Prescription," examines the role that natural healing modalities, sleep, diet and various forms of stress relief play in fostering not just good health, but overall wellbeing. Building on her previous best seller, "The Holistic RX," "The Qur'anic Prescription," is a book that should be in the library of anyone searching for natural paths to healing and good health." – **Imam Zaid Shakir**

Our teachers of spirituality emphasize that the prerequisite to true tawbah (repentance) is māl ḥalāl (purity of wealth). It is also their observation that halal food, like halal money, creates the inclination to obey one's Lord and that haram food, like haram money, creates the inclination and strong urge to disobey Allah.

Think of it as a chain of events: halal money is used to purchase halal food that is then used to feed and nourish yourself and your family. The very food you eat then provides the energy to your body to create cells, the building blocks of life. Down to this microscopic level, the very cells replicating in your body as a result of the halal food you ate and, by extension, the halal money it was purchased with, have an inclination to obey Allah and aid you in this!

Unfortunately, the opposite is also true and at times we wonder why it is so difficult for us to obey Allah. It may not occur to us to look more closely at the food we consume and the money we purchase it with as a first step to growing stronger spiritually and deepening our relationship with God. Do check the sources of your income. Do make sure you only feed your body with what is rigorously halal, tayyib (pure and wholesome), and untainted with the disobedience of God for ultimately it affects your soul and the souls of your loved ones. May Allah, Most Great, bless your family and mine with abundant provisions and protection in this life and the next. Ameen. – **Rania Awaad, MD,** Clinical Associate Professor of Psychiatry and Director of Muslim Mental Health Lab, Stanford University School of Medicine, Director, Khalil Centre Bay Area, Director, The Rahmah Foundation, Professor of Islamic Law, Zaytuna College

This book is phenomenal! If you are serious about being informed on how to improve the quality of your life, not just your health, read this book! She does a great job of legitimizing the fact that it is an Islamic obligation to take care of our health; that which Allah has given us and can easily take away. Reading this book will encourage you to read the Qur'an and leave you with your own enlightening reflections regarding gratitude and its manifestation of self-care via nutrition. – **Sheikh Abdullah Oduro,** Yaqeen Institute, Imam at the Islamic Center of Coppell

Introduction

Wake up. Pray. Sleep. Wake up. Kids. Eat. Commute. Work. Pray. Eat. Work. Pray. Commute. Kids. Eat. Pray. Work. Pray. Sleep…*Repeat*.

March 2020, Allah gave the world a wake up call. In a world of constant stress, fear and negativity, we are sucked into a world of sickness. The world started to slow down, but with our busy lives, stuck on electronics, the worldly life continues to consume our thoughts, our habits, our eating, our time for good and it has also taken a toll on all our health, putting our future at risk.

Two blessings from the Almighty that many people take for granted – health and time. (Bukhārī).

Sadly, most people will continue on that hamster wheel, like mindless cattle, giving little thoughts to their actions. This wake up call, has bought us time to reflect on our health. Unfortunately, this pandemic has also shed light on another pandemic that has been slowly consuming our lives—chronic disease.

The burden of chronic diseases around the globe is continuing to grow at an alarming rate! Each year, 57 million people die around the world and three fourths of those deaths are due to chronic diseases. One third of all deaths occur from heart disease (up 50percent from 1999) and stroke (up 32percent), with cancer (up 69percent) being the second leading cause of death.[1] It is estimated that by 2045, there will be 700 million people living with diabetes (up 148percent) all over the world.[2] Worldwide obesity has nearly tripled since 1975.[3] Obesity affects one in every three adults and almost 2 billion adults are overweight. What is even worse is that the rise of chronic illness is also affecting our children, as one in five children are obese, with 38 million children under the age of 5 either overweight or obese[4].

According to the Global Burden of Disease study for 2019 published in *The Lancet*, it was found that while global healthy life expectancy has increased between 1990 and 2019, it has not risen as much as overall life expectancy in 198 of the 204 countries assessed, which means that people are living more years in poor health.

It is not just our bodies that are suffering, but also our children's brains. If we continue our current trajectory, one in every four children will have a form of autism by 2033.[4] Let's stop and think about that for a second. With chronic disease on the rise, what will happen to humanity if all our children are sick, and continue to get sicker?

Society Leaves Us Hopeless

We all know a child, a mother, a father, a sibling, a relative or a friend who is dealing with a chronic health condition. When the dark cloud of chronic disease permeates our lives, we turn straight to the doctors, for maybe an inkling of hope and power in changing our gloomy condition.

Conventional medicine works phenomenally well for acute care but, sadly, it has its limits when it comes to chronic illness. For the most part, instead of addressing the root causes of chronic diseases, doctors may just 'name it and tame it,' putting a band aid on the problem. The hope primarily lies in the pharmaceutical or surgical procedure, all with their own set of side effects and complications. Suddenly, you are stampled with a lifelong diagnosis, the life that was once yours has now been taken over by your chronic conditions, your doctor, the pharmaceutical and insurance companies! Don't get me wrong, sometimes we *need* medication and, in some situations, medication offers so much hope for symptom improvement, as you may need to put out the fire before you can control the blaze. Beyond the acute phase, beyond meds, there is very little hope of healing or lifestyle advice so you can take back charge of your health.

How do I know? As a family physician in the United States, I can tell you that conventionally trained doctors are taught very little about what we can do to heal and prevent chronic disease. For the vast majority of doctors, we are paid not for how many patients we *heal*, but for how many patients we *see*. Living in this world, my husband has to see 110 patients a week for our paycheck not to go half. So in a 10-15 minute appointment, physicians don't have enough time to address the root causes of diseases and to teach lifestyle techniques. Additionally, we were taught the worst patients were the ones that consulted "Dr Google", did their own research and presented different options in their care. You are expected to listen to whatever the doctor tells you, without questioning, otherwise, you are stamped with a "non-compliant" label. I do believe that most physicians truly intend to help their patients, but unfortunately the conventional medicine tools in our tool belt don't include many tools for preventing, and reversing chronic disease, leaving the patient with limited hope. I too was left with little hope.

When I was diagnosed with lupus, joint pain, severe fatigue, thyroid problems, digestive issues, acne, sebhorric dermatitis, indigestion, eczema and weight issues, I was left with little hope, despite being a physician. I felt that every corner I turned, there was another chronic condition, but when I was hit with a diagnosis that could take my life away, I searched for answers. I had watched so many die of this condition, I was determined not to be part of their number. Miserable, the only solution I was given was in pharmaceuticals. Was I supposed to be on these medications all my life? The side effects alone scared me. 'May cause death.' That is what I was trying to prevent! There had to be another way. Something just didn't make sense to me.

Hopeless, I turned to the Qur'an, I turned to Allah and discovered so much hope!

Allah Gives Us Hope

All through medical school, through residency and even as a practising medical physician, the approach to chronic diseases, how we dealt with the patient, the system, the limited supply of tools in our tool belt, didn't make sense to me. In Islam, Allah tells us to take charge of our lives, to never lose hope and to continue to look for answers. Allah taught us how to take care of our bodies (as our bodies have a right over us), He also taught us to continue to be in the best form that we could be and, most importantly, He taught us the importance of preventing problems.

But when we hear words like, 'Sorry, there is nothing more we can do,' or 'You will have to live with this diagnosis the rest of your life,' or 'There is nothing you can do to fix this, this medication is the only hope you have,' how is it possible that there is nothing we can do?

Allah tells us differently. Allah gives us our hope back, Allah gives us back control, Allah swears He will continue to increase us, and it is He who cures us.

Do not lose hope, nor be sad. You will surely be victorious if you are true believers. (Qur'an 3:139)

And [remember] when your Lord proclaimed, 'If you are grateful, I will surely increase you [in favour]; but if you deny, indeed, My punishment is severe.' (Qur'an 14:7)

... And We have sent down to you the Book [the Qur'an] as an exposition of everything, a guidance, a mercy, and glad tidings for those who have submitted themselves [to Allah as Muslims]. (Qur'an 16: 89)

And We send down the Qur'an that which is healing and mercy for the believers, but it does not increase the wrongdoers except in loss. (Qur'an 17:82)

'And when I am ill, it is He who cures me.' (Qur'an 26:80)

Oh mankind, there has come to you instruction from Lord and healing from what is in the breast and guidance and mercy for the believers. (Qur'an 10:57)

… This Qur'an is an insight from your Lord – A guidance and a mercy for those who believe. (Qur'an 7:203)

Surely this (Qur'an) is only a reminder to the whole world to whoever of you will also take the straight path. (Qur'an 81:27-28)

We as Muslims pray a minimum of 17 times a day in Surah al-Fātiḥah,

Guide us on the straight path (Qur'an 1:6).

No one knows how long they will live. We don't know what tomorrow or the next hour will bring – that answer is only in Allah's hands, so take that stress off your shoulders, and entrust Allah with it. But the decisions you make today are in your hands. How are we supposed to live our lives to obtain the greatest potential?

When something we have bought fails to work properly, we go back to the instruction manual to find out what went wrong. When our bodies, our brains, our behaviour, our emotions are not working the way they should, we need to go back to the instruction manual given to us by our Maker. We must get back to the Qur'an, which is a guidance for humanity and a complete cure for the illnesses of the mind, body and soul. Let's start with the basics. It is time to actually live the Qur'an, it is time to read.

Getting Back to the Qur'an-Time to Read

Read in the name of your Lord who created. (Qur'an 96:1)

When the world falls into a hopeless abyss, it needs hope, guidance and light. Allah, glorified and exalted is He, the Most Merciful, the Ultimate Provider of Peace, the Creator, the Maker, the All-Hearing, the All-Seeing, the Nourisher, the Loving, the Giver of Life, the Bringer of Death, the All-Knowing, asked Prophet, peace and blessings be upon him, to *read*.

Allah could have asked him to *do*, but instead He asked him to *read* or *recite*. Our religion is so beautiful that Allah constantly wants us to use our minds and brains and understand, not just follow.

Anas ibn Mālik reported that the Messenger of Allah, peace and blessings be upon him, said, "Seeking knowledge is an obligation upon every Muslim.' (Ibn Mājah)

Thus, the pursuit of knowledge is obligatory on all the believers.

[This is] a Book [the Qur'an] which We have sent down to you, full of blessings that they may ponder over its verses, and that people of understanding may remember. (Qur'an 38: 29)

... Allah will exalt in degree those of you who believe and those who have been granted knowledge ... (Qur'an 58: 11)

'My Lord! Enrich me with knowledge...' (Qur'an 20:114)

The Prophet peace and blessings be upon him said, urging people to seek knowledge everywhere: 'Whoever follows a path seeking knowledge, Allah will ease his way to paradise.' (Muslim)

Through that knowledge, we gain freedom from the chains of mankind that keep us on that hamster wheel, that trap our children and our desires. When we are educated, we are empowered. Allah sent us the Qur'an and Sunnah to guide us about how we should be living our lives and has given us the best example to follow, the Prophet, peace and blessings be upon him.

Indeed in the Messenger of Allah [Muhammad] you have a good example to follow for him who hopes in [the Meeting with] Allah and the Last Day and remembers Allah much. (Qur'an 33: 21)

But let's face it, with today's busy world, it's easy to just follow the crowd. If everyone is doing it, it must be good. If our mosques and scholars are doing it, it must be in our best interest? Are we truly stuck in a life defined by society? Why are we not thinking with our brains? Why are we not reading? Why aren't we reflecting?

Do they not then reflect on the Qur'an? Or are there locks up on their hearts? (Qur'an 47:24)

(This is) a blessed Book which we have revealed to you (O Muhammad), that they may reflect upon its verses and that those of understanding would be reminded. (Qur'an 38:29)

The Qur'an is the solution to escape the hamster wheel we have all been on, and put our bodies back into balance. Time to take back your health, take back control of your time and life. I have escaped the hamster wheel and I have helped thousands of patients do the same. How did that happen?

By actually living the Qur'an and Sunnah, *alḥamdulillāh*, we naturally fall back into balance and get our lives back. I did this and so can you. When I was hopeless, when I knew I was falling apart, I read, I learned, I educated myself, I started to truly live the Qur'an and Sunnah in every breath I take, to every bite I eat, to the best of my ability. I am free of social norms, I am free of my thoughts, my actions, or my life being in someone else's hands. I have broken through the invisible chains that kept me stuck. I am now actually living the life I was meant to live, the way Allah, glorified and exalted, has intended me to live, with nothing holding me down.

My Journey and My Du'ā's Answered

Before becoming a board-certified integrative holistic family physician, I was – like most Americans – unhealthy and overweight. I had many of the same bad habits that have led most people to chronic disease. I was suffering from thyroid disease, acne, seborrheic dermatitis, weight and hormonal problems, digestive issues, severe fatigue, joint and muscle aches and even lupus (SLE), a disease that literally attacks every cell and organ of the body, eventually killing you. My husband and I were both medical residents, working 80-hour work weeks each, *and* I could do nothing but continue on that hamster wheel, like it was my new normal, just trying to stay above water. Until the day when the hamster wheel that I was on came to an abrupt and screeching *halt*!

At noon, my husband had a gut inclination, 'Can you go and check up on Abdullah? I feel like something is wrong.' Almost laughing it off, I thought twice and walked across to the daycare. I was not prepared for what would unfold next – I walked into every parent's worst nightmare.

When I went into the daycare infant room, something was off. The lights were dimmed. The daycare provider was rocking back and forth. As I approached her, she immediately started to stare. I started to talk, trying to break the awkwardness in the room, until I heard barely audible murmuring in the back of the room. I ran back to find my first born son, my gift from Allah, glorified and exalted is He, arms and legs strapped down with a receiving blanket, pacifier in his mouth and his plush green "Winnie the Pooh" blanket wrapped tightly around his mouth and nose, face red, cheeks swollen, eyes bloodshot and shiny with tears, almost suffocating to death. I quickly unwrapped his face, cradling him in my arms. 'You could have killed my child!' I screamed at the daycare provider, and ran out.

That day, Allah, glorified and exalted, saved my child. That day, I made a heartfelt solemn promise to take care of these gifts from Allah, glorified and exalted, the best I know how, but how could I take care of these gifts when I couldn't even take care of myself? I myself was falling apart!

Despite being a medical physician, I went to one doctor after another to find out how I can stop these diseases from progressing, eventually killing me and taking my family from me?

No one could answer my question or even had time to listen to my concerns. But I was persistent in looking for answers. What could I do to take back control of my life? I was told, 'Just sit back and let the disease take its course, there is nothing you can do.' But I refused to sit back and watch this disease kill me, there had to be another way. As both, a medical doctor and a patient, I was tired of a methodology that covered up symptoms and didn't answer the question of why I did get sick in the first place? They never got to the root cause of problems. I knew I had the potential to fly but was tired of being weighed down by my chronic illnesses. Hopeless, I made *duʿāʾ* to Allah, glorified and exalted is He, to guide me. And He did.

Allah, glorified and exalted is He, guided me to join a holistic medical practice. Working with board-certified physicians, mental health professionals, nutritionists, exercise physiologists, chiropractors, homeopaths, acupuncturists, and others, I quickly realized that medical school and residency hadn't taught me what I really needed to know about how to keep people's brains, bodies and souls truly healthy. I was not taught one class on nutrition and very little on stress management and, surprisingly, my colleagues and siblings in pediatrics, internal medicine, gynaecology and psychiatry were all in the same boat.

On my quest for true healing, I came to understand that inflammation is one of the primary processes behind most chronic health conditions. Lowering this inflammation is the key to renewed health, yet this is often overlooked. I discovered that the solution lies in the fields of holistic and functional medicine, which gets to the fundamental reasons of why you're feeling the way you're feeling. It uses all the effective tools available – complementary, alternative, and integrative medicine, combined with conventional treatments and unconditional love – to help get your body back into balance. Years of study in holistic and functional medicine, and applying everything I learned on myself as well as my patients, has transformed my life as a doctor and coach to people with chronic conditions. I now know how to help my patients overcome inflammation, optimize their mitochondria and radically improve their health.

Blown away with what I was seeing in my clinic, I started to write it all down, and came out with my first book, called *The Holistic Rx: Your Guide to Healing Chronic Inflammation and Disease*, which is the best of functional, integrative and holistic medicine covering over 80 conditions for all ages. When I started to educate Muslim audiences, I opened up the Qur'an and it blew my mind to another level; it had everything that I had been doing with patients and my family and exactly how we should be living our lives. When I implemented what I am teaching you here (with the sole intention that every step I take, every bite I eat and every word I speak are for Allah and Allah alone), *alḥamdullāh*, I was cured from the ailments that almost took my life away.

Alḥamdulillāh, I found my life's mission.

As a mother, I included my four sons in this mission. During the Quarantine, we wrote two children books together, *Adam's Healing Adventures* Series. I wrote

The Pandemic Prescription: Restoring Hope from Qur'an, Sunnah and Science and *The Holistic Rx for Kids: Parenting Healthy Brains and Bodies in a Changing World*. My children now host their own podcast called, The Holistic Kids' Show, where my children interview biggest names in the world of holistic, integrative functional medicine and parenting. My inlaws and I even started HolisticUrdu, MD that gets millions of views. We have made this mission a family affair. *Alḥamdulillāh!*

As you can see, this is my passion, purpose and mission on this planet. Getting back to the Qur'an and Sunnah, eating, living and breathing the way Allah intended for us has allowed me to put my body back into balance, alleviate the symptoms from within, get rid of medications for good, and take back the reins of my health. Now I can actually live my true potential. *Alḥamdulillāh!* Allah heals and Allah cures.

Allah Heals and Cures

Allah can heal and cure. Allah talks about shifa in numerous ayahs and hadith. Shifa means lightening the burden of disease, healing by undoing the excess or imbalances we may get into and bring us back within healthy limits, as each one of us is struggling with our individual imbalances.....patients I discuss here have been particularly inspirational. Once we were able to put their lifestyles and thereby their brains and bodies back into balance, shifa happens. *Allāhu akbar!*

> The Prophet, peace and blessings be upon him, said: 'There is no disease that Allah has created, except that He has also created its treatment.' (Bukhārī)

Every day, my patients inspire me and it is my passion to guide as many people as possible on the path toward true healing and real living, according to the Qur'an and Sunnah. In my twelve years of practising holistic, functional, integrative, conventional medicine, and Qur'anic and Prophetic medicine all into one, these patients I discuss here have been particularly inspirational.

One of my first patients was a twenty-one-year-old woman who had suffered from severe eczema for most of her life. The eczema caused her skin to burn, and the only way she could get any relief from the pain was to sit in a bath for eight hours a day. The pain became so unbearable that she tried to commit suicide three times. Distraught, she saw physician after physician, and as a last resort she came to me. After just a week of applying the strategies I will teach you in this book, by putting her body back into balance, and fixing deficiencies (that were brought on by these imbalances), the full body burning that had plagued her for years was gone. Tears flowed down her face as she asked, 'Why hadn't I heard about this treatment earlier?'

She had suffered hopelessly for years when the answer lay in the one thing that she could control: her lifestyle.

Another inspirational patient who changed my life is a thirty-one-year-old woman who had been diagnosed with several autoimmune diseases, including myasthenia gravis (an autoimmune disease of the muscles), Hashimoto's disease, lichen planus, psoriasis, eczema, and suspected Sjogren's syndrome, along with other chronic conditions. She was advised to start an eighth medication because of uncontrolled symptoms. Frustrated, when her doctor gave her no other option to slow down her diseases, she came to me. The results were remarkable and changed the way I looked at disease and treated patients forever.

She reflected, 'After just six months on the healing diet, I was completely off medication, I had lost weight, and my depression and anxiety had completely disappeared. I felt more like myself than I had in a very long time.' She continues to do well, exercising and generally living her life without those health problems, achieving her lifelong dream of becoming a scuba instructor – a dream others had told her to abandon!

If we give the body exactly what it needs to heal, healing is possible at any age. A couple in their seventies, who continue to inspire me every day, have healthier lives now compared to when they were younger. They suffered from chronic pain, digestive issues, unexplainable rashes, problems with weight, diabetes, high blood pressure, sleep problems and kidney disease.

Within a week of starting the diet and lifestyle according to the Qur'an and Sunnah, and fixing deficiencies, all their symptoms were gone, and they continue to lose weight, feel great and are now weaned off their medications with the help of their doctors.

I have twelve years of people's stories about reclaiming their lives and living a more fulfilling life when they put their bodies back into balance, by living life the way Allah has instructed us to live. These stories are among thousands of examples that add fuel to my fire to help spread the word of true healing and real living. My patients are improving the quality of their lives, and preventing (or recovering from) autoimmune diseases, skin problems, mood disorders, digestive issues, cancer, allergies, asthma, autism, chronic pain, weight problems along with a very wide range of nonspecific symptoms, simply by implementing evidence-based, cost-effective lifestyle changes, all according to the Qur'an and Sunnah. Even more amazing is that once you target the root cause, you can improve not just one chronic condition, but all of them simultaneously. *Allāhu akbar*!

All these stories are meant to inspire you – that at any age or background, you can have a healthier life. They inspire me to continue my work, even when I sometimes feel overwhelmed by my own busy and demanding life. I had to get this secret of healing out to the world, as this secret on how we can put our bodies back into balance is already in our hands – the Qur'an.

How to Navigate This Book

It is Allah who made for you the earth a place of settlement and the sky a ceiling and formed you and perfected your forms and provided you with good things. That is Allah, your Lord; then blessed is Allah, Lord of the worlds. (Qur'an 40:64)

Allah has created the sky and earth, the night and day, the mountains and the seas, the male and the female—all in perfect harmony. Islam is a way of life, which teaches us how we eat, drink, behave, sleep, greet, all to maintain a balance. That balance taught to us by Allah, also removes fear, allows us to think, clears confusion about social norms and helps us regain our health—mind, body and soul. Allah formed us, perfected us and He knows what is good for us and what isn't.

[This is] a Book [the Qur'an] which We have sent down to you, full of blessings that they may ponder over its verses, and that people of understanding may remember. (Qur'an 38: 29)

Time to get back in control of your life, the way Allah, glorified and exalted is He, intended! Time to *read* (*iqra*), learn and teach, so we can create a ripple effect to empower humanity, *insha'Allāh*.

The Qur'anic Prescription approaches health and healing in three parts. The first two parts are focussed on general lifestyle tips to create a balanced inner and outer world that applies to everyone, regardless of their age and background. The third part is for those who want to take their healing to the next level.

Part 1 is about realizing we have a global problem – an epidemic hitting our families and our planet today because we are disrupting Allah's balance. We can't fix a problem whose existence is unknown to us, so in Chapter 1, we dive into how the impurities and toxins around us are destroying our present and our future. It discusses how our bodies, brains and world are put out of balance by not following what Allah, glorified and exalted is He, has intended, which sabotages our decision-making skills, increases inflammation, chronic disease and planetary destruction. Chapter 2 sheds light on what the Qur'an, Sunnah and modern science have to say about the overlooked key to *Jannah* and success – the pillars of a pure (*tayyib*) lifestyle – which involves optimizing digestive health and detoxification, including what to eat and the four S's: stress, sleep, social health, and spirituality.

In Part 2 of the book, we dive deeper into the pillars of a pure lifestyle. We examine further what the Qur'an, Sunnah, and science say about each one of these vital pillars of health and wellness, combined with practical tips for the modern age to keep our bodies balanced.

Part 3 takes these principles and practical advice one step further, specifically for those suffering with an ailment. It offers a simple, easy-to-follow, holistic, functional and integrative prescription for putting the body back into balance, thereby lowering the body's response (inflammation), optimizing the mitochondria (the powerhouse of the cell), the ability to make better decisions, and achieving lasting optimal health and happiness, the Qur'anic way. *Insha'Allāh*, you will be able to see benefits right away, not just for one condition, but for all of them simultaneously! What's even more exciting – it's cost-and time-effective and you are doing it for Allah, glorified and exalted is He, increasing your reward with Him!

Bismillāh, You Got This!

Remember Allah, glorified and exalted is He, loves you more than anyone has ever loved you and He is closer to you than your own jugular vein, *Subḥānallāh*! You're a gem, inside and out, no matter your age or background! You are a beacon of inspiration to those around you. Look at all that you have accomplished despite being less than 100 percent! When you're in good health, you're free to get off the hamster wheel, break the chains of modern life and actually live your life the way you were meant to. Imagine everything you'll be able to accomplish when you're feeling your best. There's no limit to what you can do. Now imagine what the Muslim *ummah* can accomplish when we are all feeling our best, when we are living by the Qur'an and Sunnah and are actually become a people who praise Allah!

> The Prophet Muhammad, peace and blessings be upon him, has said that Allah, glorified and exalted is He, said: *'If you come to Me walking, I will come to you running.' (Bukhārī)*

The hope lies in educating *yourself*! Once we start to take care of our lives and the environments we live in – according to the Qur'an and Sunnah – we can put our bodies and the world back into balance, improve morbidity and mortality from chronic disease worldwide, bring peace and unity, fix our food system, improve our economy, protect our planet, and even survive another pandemic, *insha'Allāh*. This book empowers you to optimize your health and well-being. It combines the Qur'an, Sunnah and science to help you live your purest (*ṭayyib*) life, to keep you and your family's lives in balance, saving our communities, children and planet.

> *... Verily Allah will never change the condition of a people until they change what is in themselves ...* (Qur'an 13: 11)

It is the choices you make that will create a brighter future for everyone. Let this journey towards balance and health begin – one step at a time, at your own pace. The All-Knowing and All-Hearing will make it easy for you, *insha'Allāh*.

So remember Me; I will remember you. And be grateful to Me and do not deny Me.
(Qur'an 2:152)

Let's remember Allah, be grateful and educate ourselves, because we and our families are worth it! Let's take care of the gifts Allah, glorified and exalted is He, gave us – our health, our families and our planet. Let's start in Allah's name (*bismillāh*), and make an intention that we are doing this for Allah alone, glorified and exalted is He, and be thankful for all His blessings.

May Allah, glorified and exalted is He, help you with this journey, *āmīn*.

PART 1

Spinning Out of Control

The Threat of Today's Crisis on Our Future

Our Present, Future, Economy and Suffering World

Who created you, proportioned you, and balanced you? (Qur'an 82:7)
Verily, We have created the human from a quintessence of clay; then We placed him as a drop in a fixed resting place. We then made the drop into a clot and that into a fetus. We then made bones and clothed the bones with flesh and from that brought forth another creation. Therefore, blessed is God, the very Best of those who create. (Qur'an 23:12-14)

The human body is one of Allah's greatest miracles. The average human body contains around 37.2 trillion cells. About 300 million cells die every minute in our bodies, producing 25 million new cells each second. The heart beats more than 3 billion times in an average human lifespan. Human cells make up only 43 percent of the body's total cell count. The human genome is made up of 20,000 instructions called genes.[1] There are more bacteria in a human mouth than there are people in the world, with most of the bacteria present in the digestive tract.[2] If we add all the genes of our bacteria, we can then talk about 2–20 million microbial genes.[3] We have more than 10,000 different microbe species researchers have identified living in the human body. 3.3 million of non-redundant genes in the human gut microbiome. We have 60 thousand miles of blood vessels running through our body and messages from the human brain travel along our nerves up to 200 miles an hour, taking in the world around us.

Our bodies are protected by a series of miraculous defence systems working nonstop to keep our cells, organs and every bodily activity functioning smoothly, in order to keep us healthy. Maintaining and optimizing these defence systems are key to keeping our bodies in balance. But what happens if these beautiful systems stop working correctly? The answer is: an epidemic.

A epidemic of chronic disease. Our health, our future's health, the future of humanity and the future of this world will be at stake.

3

Our Suffering Present

People are getting sicker and sicker and chronic diseases are on the rise. According to the National Council on Aging, chronic diseases include heart disease, depression, hypertension, diabetes, arthritis, dementia, chronic kidney disease, high cholesterol and chronic obstructive pulmonary disease. Six in ten adults have a chronic disease and four in ten adults have two or more chronic health conditions. About 80percent of older adults have at least one chronic disease, and 77percent have two or more chronic health conditions.

Every 40 seconds someone dies of a heart attack[4] or suicide.[5] Cancer is the second highest cause of death worldwide,[6] taking the lives of 10 million people each year. Heart disease, cancer and strokes account for more than half of all deaths each year. 20 million people die from heart-related diseases. The World Health Organizations and Centers for Disease Control state that chronic diseases are the leading causes of death and disability, being responsible for seven out of ten deaths every year.[7]

According to a study published in the British scientific journal, *Age and Ageing*, the number of seniors with four or more chronic diseases is expected to double by 2035. It is projected that ten years from now, 83 million Americans will have three or more chronic conditions, compared to 30 million in 2015; 50 million people have Alzheimer's disease and 60 percent of Americans are overweight or obese.[8] Roughly 40 percent of adults worldwide are considered obese or overweight. About 75 percent of visits to the doctors are related to chronic diseases, and almost half of the US population have diabetes or prediabetes,[9] which kill at least 1.6 million globally each year, a disease largely dependant on lifestyle. National Public Radio News reported that they found an overall 52.4 percent decline in sperm concentration and a 59.3 percent decline in the total sperm count over a 39-year period.[10] Chronic health conditions are extremely common, are slowly killing us, and have an enormous impact on people's lives. What is even worse is that studies have found that health in Muslim majority countries is substantially worse than in non-Muslim majority countries.[11] Data from the International Diabetes Foundation projects that there will be an increase of diabetes by 2045, an increase by 142.8 percent in Africa, 55.4 percent in South America, and 96.4 percent in the Middle East and North Africa; 80 percent of all individuals with insulin resistance live in developing countries, half of all adults in China and India are insulin resistant. According to the International Diabetes Federation, the number of cases of insulin resistance worldwide has doubled in the past three decades and will likely double again in less than two more.

In 2021 *JAMA Psychiatry*, found that Muslim adults in the US were twice as likely to report a history of suicide attempt compared with individuals from other faith traditions. (Awaad R, El-Gabalawy O, Jackson-Shaheed E, Zia B, Keshavarzi H, Mogahed D, Altalib H. Suicide Attempts of Muslims Compared With Other

Religious Groups in the US. JAMA Psychiatry. 2021 Sep 1;78(9):1041-1044. doi: 10.1001/jamapsychiatry.2021.1813. PMID: 34287614; PMCID: PMC8295887.)

What is astonishing is that Allah's Messenger (peace and blessings be upon him) predicted this:

Of the signs of Judgement Day is that obesity will spread amongst the people. (Bukhārī)

Our Suffering Future

Unfortunately, it's not just adults who are suffering, it is also children – both in their physical and mental health. This will be the first generation of kids not to outlive their parents, as our children are living shorter and sicker lives. What is very concerning is that chronic diseases have quadrupled among children since the 1960s. Obesity rates have doubled in more than seventy countries since 1980 and has tripled in children.[12] Especially in Arab countries, adolescent obesity has reached a critical level.[13]

Fifty-four percent of American children have a diagnosed chronic health condition, an estimate which will rise to 80 percent by 2025. Many kids have overlapping comorbid diagnoses. There is a rise in inflammatory conditions like allergy and autoimmunity linked to poor diet.

Seventy percent of obese children have at least one cardiovascular risk factor, and 39 percent have two or more risk factors. Cancer is one of the leading causes of death in children between the ages of 5 to 14. One in ten children have asthma. One in thirteen children have food allergies. Given current trends, one in every three children born in 2000 will develop diabetes over the course of a lifetime.[14]

Mental health has gone up, with increasing rates of depression, suicide, behaviour problems, ADHD and neurodevelopmental disorders in children, much of which is linked to diet.[15] One in six American children has at least one neurodevelopmental disorder like autism, ADHD, dyslexia, specific learning disorders, communication disorders, sensory processing disorders and more. Serious depression is worsening, with the suicide rate among teenage girls reaching a forty-year high, increasing thirteen years in a row, hitting those that live in less populated and rural areas the hardest,[16] and suicide risks have soared to 56 percent between 2007 and 2016[17] despite a whopping 400 percent increase in antidepressant prescriptions in the US since the 1990s.[18] The number of teenage girls, out of a hundred thousand, who are admitted to hospital every year because of cutting or harming themselves (which was stable until 2011) has started to go up to about 62 percent for older teen girls and 189 percent for pre-teen girls, i.e. it has nearly tripled! We are also seeing the same patterns for suicides. Suicide among older teen girls (15-19 years) is up 70 percent compared to the first decade of the century. In 2018, autism was found in one in thirty-six children and, if we continue at the current trajectory, one in every four will have autism by 2033.[19]

The environment our children are living in is compromising their ability to lead successful lives, as their lifestyle is affecting their brain development and is leading to mental health issues. Kids that ate ultra-processed foods had 10 percent smaller brains and seven points lower IQ. With the most resources in the world, the United States is ranked thirty-first in reading and mathematics on a global level. Good mental health has been linked to a healthy diet.[20]

Our Suffering Economy and Environment

Chronic disease has a huge cost on our health and pockets, as it is now the single biggest threat to global economic development. Chronic disease accounts for 86 percent of our nation's health care costs.[21] For obesity and diabetes, the total cost for chronic health conditions, indirect and direct causes is 3.7 trillion dollars every year, and it is estimated to get to 95 trillion dollars over the next thirty-five years (direct and indirect causes due to obesity, diabetes, mental health issues, lost productivity due to chronic conditions, disability and direct health care costs).[22]

Forty-eight percent of our government's mandatory spending will be on Medicare to deal with chronic illness just as it relates to our food, as one third of the money allocated for Medicare is just for diabetes!

O children of Adam, take your adornment at every mosque, and eat and drink, but be not excessive. Indeed, He likes not those who commit excess. (Qur'an 7: 31)

Considering the food Americans waste, 40 percent of the food produced, leaves a huge global impact that costs more than $2.6 trillion a year.

Our Suffering World

As for the pure land, vegetation comes out by its Lord's will, but poor land produces in agony. We explain Our messages in various ways to those people who are grateful. (Qur'an 7: 58)

Evil has appeared on land and sea because of what the hands of people have earned [by oppression and evil deeds], that Allah may make them taste a part of that which they have done, in order that they may return. (Qur'an 30: 41)

Our world is suffering: climate change is real. Climate change and global warming, change that is happening to our planet, leading to unpredictable weather, droughts, rising sea levels, and global warming that leads to shrinking glaciers and melting ice, harsher winters, flooding and other serious problems. Climate change is also impacting our food, animal and plant species. Studies have shown that a third of all animal and plant species on the planet could face extinction by 2070,[23] and we have already lost 90 percent of the plant varieties and half of the livestock.[24] Forty-four of the world's 538 species are already extinct at one or more sites that they had inhabited before. We are losing 1 percent of consumable food calories per year of the ten top world crops.

The food system, food waste and our industrial agriculture is the single biggest cause of climate change (yes, even more than fossil fuels), as it contributes to about 56 percent of non-carbon dioxide emissions and contributes to up to 29 percent of total greenhouse gas emissions. With the use of these chemicals and industrial farming, fertilizing itself requires a large amount of energy, as it is the biggest consumer of natural gas from fracking, releasing 40–50 percent more methane. When we add chemicals to our soil, it destroys the earth, it causes nitrous oxide and when combined with methane, now you have a greenhouse gas that is three hundred times more potent than carbon dioxide! It contributes to about a third to 40 percent of all greenhouse gasses in the environment, because when we destroy the soil, it is unable to hold water and carbon, and releases greenhouse gasses, some 600 million tons of CO_2 equivalent into the air every year!

But what is scary is that because of all the impurities in our lives and what we dump in our environment – 200 million tons of fertilizer globally every year[25] – we have lost so much. We have lost half of livestock species, 90 percent of edible plant species, 75 percent of pollinator species, all of which are disappearing at the rate of mass extension.

We are losing about 2 billion tons of topsoil a year.[26] Dirt is lifeless, with limited nutrients to feed the plants, so needing tons of fertilizer, and other chemicals to even cause food to grow. Soil is different. Only two square centimeters of soil will have more microbial diversity then anything in the universe, which eliminates the need for chemicals. But with chemical and industrial farming, with the loss of about a third of soil in the last 150 years, and the loss of our natural ecosystems (leading to loss of nutrients, minerals and biodiversity), desertification increased, killing our marine life including phytoplankton and the coral reef, depleting our sources for fresh water, all leading to disease and imbalance. All the chemicals we are dumping into the soil and water can destroy them, leading to marine death and decreased biodiversity of the planet. Unfortunately, the development of agriculture has led to the decrease of food diversity, leading to disease.

We need the oceans to help us protect climate change, as coastal plants can store 20 times more carbon than rainforests on land; 93 percent of all the world's CO_2 is stored in the oceans with the help of marine vegetation, algae and coral. Losing just 1 percent of this ecosystem is equivalent to releasing the emissions of 97 million cars. Unfortunately, the industrial crops of corn and wheat are reliant on 400 billion pounds of nitrogen fertilizer globally a year, that ends up in our water bodies leading

7

to about 400 marine dead zones around the world, as big as the size of Europe combined, that 500 billion people depend on for food. Every year approximately 25 million acres of forest are lost (land deforestation) and bottom trolling wipes out an estimated 3.9 billion acres. If we continue on the current trajectory, we will lose 90 percent of our coral reefs by 2050 and the oceans will be completely empty by 2048!

The UN informs us that we have only about sixty harvests left, then what? Without any life in our oceans… what will happen to humanity? No soil, no plants, no animals, no food, no humans – that is something to think about!

And when it is said to them, 'Do not cause corruption on the earth,' they say, 'We are but reformers.' Unquestionably, it is they who are the corrupters, but they perceive [it] not. (Qur'an 2: 11–12)

We believe we are making the earth better for everyone, but we are only destroying it.

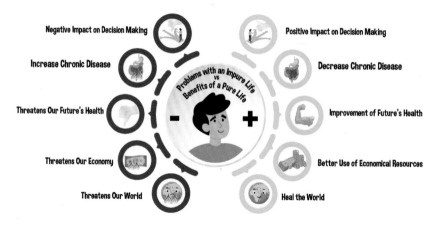

PICTURE 1.1   PURE LIFESTYLE VS IMPURE LIFESTYLE

From Hopelessness to Hope

What comes to our minds when reading these statistics? If – like me – you are stunned and feeling hopeless, then it's easier to stick our heads in the ground and pretend everything is okay, when clearly we are getting sicker as human beings along with the planet. Well, this is *not* genetic or better diagnosis. Something is happening to our children epigenetically.

We are getting sicker day by day. Conventional medicine is great, but when it comes to healing and preventing chronic disease, we need to dig a little deeper, we need to look past drug treatments, as they alone will not keep us healthy and happy.

There is so much hope, we just need to understand what is causing this problem – the imbalances around us that lead to problems. Why are we suffering? Why is our planet suffering? The answer is simple: we are out of balance and inflamed.

And if God touches thee with affliction, none can remove it but He: if He touches thee with happiness He has power over all things. (Qur'an 6: 17)

The hope lies in educating *ourselves*! Once we start to take care of our lives and the environments we live in – according to Qur'an and Sunnah – we can put our bodies and world back into balance, improve morbidity and mortality from chronic disease, fix our food system, improve our economy and even save our planet, by returning to the Qur'an and Sunnah for guidance. Once we start taking care of the trusts that Allah, glorified and exalted is He, has given us, He can heal us and the planet, but we must do our part. When our bodies are out of balance, their response is heightened inflammation.

The Role of Inflammation in Chronic Illness

The first step of your healing journey is to understand what's fueling your symptoms – that is, why you're feeling the way you do and why the *ummah* is suffering.

When you go to your doctor, let's say for a headache, you are given an anti-inflammatory. But what about for eczema? An anti-inflammatory. For pain? An anti-inflammatory. Allergies? An anti-inflammatory. Autoimmune condition like lupus? An anti-inflammatory. Cancer? An anti-inflammatory. See the pattern?

It doesn't matter what the chronic conditions or symptoms are: depression, mood disorders, thyroid disease, autoimmune disorders, digestive issues, skin disorders, cancer, autism or more general symptoms like chronic pain, fatigue, sinus issues, allergies or even the simple fact of constantly making the wrong decisions or craving the wrong type of food. These seem like different problems, but they have one thing in common: your body is out of balance. This leads to the body's response – inflammation – the mechanism behind most of your chronic conditions and symptoms. Even before your diseases become noticeable, inflammation starts brewing in your body, so by the time you begin to feel symptoms, the damage has already started.

Doctors know that the underlying mechanism is inflammation, but doctors have never been taught to address why someone is getting sick in the first place and what is causing the imbalance. So, by putting your body back into balance, you can lower inflammation, help your body function better, healing not one symptom, but all of them simultaneously.

What is Inflammation?

Inflammation means 'fire inside' and it's your body's natural defensive response to your body's immune system trying to fight off problems or even heal wounds. Without inflammation, we would be in danger as we would have no way to fight microbial invaders or repair any damage in the body. But you want just about the right amount of inflammation, as too much or too little can both cause problems. There are two forms of inflammation: acute and chronic.[24]

A healthy inflammation response, or acute inflammation, lasts for a short time, and is a good sign that your body and its defences are working properly. But if the switch in our immune system stays 'on' for too long, it can be too much of a good thing. Modern life's constant daily exposures to triggers like chronic stress, toxins, impure and toxic food, allergens, low grade infections, etc., can all start to drive disease, destroying our miracle of a body. So this takes a little longer to kick in and takes time to develop. When the immune system is properly functioning, it can keep this fire under control, but with constant exposures to triggers, the inflammatory molecules (like cytokines) get out of control, destroying everything in their path, damaging tissues and organs, leading to chronic diseases of every stripe.[25]

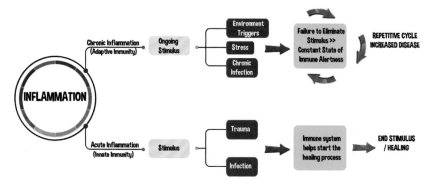

PICTURE 1.2   ACUTE AND CHRONIC INFLAMMATION

Inflammation and Our Genes, Brains and Body

Every thought, action and bite we take can influence everything down to our genetic code, altering the activity of our DNA through a science called epigenetics. Epigenetics is the study of change in our gene function without physical mutations to the DNA structure— in other words, we can control our genes. Adults and children all have around 25,000 genes that control the production of proteins in the body. The human genome is made up of about 1 percent that codes for genes, while the rest of the 99 percent does not code for genes, also known as 'junk DNA'. Science has proven that this is where the information resides which tells the genes how they are going to be expressed—determining when and where genes are turned on and off, depending on our lifestyles and experiences.

Some conditions have a genetic component, but many researchers have determined that less than 10 percent of those with the genes for an autoimmune disease will actually develop it. Genes may load the gun, but the environment pulls the trigger— we can turn on and off our genes with the decisions they make each day and the experiences they have. Those control mechanisms, above our genes, are controlling factors that regulate how we look, act and feel in direct communication with our environment and lifestyle. How our families live, their medications, the internal and external environments and lifestyles, digestive health including our microbiome (our gut's bacteria), nutrition, toxins, stressors, trauma, exercise, sleep, optimism, and spiritual health, or any other life experiences, can turn on and off these genes, all alter how their genes are expressed. Genes can actually shape the behaviour of the individual—all determined through our lifestyle.

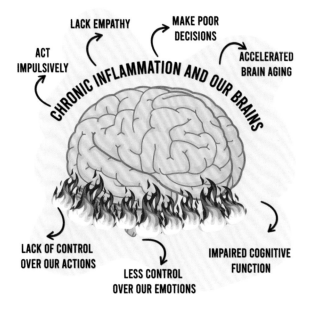

PICTURE 1.3 INFLAMMATION AND OUR BRAINS

Chronic inflammation can also affect our brains. Studies have shown that inflammation was found to decrease the strength of the connection between the prefrontal cortex and amygdala,[27] and leads to a heightened response when it is presented with something that is maybe threatening.[28] Behaviour and inflammation are connected, as chronic inflammation can influence our behaviour and that of our children.

Subḥānallāh, if that wasn't enough, inflammatory precursors like kynurenic acid, quinolinic acid and picolinate are made because inflammation disrupts our brain chemistry, so we can't make serotonin. Extra precursors are present that lead to further inflammation. Research has also shown that inflammation is strongly linked with accelerated brain aging and impaired cognitive function.[29] Chronic inflammation can lead us to act impulsively, lack empathy, make poor decisions, and have less control over our emotions and actions.

Mitochondria are a key energy source for our bodies and are the powerhouse of the cell. They are little factories (each cell holds hundreds or thousands) in our cells that take the food we eat and convert them to energy (adenosine triphosphate or ATP) and this energy is used to support our bodily functions. Healthy mitochondria are essential for our overall health and well-being.

Mitochondria are able to perceive signals of inflammation, then activate and manage the innate immune system. Mitochondria can be damaged through uncontrolled oxidative stress that can degrade their protein, membranes and DNA.

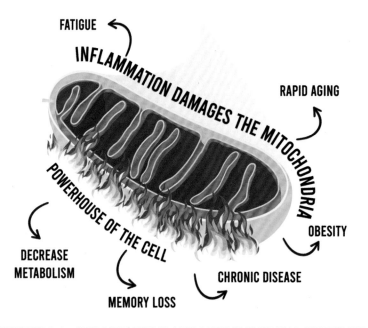

PICTURE 1.4   INFLAMMATION AND MITOCHONDRIAL FUNCTION

When our mitochondria aren't working properly, our metabolism decreases, leading to obesity, as inflammation interferes with the job of the mitochondria to burn fat and makes fat loss very difficult. It can affect every part of the body, and overall body inflammation can lead to autoimmunity and cancer. Unfortunately, we are seeing more and more of it.

Lowering inflammation, by addressing the root cause and putting our bodies back into balance will optimize the function of the mitochondria and allow each cell of the body to function optimally.[30]

Are You Inflamed? Is Your Body Out of Balance?

Symptoms of inflammation include general symptoms like fever, congestion, stiffness, dry eyes, irritability, fatigue, mood disorders, concentration issues and more specific symptoms like allergies, depression, anxiety, headaches, weight issues, and chronic pain. Everyone is different, so your symptoms depend on the body part that is inflamed.

Standard medicine holds that such diseases can be managed but rarely cured. In contrast, the holistic, functional and integrative approach (according to the Qur'an and Sunnah) is effective in treating all chronic conditions, because it addresses the underlying mechanism: chronic inflammation. As inflammation is the body's response, it is important to find out the individual root cause that is leading to this increased inflammatory reaction and subsequently to the symptoms.

Inflammation of the brain and body causes inflammation of our behaviour and emotions. When we put our body and mind back into balance, we can help save the present and future as well as the planet.

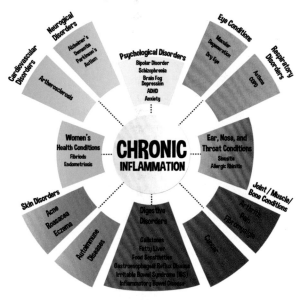

PICTURE 1.5 CHRONIC INFLAMMATION AND DISEASE

Why Our Bodies are Inflamed, Out of Balance and Disrupting Allah's Harmony

Thus, have We made of you an Ummah [community of believers] justly balanced. (Qur'an 2: 143)

And the earth – We have spread it and cast therein firmly set mountains and caused them to grow therein [something] of every well-balanced thing. (Qur'an 15: 19)

Allah, glorified and exalted is He, has made everything in perfect balance and harmony – the sun and the moon, the water and the land, man and woman. It is when we disrupt this balance that humankind and our planet suffer. That is exactly what is happening now – we are disrupting Allah's perfect balance.

Everything good that happens to you (O Man) is from God, everything bad that happens to you is from your own actions. (Qur'an 4: 79)

We send signals to our environment and to our bodies that influence our genetic make-up. Every bite we take and every thought we have can change the expression of these genes and the activity of our DNA, analysed though a science called epigenetics, as discussed above. Genes may load the gun, but the environment pulls the trigger. Epigenetics tells us that we can turn our genes on and off by our lifestyles. So how we live, our medications, our internal and external environment and lifestyles, digestive health, including our microbiome (our gut's bacteria), nutrition, toxins, stressors, trauma, exercise, sleep, optimism, and spiritual health, can all alter how our genes are expressed, and are able to turn on and off these genes!

More than 90 percent of the genetic switches in our DNA that are associated with longevity are significantly influenced by our lifestyle choices.[31]

According to the Organization for Economic Cooperation and Development (OECD), the United States spends more on health care than any other country, but this hasn't translated into longer lives, as we rank forty-sixth in life expectancy compared to the rest of the world,[32] with most Muslim countries with even lower life expectancies. Everyone knows at least the basics about what or what not to do, but why aren't we doing those or learning more?

So whatever good happens is from Allah, and whatever bad happens is from our own selves, because of our lifestyles, and how we choose to live can influence the release of pro-inflammatory cytokines, thereby potentially increasing the likelihood that we will develop chronic conditions. These changes can then be passed on to our offspring.

What is going on? Why are we all out of balance? Why are we all getting sicker? Our bodies are one interconnected ecosystem. Our lifestyles are the key to that answer, which are putting our bodies out of balance, influencing our genes and increasing inflammation. How do we change? First by intimately influencing our minds and the decisions we chose to make every day.

We are Making the Wrong Decisions

You are what your brain is.

What we wear in the morning, what we eat, the decisions we make and how we feel is dictated by our brains. The average brain is believed to generate tens of thousands of thoughts per day, with brain information travelling more that 250mph! The human brain is made up of over 100 billion brain cells and over 50 trillion synapses. A 2019 study from John Hopkins University shows that chronic inflammation in middle life is linked to later cognitive decline and Alzheimer's disease, reinforcing that inflammation can lead to decline in brain capabilites.

Brain development is very rapid in the womb; it accelerates in the first two to three years and continues to sculpt for the next 20 years or so. A newborn's brain triples in size in the first year of its life. It then starts to structurally deteriorate as early as the 30s, and after the age of 40, parts of the brain (like the hippocampus) shrink about 0.5 percent per year. What determines how fast our brains decline? Our lifestyles, medical conditions, the environment we live in and our genetics.

There are two critical players that are involved in our decision-making skills (or neuroeconomics) – the prefrontal cortex and our amygdala.

The prefrontal cortex, the more developed part of the brain, is responsible for rational decision-making skills; it examines the pros and cons and helps us think through our actions after taking a look at the whole picture. By contrast, the amygdala is the reactive part of the brain; it is responsible for primitive, impulsive, fight-or-flight reactions or decisions. To make a thought-out rational decision, we need to have both of these working together. Unfortunately, because our lifestyles are out of balance – impure food, increased stress, lack of sleep, lack of exercise, negative social environments, lack of nature and excessive screen time – the prefrontal cortex and the amygdala are becoming disconnected, leading to poor decisions, decreased empathy and the fostering of an 'everyone is against us' mentality.

O mankind, eat from whatever is on earth [that is] lawful and pure and do not follow the footsteps of Satan. Indeed, he is to you a clear enemy. (Qur'an 2:168)

Anything that heightens the inflammatory response leads to chronic inflammation which can compromise the access of the prefrontal cortex, threatening the ability to use it effectively, to change and compromise our thinking and decisions.

Changing our lifestyles, specifically our diets, can change our brains, helping us to make better decisions. So it is time you took charge of your brain and body, otherwise someone else will. It's time to take back your brain and your life by putting your lifestyle back into balance!

Our Decisions Putting Our World Out of Balance

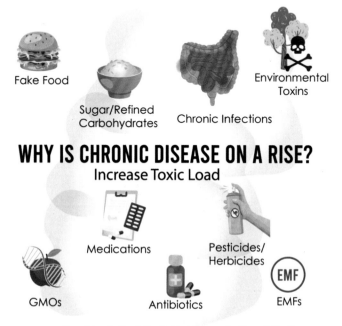

Fake Food

Sugar/Refined Carbohydrates

Chronic Infections

Environmental Toxins

WHY IS CHRONIC DISEASE ON A RISE?
Increase Toxic Load

Medications

Pesticides/ Herbicides

GMOs

Antibiotics

EMFs

Too Much Bad Stuff, Not Enough Good Stuff

PICTURE 1.6   WHY CHRONIC DISEASE IS ON A RISE?

Our Food and Digestive Health Are Out of Balance – Eating the Wrong Food and Overeating

What is the difference between someone with a chronic condition and someone without one? The environment. The biggest connection between our insides and our outsides is our mouths, and what we put through our guts or digestive tracts. Science shows that the gut encompasses our total health. The majority of our immune system (70–80 percent) and 100 trillion bacteria (that dictate our health, our decisions and even affect our genes) are in our guts.

The million-dollar question everyday is, 'What am I going to eat today?' Especially with all the confusion surrounding food: something is good one day, terrible the next, and then good again the day after that. With all this confusion, it's tempting to pick up the quickest convenience food. Let's face it, confusion sells – given how Big Food operates. Our processed, industrialized, westernized global diet is the biggest killer on the planet; it is responsible for taking the lives of eleven million people every year, and an estimated 2.1 billion adults are overweight, while 820 million people are globally undernourished.

The Wrong Impure Food We Eat Is Making Us Sick

The food we eat is not the same food our ancestors ate, or what the Prophet, peace and blessings be upon him, ate. It has drastically changed over the last forty years. In the first part of the twentieth century, chemically-altered food substances replaced pure foods; real food was replaced with bioengineered food that lacked nutrition, costing billions, and manipulating the world's diet making it a global challenge.

The food we eat, e.g., impure and processed foods, is the single biggest cause of death worldwide, as 70 percent of deaths are from non-communicable diseases, even worse than smoking or any other cause. Globally, one in five deaths in 2017 was associated with a poor diet.[33] For every 10 percent of our diets that comes from processed, artificial, impure foods, our risk of death goes up by 14 percent for 'all cause mortality.'[34] Politics and money are at the centre of our food system and policies, and they protect and encourage Big Ag and Big Food's control of our food system, in their favour, as 60 percent of all vegetable seeds are controlled by four big companies. If genetically-modified organism (GMO) seeds are not the only problem, food additives have made their way into our foods to improve taste and extend shelf life. Today, there are an estimated 10,000 chemicals we commonly use in our food, whereas in 1958 there were only around 800 chemicals. At least a thousand of these current food additives have never been reviewed for their safety by the Food and Drugs Administration (FDA).

Not Eating Pure Foods Is Putting Us Out of Balance

Allah has created for us over 250,000 plants to eat, each with its own nutritional benefit. Unfortunately, only 2 percent of our farmland is used to grow fruits and vegetables, while 59 percent of our farmland is used to grow commodity crops like corn, soy and wheat. Sixty percent of the world's calorie intake is dominated by three crops – wheat, rice and corn – that are turned into ultra-processed food, i.e. cheap sources of energy that are relatively low in nutrition and consumed more by the poor, young, or less educated.[35] Sixty-seven percent of all farmland is used to grow food for family-farmed animals and 53 percent of all farmland grows soy and corn.[36]

17

With this giant shift in nutrition to a dietary lack of diversity, more than 90 percent of Americans lack one or more nutrients at levels that create vitamin and nutrient deficiencies, like B vitamins, magnesium, Vitamin D, selenium, Vitamin K2, Vitamin E and potassium which are not found in the modern diet.[37]

In fact, the primary cause of disease is the lack of vegetables and fruits in our diet that leads to nutritional deficiencies, creating an imbalance in the body. Globally, 78 percent of the world's population doesn't eat the minimum of five servings of fruits and vegetables a day.[38] In the 2019 issue of *The Journal of Nutrition*, it was reported that only 18 percent of individuals in low and middle income contries meet WHO recommendations of consuming 400 g/d of fruits and vegetables, which equates to ~5 servings/day. We are producing nutrient-poor and high-calorie foods that leave our bodies malnourished but overfed. Unfortunately, the agricultural system doesn't even produce enough for everyone to have their minimum requirement of fruits and vegetables.

In 2019, *The Lancet* published the dietary risk-factors existing in 195 countries based on the effects of diet on health, covering a twenty-seven year period. They concluded that a diet without enough healthy foods and with too many bad foods accounted for 11 million deaths and 255 million years of disability. Most strikingly, it was found that the lack of protective foods (or real unprocessed foods) was as important, or even more important, in determining a risk of death than the overconsumption of processed foods.[39]

Overeating

But those who disbelieve enjoy themselves and eat as grazing livestock eat, and the Fire will be a residence for them. (Qur'an 47: 12)

Our food system no longer belongs to the people, but to politicians, Big Ag and Big Food, that dominate our food system, and support foods that lead to overeating and undernourishment. For the first time ever, as our bodies are constantly being fed, the stage is set for disease, and most Americans eat all day long.[40]

For the first time in history, there are more overweight than underfed people on Earth,[41] mostly in the low–middle income countries. The World Health Organization (WHO) has formally recognized obesity as a global epidemic.[42] We are eating the wrong, energy-dense, nutrient-poor foods, overeating, and eating all the time. Fast food chains that are viewed as low-class in the US are marketed in poorer countries as high-class food. These foods are not leading to just sickness, but are making us addicted.

The American Journal of Clinical Nutrition explored the science of ultra-processed foods and food addiction that might be contributing to overeating and obesity. In one study,[43] involving more than 500 people, it was found that foods like pizza, chocolate, potato chips, ice cream, french fries, cheeseburgers and cookies, elicited 'addictive-like' eating behaviours, intense cravings, loss of control and the inability to cut back despite experiencing harmful consequences and desperately wanting to stop eating them. In one study[44], it was noticed that when some tried to cut back on these highly processed foods, they experienced symptoms that were similar to withdrawal effects seen in drug abusers. Other researchers found that people who frequently consume junk food can develop a tolerance to them over time, so they need more and more amounts to derive the same enjoyment. The researchers in these studies argue that overeating is driven in part by the food industry which markets more than 20,000 new products every year. This overeating and eating all the time impairs our mitochondrial function, disrupts our circadian rhythm and decreases our ability to burn fat.

This was evident when I travelled to Asia, as India is now the diabetes capital of the world and, when I went for *Hajj*, I noticed the Arab world being flooded with processed foods and soft drinks. As we prayed during Arafat for health, they were passing out soda and processed foods. The Middle East and North Africa have the second highest increase in diabetes globally – the number of people with the disease is projected to soar to more than 95 percent by 2035.[45] This disease has hit the heart of the Muslim world, and we need to speak up as Muslims to get these large coorporations that are destroying our health inside the Haram.

Foods Disrupts the Digestive Health Leading to Inflammation

These unhealthy foods change our biochemistry with every bite we take, and constantly influence how we feel, as these energy-dense, nutrient-poor foods destory our health and brains, even down to our microbiome and genes. Poor dietary choices lead to inflammation, and make us impulsive, as these foods promote overeating by stimulating brain-reward pathways and appetite, leading to weight gain and keeping our fat cells hooked, disassociating us from the prefrontal cortices and preventing us from making good decisions. In other words, our mental health is highly associated with the health of our gut and food choices.

Through putting impure, artificial, GMO foods into our bodies, we are disrupting the "bugs" in our gut and throwing off our immune system. Impurities can also lead to an imbalance in our gut bacteria and breaks in the blood-brain barrier (also known as breaches in the blood-brain barrier), which lead to so many chronic diseases, including depression, anxiety, autism, autoimmunity, Alzheimer's and even cancer.[46]

Science has proven how dangerous impure foods are to our bodily *and* spiritual health: they increase inflammation, our appetites and the amount of food we eat (that leads to leptin resistance, a hormone that helps to tell us when we are full), and lead to prediabetes and weight gain (leading to insulin resistance, a hormone that helps us balance glucose or sugar in the body). Insulin resistance is present in almost every chronic disease. Inflammation also affects our children: we need to stop it now by changing what we can control, our food and our environment. We can change our food system, and even our planet. These foods hurt us and deplete the soil, water, and oil resources and are the largest source of greenhouse gases.

The Problem with Our Food System

So what is going on? Though we like to place the blame on the patients, what we don't see is the intricate web of government policies that determines the foods we eat, namely, highly processed ones, or those we don't eat, e.g., fruits and vegetables, and how these foods are grown, produced, marketed and distributed.

Our food system and the education we receive about food are manipulated such that citizens are no longer the centre of our food system, instead the corporations – processed food companies, seed companies and chemical fertilizer companies – now control everything from the growing of food to how it ends up on our plates.

These corporations are purposely targeting our kids with colourful advertising, including minorities and are now selling bad food to the rest of the world.

> *[And they should consider that] when those who have been followed disassociate themselves from those who followed [them], and they [all] see the punishment, and cut off from them are the ties [of relationship]. Those who followed will say, "If only we had another turn [at worldly life] so we could disassociate ourselves from them as they have disassociated themselves from us." Thus will Allah show them their deeds as regrets upon them. And they are never to emerge from the Fire.* (Qur'an 2:166–7)

The US government supports the production and sales of foods that are biologically addictive and foods that lead to sickness and disease, providing too much of the food that hurts us, and not enough of the food that benefits us. A food monopoly of $15 trillion dollars is made up of Big Food companies, fertilizer companies, Big Seed companies and Big Ag Companies. Eighty percent of American schools have contracts with soda companies and half of these schools serve fast food at lunch.

Food science has never been more complicated, as large companies engineer foods in their chemistry labs with unpronounceable names. Food companies add addictive and toxic substances, calling them food, but they are better thought of as similar to drugs.

Our Environment and Detoxification Pathways Are Out of Balance

Now, behold! Your Lord said to the angels: I am placing upon the earth a human successor to steward it. (Qur'an 2:30)

Eat and drink of that which Allah has provided and do not act corruptly, making mischief on the earth. (Qur'an 2:60)

And do good as Allah has been good to you, and seek not mischief in the land. Verily, Allah likes not the mufsidūn [those who commit great crimes and sins, oppressors, tyrants, mischief-makers, corrupters]. (Qur'an 28:77)

We are exposed to more and more chemicals, pesticides, pharmaceutical drugs and radiation than ever before – with more than one hundred thousand new chemicals in the past few years slowly penetrating our everyday lives, most invisibly. Our bodies are not meant to handle the enormous amount of artificial pollutants we are exposed to daily, inside and out. Slow regular exposure can cause the toxins to accumulate in our bodies, and we depend on our livers to remove these toxins.

This planet is our trust, but we are destroying ourselves and the environment that we all call home. We are filling our world with chemicals. We are dumping 5.4 billion pounds of pesticides and over 200 million pounds of fertilizer worldwide every year. We have disrupted the soil, and need more fertilizers and pesticides to grow crops, depleting the minerals and diversity of the soil.

A pesticide named Glyphosate is an active ingredient in Roundup, a broad spectrum of herbicide that is widely used in the United States. With the rise in GMO seeds came the rise of pesticides, known as "Roundup Ready Crops", meaning the crop can be sprayed with more and more pesticide without killing it. The World Health Organization (WHO) relabeled Glyphosate as a "possible carcinogen". It is toxic to our gut organisms, impairs the mitochondria from functioning properly and disrupts hormone balance.

Electromagnetic fields (EMFs) are gaining new attention as we swim in a sea of EMFs all day long from cell towers/mobile phone masts, computers, microwaves, Bluetooth devices and most importantly from your cell/mobile phones. The negative health effects of EMF exposure include cellular dysfunction, increased intracellular calcium that generates oxidative stress causing unrepaired DNA damage that increases the levels of nitric oxide (NO), excessive amounts of which are dangerous, and superoxide genetic mutations and disease.[47] So it makes it all the more important to eat well in order to optimize the body's mechanism of repair and regeneration.

Our Mental Health and Emotions Are Out of Balance

Living in a world of constant stress, lack of exposure to nature, lack of exercise, constant negativity, having minds that are constantly on the go, inability to sleep, and negative social relationships can lead to disease and, most importantly, chronic stress, which kills brain cells in the prefrontal cortex and makes them grow in the amygdala for a "fight or flight" type of response.

Due to our chaotic lives, our minds no longer know how to stay still, limiting the time and space we have for daily reflection. We are living in a world where our minds can't even stay still during prayer, increasing chronic stress further.

Lack of Nature

Americans spend about 87 percent of their time indoors and another 6 percent in their cars.[48] We have evolved to benefit from dirt and nature, but by staying away from them there has been an increase in asthma, autoimmune disorders, and food allergies, and this could be due to the lack of exposure to nature and its rich microbial enviroments that can be found in soil.[49]

Lack of Sleep

A third of American adults get less than the recommended hours of sleep.[50] When we fail to get enough rest, our bodies may not complete some important tasks, increasing the chance of developing problems due to excess toxins, inflammation, and hormone imbalances. One week of sleep deprivation can alter the function of 711 genes, including the ones involved in metabolism, immunity, inflammation and even stress.[51] Lack of sleep can contribute to bad decision-making, negative emotions, and even addictive behaviours.

Many turn to sleep aids, with their unrelenting side effects that may increase the risk of depression, dementia, cancer and even infections, as they have been linked to 400,000 US deaths per year.[52]

Lack of Real Social Connections

In our new age of internet and social media, around 70 percent of the world's population owns a cell or mobile phone.[53] Unfortunately, our digital life is disconnecting us from those who matter most. Studies have shown that the average user spends more than two hours on social networking sites a day and another survey has shown that Americans are staring at a screen 42 percent of the time.[54] We are becoming addicted to the internet, promoting mindless activity, which is disconnecting us from our higher-level brain functions. The longer we spend on devices, the less we benefit and the more corporations benefit. A study from 2018 showed that having a phone present during a conversation between two strangers was linked to greater distraction[55] and lower levels of perceived empathy.[56] Men between the ages of 19–32 showed greater loneliness and depression the more social media they used. [57]

Increased Negativity

And [remember] when your Lord proclaimed, "If you are grateful, I will surely increase you [in favour]; but if you deny, indeed, My punishment is severe." (Qur'an 14:7)

We live in a world where we wake up to negativity: our social media is filled with negativity; our social and work environments are negative; our family lives are negative; and we go to sleep focussed on all the things that are going wrong in our lives. We are losing our sense of self and self-worth. Our identities are being sold to us: telling us what we are supposed to have, what we should be looking like and what we need to achieve – and this leaves us feeling inadequate.

The lens through which we view the world is clouded, with instant access to everything at our fingertips. We live in peaceful environments, enjoy lower rates of poverty and crime rates have fallen in the US from the 1990s to the 2000s[58], but the news, social media and TV are saying something else. Among college students, only fifteen minutes of exposure to news was enough to increase symptoms of anxiety.[59]

Through the science of neuroplasticity, the ability to form and organize synaptic connections, with constant negativity or fear, our brains rewire to respond to this negativity, threating our ability to employ the prefrontal cortex, leading to disease and despair.

Chronic stress disconnects the two sections of the brain, leading to decreased empathy, impulsive behaviour and poor decision-making. The lack of social connection, sleep, nature and gratitude increases the activation of the amygdala. Unfortunately, chronic stress and unhappiness lead to looking for quick fixes or instant gratification, like checking our messages and emails to give us a dopamine burst, resulting in the chronic use of short-term fixes that may cause chronic stress, inflammation and disease. We have fallen into this digital world that exacerbates chronic stress and inflammation.

This digital life has disconnected us, and some studies have proven that excessive screen time results in a lack of secure attachments, limited family time, sleep disruptions, mood disturbances, increasing obestiy and harming our overall physical and mental health.

We are more out of balance than we have ever been before. So to put it simply, when we live impurely, we intoxicate the earth, we disrupt Allah's balance and alter our genes. Allah, glorified and exalted is He, has told us that these impurities are going to be in such abundance that they will start to look pleasing to us. But then we must educate ourselves that the pure and the impure are not the same.

Islam and Balance

Say: Impure and pure are not equal, even though the abundance of impure may be pleasing to you. Have fear of God, you who are endowed with understanding, so that you may succeed. (Qur'an 5: 100)

Should not He who has created know? And He is the most kind and courteous [to his slaves] All Aware [of everything]. (Qur'an 67: 14)

The Qur'an is a timeless guidance to all of mankind. Allah, glorified and exalted is He, knows that the human body needs balance. Allah, glorified and exalted is He, has constantly given us the keys to success in all aspects, for those who understand. So to succeed at anything, we need to get back to the equation that Allah, glorified and exalted is He, has given us:

Those who follow the Messenger, the unlettered prophet, whom they find written in what they have of the Torah and the Gospel, who enjoins upon them what is right and forbids them what is wrong and makes lawful for them the pure things and prohibits for them the impure things and relieves them of their burden and the shackles which were upon them. So they who have believed in him, honored him, supported him and followed the light which was sent down with him – it is those who will be the successful. (Qur'an 7: 157)

The Equation is Simple

Follow the Messenger, peace and blessings be upon him + Live Purely, Prohibit the Impure = Success

(*falāḥ* is success in this life and the Hereafter)

Pure food, pure environment, pure thoughts, pure words, pure friends, pure sleep, positive thoughts, a pure lifestyle (pillars of optimal health) = success and health

The key to a balanced life is to live a *tayyib* life. To live purely, uncontaminated, all naturally with what Allah, glorified and exalted is He, has provided us, to live in balance.

But then He has given us another equation to success:

Say, "Not equal are the pure and the impure, although the abundance of impure might impress you." So fear Allah, O you of understanding, that you may be successful. (Qur'an 5:100)

Fear of Allah, glorified and exalted is He + Understanding = Success

In order to succeed we must have God- consciousness and understand.

And whoever is blind in this [life] will be blind in the Hereafter and more astray in way. (Qur'an 17: 72)

Time to lift the veil from our eyes, open our minds and actually think and reflect about what we are doing to our bodies and our planet – the gifts that Allah, glorified and exalted is He, has given us, our *amānah* or trust. So let's dive in a little deeper to understand better the importance of a *ṭayyib* or pure lifestyle, that we may put everything back into balance, to purify our hearts, to heal our bodies and our planet for ultimate *falāḥ* (success) in this life and the Hereafter.

A *Ṭayyib* Lifestyle Balances Us and Reinstates Hope

O you who have believed, eat from the good things which We have provided for you and be grateful to Allah, glorified and exalted, if it is [indeed] Him that you worship. (Qur'an 2: 172)

When I learned this *āyahs*, it changed my world. This was how I was able to help people get back to balance. So we need to take a deeper dive into what exactly is *ṭayyib*, and why it is the overlooked key to heaven and success. Why does Allah connect it with gratitude and whether we truly worship him?

The Overlooked Key to Heaven and Success – *Ṭayyib*

Over and over in the Qur'an, Allah refers to *ṭayyib*, so let's dive into this overlooked key to heaven, success and consequently our health – a key piece in putting our bodies back into balance.

What is *Ṭayyib*?

Ṭayyib is a very comprehensive word that has an important place in the Qur'an and Sunnah. In Surah *al-Baqarah*, Allah, glorified and exalted is He, has clearly defined "*ṭayyib*". Allah, glorified and exalted is He, clearly and unequivocally commands us to eat of that which is *ṭayyib* from what He has provided for us. So, the word "*ṭayyib*" itself means to be pure, good, clean, wholesome, gentle, excellent, fair and lawful. Its opposite, *khabīth*, means impure, genetically modified, artificial in terms of colours and preservatives, toxic, etc. This concept is often paired together with "halal", as in "halal and *ṭayyib*", as well as used alone.

In my thirty-seven years on this planet, I was always taught to ask if the food is "halal" but never if it was "*ṭayyib*".

Allah, glorified and exalted is He, describes what is *tayyib* as a strong tree and its opposite, what is *khabīth* (impure), as a weak tree which lacks resilience and can be uprooted at any moment from the surface of the earth.

Have you not considered how Allah presents an example, [making] a good/pure word like a good/pure tree, whose root is firmly fixed and its branches [high] in the sky? It produces its fruit all the time, by permission of its Lord. And Allah presents examples for the people that perhaps they will be reminded. *And the example of a bad word is like a bad tree, uprooted from the surface of the earth, not having any stability.* (Qur'an 14: 24–26)

Living a *tayyib* life puts your body back into balance and increases resilience to whatever life may throw at you. Allah, glorified and exalted is He, will help you stay firm, emotionally, mentally, physically and spiritually, *insha'Allāh*.

Allah keeps firm those who believe, with the firm word, in worldly life and in the Hereafter. And Allah sends astray the wrongdoers. And Allah does what He wills. (Qur'an 14: 27)

Diving into the *Ṭayyib* – Surah al-Baqarah Verses 166–172

In trying to understand the concept of *tayyib*, this passage of the Qur'an sheds light on its importance, what society will say, and what to do to succeed, if we truly believe in Allah:

[And they should consider that] when those who have been followed disassociate themselves from those who followed [them], and they [all] see the punishment, and cut off from them are the ties [of relationship]. Those who followed will say, "If only we had another turn [at worldly life] so we could disassociate ourselves from them as they have disassociated themselves from us." Thus will Allah show them their deeds as regrets upon them. And they are never to emerge from the Fire. O mankind, eat from whatever is on earth [that is] lawful and good and do not follow the footsteps of Satan. Indeed, he is to you a clear enemy. He only orders you to evil and immorality and to say about Allah what you do not know. And when it is said to them, "Follow what Allah has revealed," they say, "Rather, we will follow that which we found our fathers doing." Even though their fathers understood nothing, nor were they guided? The example of those who disbelieve is like that of one who shouts at what hears nothing but calls and cries cattle or sheep – deaf, dumb and blind, so they do not understand. O you who have believed, eat from the good things which We have provided for you and be grateful to Allah if it is [indeed] Him that you worship. (Qur'an 2: 166–172)

Let's examine this passage. In verses 166–168, Allah, glorified and exalted is He, paints a picture of people standing next to Hellfire, with multiple regrets (*ḥasarāt*) for following social norms blindly. They wished they had dissociated themselves from these people. After painting this picture, this passage then takes the reader to the solution on how we can prevent that outcome. Allah, glorified and exalted is He, says, *O mankind, eat from whatever is on earth [that is] lawful and good and do not follow the footsteps of Satan. Indeed, he is to you a clear enemy* (Qur'an 2: 168). Then in verse 170, Allah, glorified and exalted is He, says, they will ignore revelation and stick to what their forefathers have done, showing the herd mentality of cattle. They are deaf, dumb and blind, and will never understand.

Isn't that what is happening now? We are stuck in our ways too, despite all the evidence at hand, and that we know better and know more than our forefathers, but this self-satisfaction keeps us stuck, and doesn't allow us to unlearn what we think we know and relearn what we need to know. We are stuck with a herd mentality, not thinking, chewing all day long, going along in the direction that everyone else is following. If a commercial tells us something is good, we move our mouths without using our brains and continue to eat like cattle. Then Allah, glorified and exalted is He, says, in verse 172 that, *Eat from the good things (tayyib) which We have provided for you and be grateful to Allah if it is [indeed] Him that you worship.* Allah uses the word "'*in kuntum iyyāhu taʿbudūn*," meaning if you truly worship Allah or if you are truly enslaved to Allah. So the question is, who are we enslaved to? We are enslaved to our desires, when our purpose on this planet is really to worship Allah.

And I did not create the jinn and mankind except to worship Me. (Qur'an 51: 57)

In *āyahs* 172, as well as in many other places in the Qur'an, Allah, glorified and exalted is He, has equated eating pure foods with truly believing in Allah. So if we don't eat pure foods, what does that say about us as Muslims? Who are we truly following? The answer lies in *āyahs* 168:

O mankind! Eat the lawful and good things out of what is in the earth, and do not follow the footsteps of the shaytān; surely he is your open enemy. (Qur'an 2: 168)

We are following Satan (the *Shaytān*) as not eating pure food opens doors that may lead us down the wrong path, a path away from Allah. If we go down that path, the path of impurity, we are opening doors in our heart for Satan to enter. We are no longer slaves of Allah, but slaves of the sugar companies, the fast food companies, the pesticide companies (Monsanto), the pharmaceutical companies, and even the materialistic goods companies. It's time to get back to the Qur'an, back to a *tayyib* life, back to Allah.

The Two Keys to Optimal Success – Halal and Ṭayyib

Living pure (*tayyib*) lives is one of the overlooked keys to ultimate success (*falāḥ*) in this world and in the Hereafter. But what is important to realise is that this is found all over the Qur'an, and He has equated it to being believers who truly worship Allah.

O mankind! Eat the lawful and good things out of what is in the earth, and do not follow the footsteps of the shaytan; surely he is your open enemy. (Qur'an 2: 168)

"O you who have believed, eat from the good things which We have provided for you and be grateful to Allah if it is [indeed] Him that you worship. (Qur'an 2: 172)

And eat of what Allah has provided for you [which is] lawful and good. And fear Allah, in whom you are believers. (Qur'an 5: 88)

Those who follow the Messenger, the unlettered prophet, whom they find written in what they have of the Torah and the Gospel, who enjoins upon them what is right and forbids them what is wrong and makes lawful for them the good things and prohibits for them the impure things and relieves them of their burden and the shackles which were upon them. So they who have believed in him, honored him, supported him and followed the light which was sent down with him – it is those who will be the successful. (Qur'an 7: 157)

Then eat of what Allah has provided for you [which is] lawful and good. And be grateful for the favour of Allah, if it is [indeed] Him that you worship. (Qur'an 16: 114)

Allah's Equation for Success

Those who follow the Messenger, the unlettered prophet, whom they find written in what they have of the Torah and the Gospel, who enjoins upon them what is right and forbids them what is wrong and makes lawful for them the pure things and prohibits for them the impure and relieves them of their burden and the shackles which were upon them. So they who have believed in him, honored him, supported him and followed the light which was sent down with him – it is those who will be the successful. (Qur'an 7: 157)

In the Qur'an (7:157), Allah, glorified and exalted is He, provides humankind with a formula for success:

Following the Messenger, peace and blessings be upon him + living *tayyib* (purely) + prohibiting the impure = Success

This is significant! Allah, glorified and exalted is He, has made following the unlettered Prophet, peace and blessings be upon him, *equal* to living a *tayyib* life and staying away from impurities. This means that if we don't follow one or the other we will not be successful. If we claim to follow the Prophet, peace and blessings be upon him but eat artificial or GMO-ridden food, or live an impure lifestyle, we will not be successful, and vice versa. This describes exactly what is happening to the Muslim *ummah* currently.

Allah's Command to His Messengers

> *O messengers, eat from pure things and act righteously, for I know what you do.* (Qur'an 23:51)

Allah has directly connected the way we eat to our actions. He commanded His messengers that, in order to do good, they must eat pure food, just like He has commanded all believers with the same.

The Relationship between *Tayyib* and Allah's Anger and then Hope

> *Eat of the good things We have provided for your sustenance, but commit no excess therein, lest My wrath should justly descend on you, and those on whom descends My wrath do perish indeed.* (Qur'an 20: 81)

In Surah *Tāha*, after instructing the children of Israel, Allah, glorified and exalted is He, then turns to educating the general population regarding the consequences of breaking His laws. Allah, glorified and exalted is He, instructs us all to eat *tayyib* foods that Allah, glorified and exalted, has provided and not to cross any of the limits He set, otherwise, Allah's anger will come down, seize and overwhelm us. And whoever Allah's anger comes down upon, will fall hard and fast.

But then Allah, glorified and exalted, gives us hope:

> *But indeed, I am the Perpetual Forgiver of whoever repents and believes and does righteousness and then continues in guidance.* (Qur'an 20: 82)

We recite Surah *al-Fātiḥah* several times a day, asking Allah to save us from His wrath: *The way of those on whom You have bestowed Your Grace, not the way of those who earned Your Wrath, nor of those who went astray.* (Qur'an 1: 7)

In Surah Ṭāha, Allah, glorified and exalted is He, gives us hope that He will completely forgive our sins. Allah, glorified and exalted is He, has shown us the path, it is up to us to walk *down* it or not, and He mentions this right after He talked about eating *ṭayyib*.

Artificial foods, fake foods, harmful foods, and GMO foods are by definition not *ṭayyib* as these foods inflict harm on the body, as has been documented in medical research for years. First and foremost, Allah, glorified and exalted, has directly related success in this life and the next to eating and living a *ṭayyib* life. Allah, glorified and exalted is He, has described to us the seriousness of breaking His law, but if you repent, He is All-Forgiving.

Allah, Glorified and Exalted, is Pure and Accepts Only What is Pure – Ṭayyib as a Prerequisite

This Day [all] Tayyib/Pure food has been made lawful... And whoever denies the faith, his work has become worthless, And he, in the Hereafter, will be among the losers. (Qur'an 5: 5)

Abū Hurayrah reported that the Messenger of Allah, peace and blessings be upon him, said, "O people, Allah is pure and He accepts only what is pure. Verily, Allah has commanded the believers what He has commanded His messengers. Allah said, '*O messengers, eat from good things and act righteously, for I know what you do*' (23: 51). And Allah said, '*O you who believe, eat from good things We have provided for you.*" (2: 172) (Muslim)

Working for Allah, glorified and exalted is He, goes hand-in-hand with the lifestyle we choose. In these two areas, Allah, glorified and exalted is He, and His Prophet, peace and blessings be upon him, have dictated that we eat pure food otherwise the work that we do will not be accepted and we will be among the losers.

In the above hadith, the Prophet, peace and blessings be upon him said, that Allah, glorified and exalted, is pure, and accepts only what is pure. In the next sentence he quotes the Qur'an about the qualities of the one who is pure – that he eats pure food. Through His messengers, Allah, glorified and exalted is He, has told us what He wants us to do: to eat pure food and to act righteously, and then quoting 2: 172, He states that we should only eat that which is pure. In this verse and in the above hadith, a large emphasis is put on eating and living in a pure way and working righteously. One needs to be pure for one's righteous acts to be accepted. This is a prerequisite for our good deeds to be accepted.

Ṭayyib: the Hidden Key to Taqwā

And eat of what Allah has provided for you [which is] lawful and pure and fear Allah, in whom you are believers. (Qur'an 5:88)

31

Allah has sent this book, the Qur'an as *"a guide for those who are mindful of Allah"* (Qur'an 2:2), i.e. for the *muttaqīn*.

Taqwā consists of balancing our love for Allah with not breaking His commands. When we truly have *taqwā*, we are in balance and harmony with everything around us. How we live our lives determines the state of our *taqwā*.

One of the keys to obtaining *taqwā* is described in Surah *al-Mā'idah*. In *āyahs* 88, Allah tells us that one of the ways of expressing our *taqwa* and putting It Into action is to eat halal and *tayyib*.

The root meaning of the word *taqwā* is to avoid what one dislikes. It was reported that 'Umar ibn al-Khaṭṭāb asked Ubayy ibn Ka'b about *taqwā* and Ubayy said: 'Have you ever walked on a path that has thorns on it?' 'Umar said, 'Yes!' Ubayy said: 'What did you do then?' He said: 'I rolled up my sleeves and struggled.' Ubayy said: 'That is *taqwā*.'

Taqwā has to do with prevention; building a barrier from sins. In this *āyahs*, Allah has combined it with halal and *tayyib*, pure food, again, equating those who uphold both with true believers.

Allah has commanded the believers as he commanded His messengers.

O messengers, eat from good things and act righteously, for I know what you do. (Qur'an 23:51).

The Ṭayyib and The Pandemic?

In the middle of this pandemic, when we have limited answers and need hope, we must turn to the Qur'an and look for what Allah says that we should do. Allah describes a city:

And Allah presents an example: a city which was safe and secure, its provisions coming to it in abundance from every location, but it denied the favours of Allah. So Allah made it taste the envelopment of hunger and fear for what they had been doing.... Then eat what Allah has provided for you [which is] lawful and pure. And be grateful for the favours of Allah, if it is [indeed] Him that you worship. (Qur'an 16:112-114)

This verse depicts exactly what is going on right now. We undoubtedly take for granted the blessings and bounties bestowed on us. We stuff our bodies and our children's bodies with artificial and toxic food and chemicals, keep spraying the earth with toxins, live with chronic stress, lack of sleep and negativity without thinking about the consequences of it all. Have we stopped to think that our bodies and the resources of earth are gifts from Allah and that we should be grateful to Allah for them?

Taking care of our bodies and the earth is a true act of gratitude. But by polluting our bodies and earth we become truly ungrateful. We are now suffering more than ever from the consequences of feeding toxins to our bodies and throwing toxins on our planet.

Allah, Glorified and Exalted, Knows Impurity Surrounds and Tempts Us

Say: Evil and good are not equal, even though the abundance of evil may be pleasing to you. Have fear of God, you who are endowed with understanding, so that you may triumph. (Qur'an 5: 100)

Allah, glorified and exalted is He, knows that we are bombarded all around us with impurities. But He constantly tells us to use our brains and understanding.

Ṭayyib and Being a Believer, If You Truly Worship Allah

O you who have believed, eat from the pure things which We have provided for you and be grateful to Allah if it is [indeed] Him that you worship. (Qur'an 2:172)

And eat of what Allah has provided for you [which is] lawful and pure and fear Allah, in whom you are believers. (Qur'an 5:88)

Then eat of what Allah has provided for you [which is] lawful and pure. And be grateful for the favour of Allah, if it is [indeed] Him that you worship. (Qur'an 16:114)

Over and over again, Allah has connected food to our belief in Him and whether we worship him alone.

Conclusions from the Qur'an and Sunnah

From all the verses in the Qur'an and evidence from the Sunnah, we can conclude that eating pure foods that Allah has created, and living a pure lifestyle, are directly linked to our faith and true success in this life and the next and eating anything impure (artificial, GMO, toxic) is not only prohibited but also opens the doors for the Shayṭān and wrongdoing.

33

And We shaded you with clouds and sent down to you manna and quails, [saying], "Eat from the pure things with which We have provided you." And they wronged Us not - but they were [only] wronging themselves. (Qur'an 2:57)

"Eat from the pure things which we have provided you". And they wronged Us not, but they were [only] wronging themselves. (Qur'an 7:160)

So living a pure lifestyle is key to balance, health and true success in this life and the next.

When we combine this with science, we see that impure life leads to sickness, disease and destruction of our health, future and planet. It is a simple equation:

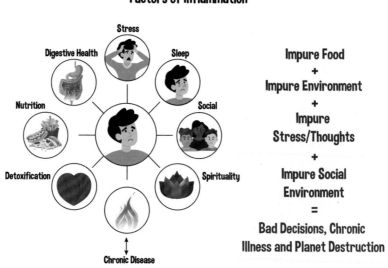

PICTURE 2.1 FACTORS OF AN IMPURE LIFE

Simple Math	
Impure Lifestyle and Effects on Our Life	**Pure Lifestyle and Effects on Our Life**
Impure Food +	Pure Food +
Impure Environment + Impure Stress/Thoughts + Impure Social Environment = *Bad Decisions* *Chronic Illnesses* *Destroying the World* *Footsteps of the Shayṭān* *Out of balance life and body*	Pure Environment + Pure Stress/Thoughts + Pure Social Environment = *Making Good Decisions* *Healing/Preventing Chronic Illness* *Healing the World* *Linking it to True Faith and Success* *True Taqwā* *Balanced life and body*

Ṭayyib Lifestyle Heals

So by optimizing and purifying our lifestyles (the pillars of optimal health), we can put our bodies and planet back into balance and heal from the inside out. An impure lifestyle leads to an imbalanced life. We talked in the last chapter about how this imbalance causes the body's response of inflammation, leading to chronic disease of all stripes in all ages, threatening our economy, with intensive farming among other things, destroying our world and hurting our future.

So what are the keys to a healthy lifestyle? Let's examine the main fundamental pillars of health.

1. Digestive Health and Detoxification
2. The Four S's (Stress, Sleep, Social Health and Spiritual Health)

Digestive Health and Nutrition – Digestive Health and Detoxification

Digestive Health and Nutrition

When Allah, glorified and exalted, talks about food, He says the food needs to be pure. We need to eat less of it and it needs to be nutrient-dense.

The Prophet (peace be upon him) said: 'The child of Adam fills no vessel worse than his stomach. Sufficient for the child of Adam are a few morsels to keep his back straight. If he must eat more, then a third should be for his food, a third for his drink, and a third left for air.' (Tirmidhī and *Musnad* of Aḥmad)

O mankind, eat from whatever is on earth [that is] lawful and good and do not follow the footsteps of Satan. Indeed, he is to you a clear enemy. (Qur'an 2: 168)

By focusing on pure foods, we can heal our bodies and our earth.

Detoxification and Our Environment

"Evil has appeared on land and sea because of what the hands of people have earned [by oppression and evil deeds], that Allah -may make them taste a part of that which they have done, in order that they may return" (Qur'an 30: 41)

Tayyib food and a tayyib lifestyle are key to optimizing your body's ability to get rid of toxins, lower inflammation and balance your hormones. A tayyib lifestyle can help save our world, replenishing the soil, our food and our communities from the inside out.

The Four S's

Stress

O mankind! There has come to you a direction from you Lord, and a healing for (the disease in your) heart, and for those who believe, a guidance, and mercy. (Qur'an 10:57)

He guides to Himself those who turn to Him in penitence – Those who have believed and whose hearts have rest in the remembrance of God. Verily in the remembrance of God, do hearts find rest. (Qur'an 13:27–28)

With stress causing more than 80 percent of the complaints presented to primary care, discussing stress management is essential in the healing and prevention of disease. This is a part of mind-body medicine, a branch of integrative medicine that looks at our thoughts, feelings, and emotions and how they affect physical health and how physical health affects spiritual and emotional well-being and also refers to overall psychological well-being.

When mind-body techniques, such as a change in mindset, mindfulness and meditation, spending time in nature, exercise, prayer and *duʿāʾ*, the remembrance of Allah, glorified and exalted is He, learning to breathe, etc. are practised daily and properly, they can have a powerful positive effect on our lives and well-being. We can also reframe the stress as a test from God, and in remembrance and prayer, and even spending time in nature, we can release that stress to a higher power. By incorporating these techniques, we can teach our body different kinds of responses to a situation so that the body doesn't turn on the damaging hormones, maintaining a balanced inner world and preventing or helping heal any chronic illness we may have.

Sleep

It is Allah Who receives the souls at the time of their death, and those that do not die during their sleep. He keeps those [souls] for which He has ordained death and sends the rest [back to their bodies] for a term appointed. (Qurʾan 39: 42)

Our bodies do consume much energy during the eight or nine hours of sleep they require, which leaves more available energy for toxin removal, hormone manufacture, and fighting infection.

Social

And (remember) the Day when the wrongdoer will bite on his hand, he will say: 'Oh! Would that I had taken a path with the Messenger. Ah! Woe to me! Would that I had never taken so-and-so as a friend! He indeed led me astray from the Reminder (the Qurʾan) after it had come to me.' (Qurʾan 25:27)

The example of the believers in their mutual love and mercy is like the example of a body. If one part of it feels pain, then all of it is affected by sickness and fever. (Bukhārī, Muslim)

Prophet Muhammad, peace and blessings be upon him, said: 'The believers are to each other like a solid building, they strengthen each other.' (Muslim)

Prophet Muhammad said: 'A person visited his brother in another town and God sent an angel to wait for him on his way. The angel said, "Where do you intend to go?" The man answered, "I intend to go to my brother in this town." The angel said, "Have you done any favour to him, the repayment of which you intend to get?" He said: "No, I love him for the sake of God, the Exalted and Glorious." Thereupon the angel said, "I am a messenger to you from God to inform you that God loves you as you love him."' (Muslim)

The social environment and limiting of tech devices are important for overall health as the feelings of being loved releases a flood of potent hormones into our blood streams, which makes us feel better emotionally with the added benefit of significantly strengthening our immune systems. Receiving love from those around us helps the body heal itself. So keep people around you that will lift you up and not drag you down.

Spiritual Health

And [remember] when your Lord proclaimed, 'If you are grateful, I will surely increase you [in favour]; but if you deny, indeed, My punishment is severe.' (Qur'an 14:7)

As we are all composed of minds, bodies and souls, healing the soul is an important aspect in the prevention and healing of disease. Scientific studies indicate the positive relationship between spirituality and health. When the thinking mind stops and spiritual energy begins to flow through you, it causes healthy changes in the physical body, especially if you practise them daily. Spirituality affects the physical body by improving blood circulation, decreasing blood pressure, improving digestion and detoxification, turning unhealthy genes off and helping to improve the overall immune system. So focus on ten things you are thankful for every morning and evening. Allah, glorified and exalted is He, and more recently science have proven that positivity heals from the inside out!

Allah, glorified and exalted is He, emphasizes the importance of being a people of *Alhamdulillah*! He uses the strongest language in the Qur'an, as He promises and swears to it that He will increase for us if we are grateful. The beauty of this is that Allah, glorified and exalted is He, doesn't specify what He will increase us in and who we need to be thankful to.

Putting Out the Fire Using the Qur'an and Sunnah!

Your body has a right over you... (Bukhārī)

Our bodies have a right over us. So we need to take care of them and of the earth the best we know how. To be truly effective at preventing, managing and/or overcoming a chronic condition or symptom, we need to address these processes at every level, we need to focus on a *tayyib* lifestyle at every level. Chronic inflammation burns in the body, slowly destroying it the way fire destroys a building. Unless the fire is put out (i.e. to calm the inflammation), we're simply allowing the building to smolder, compromising our bodies further.

Conventional medicine doesn't put out the fire of chronic illnesses but simply puts a Band-Aid on the blaze without turning off the ignition. This approach will only work superficially to keep symptoms at bay but will rarely address the root cause of the blaze. In order to effectively manage the symptoms – and, better yet, overcome the condition – we need to put out the fire once and for all, get our body and it's hormones back into balance, allow the body to stop fighting an uphill battle, and set ourselves on the path to recovery. Addressing the root causes of inflammation and optimizing our mitochondria will help us overcome not one but multiple chronic conditions and balance our hormones all at the same time.

Everyone is different, and what is an imbalance for one person may be a balance for another. So find out what is making you out of balance. Once you have dealt with the individual root cause, by living a *tayyib* life, you put your body back into balance and you can optimize healing and prevent chronic disease.

We Have Control and So Much Hope

Everything good that happens to you (O Man) is from God, everything bad that happens to you is from your own actions. (Qur'an 4:79)

Healing/pure foods, positivity, and a *tayyib*/pure lifestyle not only communicate with our genes, but they also affect us physically and spiritually. Let's try our hardest to live *tayyib* (pure) lifestyles, eat less and be more grateful.

Pure Digestive Health and Detoxification

+

Pure Four S's

= HEALING

Allah, glorified and exalted is He, doesn't test us with more than we can tolerate. Take one step towards Allah, glorified and exalted is He, and He will run towards you.

It is You we worship and You we ask for help. Guide us to the straight path. (Qur'an 1:5–6)

39

PART 2

The Pillars of a *Ṭayyib* Lifestyle

Digestive Health and Detoxification-Pure Food and Environment

It is Allah Who made for you the earth a place of settlement and the sky a ceiling and formed you and perfected your forms and provided you with good things. That is Allah, your Lord; then blessed is Allah, Lord of the worlds. (Qur'an 40:64)

He it is, Who has made the earth subservient to you [easy for you to walk, to live and to do agriculture on it], so walk in the path thereof and eat of His provision... (Qur'an 67: 15)

Digestive Health and Nutrition – The Qur'anic and Scientific Perspectives on Food

O mankind, eat from whatever is on earth which is lawful and pure and don't follow the footsteps of Satan. Indeed he is to you a clear enemy. (Qur'an 2:168)

This Day [all] Tayyib/Pure food has been made lawful...And whoever denies the faith- his work has become worthless, and he, in the Hereafter, will be among the losers. (Qur'an 5:5)

Let people then consider their food. (Qur'an 80:24)

Food is fun. Food is family. Food is joy. Food is power. Food is information. Food influences our microbes. Food is energy. Food provides instructions for every bodily function. Food influences our genes (called nutrigenomics). Food gives us the ability to take back control of our health. Food transforms our biology. Food nourishes the earth. Food activates our potential for healing or creates imbalances that lead to disease.

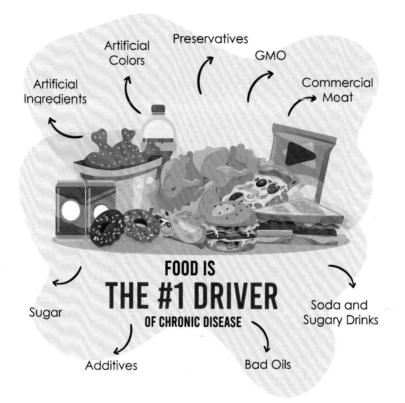

PICTURE 3.1   FOOD IS THE NUMBER ONE DRIVER OF CHRONIC DISEASE

But not just any food, pure quality foods packed with nutrients are the foundational building blocks to a flourishing world.

Food is Also Confusing!!!

One day one food is good, then the next day it's terrible and then it's good again. We have been in "food wars" for as long I can remember. One group against another group. So why is this the case? It is because nutrition research is not precise, very hard to carry out, and very difficult to control. If researchers wanted a "perfect" study, then they would have to have two or more groups of people who only eat what they want them to eat and follow this process for years, which is very difficult to do. So most of the research we have on nutrition is obtained through questionnaires and surveys, which rely on inaccurate reports while some studies are funded by parties that have a conflict of interest. Research has shown that if a study is paid for by a company, it is eight times more likely to be in the company's favour.[1] For instance, the American Heart Association receives much of its funding from pharmaceutical and food industries. It is a confusing world out there, and what is acceptable in society will continue to change, and the research we have in front of us more often than not is cherry-picked to support particular theories.

Allah, Glorified and Exalted is He, Clears the Confusion

Islam is more than just the religion of peace, it is a way of life. Allah has dictated how we should eat, drink, sleep, pray, treat others, and even use the bathroom. Allah has told us how to live our lives in order to attain true success. Allah knows that the social norms will continue to change, so we need to adhere to the baseline that Allah has given us.

Just like with everything, we need to focus on the elements we can add to our lives which will help us, and not hurt the bodies that Allah has blessed us with, and the same applies to food. We must focus on the foods that can help us, not hurt us; foods that will help us feel more energetic, keep our backs straight, help us lose weight, heal chronic diseases and obtain success in this life and the next.

Whenever Allah, glorified and exalted is He, and his Prophet, peace and blessings be upon him, talk about food, they specifically refer to *tayyib* (pure) quality, small quantity and nutrient-dense foods.

1. Pure quality food keeps the gut healthy;
2. Small quantities of pure foods can regulate glucose, decrease insulin resistance and balance hormones;
3. Nutrient-dense foods provide the body with the strength it needs to heal inside and out and create resilience.

Our Prophet, peace and blessings be upon him, gave us an excellent example in everything, especially when it comes to food. When these foods are put next to science, they are all anti-inflammatory foods!

Inflammation is the driver of chronic disease. So with that in mind, it makes sense to eat less of the food that increases inflammation, eliminating/limiting the foods that increase it, whether you have a diagnosed chronic condition or just want to prevent that.

The Qur'anic/prophetic way of life puts our body back into balance, the way Allah, glorified and exalted is He, intended. Our bodies use pure quality food which contain biological instructions that promote health, lower inflammation, balance

The Quranic Perspective on Food

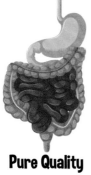
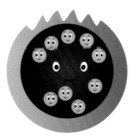
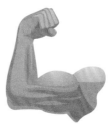

Pure Quality
Heals the Gut

"O People of faith, eat of the pure things we have given you and be grateful, if it (indeed) Allah that you worship" (Quran 2:172)

Small Quantity
Balances Insulin, Glucose and Hormone

"Eat and drink, but not to excess" (Al - Araf 7:31)

Prophetic Food
Nutrient Dense

But instead...

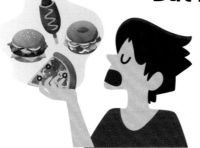

"But those who disbelieve enjoy themselves and eat as grazing livestock eat, and the Fire will be a residence for them." (Qur'an 47:12)

PICTURE 3.2   THE QUR'ANIC PRESPECTIVE ON FOOD

hormones, optimize brain function, improve the gut microbiome, and even optimize gene expression. Pure quality foods remove interference within the body and sends signals that turn gene expression on and off in just the right and appropriate way.

Pure foods can reverse climate change, build our soils thereby increasing nutrients, biodiversity, restoring the ecosystem and protecting our water. These pure foods contain 25,000 or more phytochemicals in the planet kingdom identified to date and are critical for overall health. These foods also influence all of the 37 billion chemical reactions that occur in our bodies every second. Not getting these foods can lead to chronic diseases of all types. But we can benefit from these foods only if they are of pure quality, small in quantity and dense in nutrients.

Pure Quality Foods and Our Guts

The worst vessel that the son of Adam can fill is the stomach... (Tirmidhī and Aḥmad)

Allah, glorified and exalted is He, mentions over and over again the importance of what we put in our mouths. We all know the above hadith, but have we ever seriously thought about it? Why is the stomach the worst vessel that the son/child of Adam can fill?

Now science has proven what Allah, glorified and exalted is He, has told us all along - Your gut is the gateway to your health and everyday decisions and so, restoring digestive health is very important for your overall well-being.

Why is the gut the worst vessel we can fill? Being the gateway to your health, our gut is the first to come into contact with the universe and is the first line of defence between us and the universe. Our gut houses about 70–80 percent or even more of our immune system,[2] just as it houses trillions of microorganisms that are in charge of our health and decisions!

To keep us in good health, and to keep us thinking appropriately, our guts rely on carefully maintaining a diverse and symbiotic relationship with trillions of microorganisms, as they influence everything down to the expression of our genetic code. It is empowering to think that every bite of food, every interaction with our environment, and every lifestyle choice creates a ripple effect that reaches into the microbiome and our genes.

The Role of Our Digestive Systems and Microbiome

Our digestive systems are very important in performing vital tasks to keep us all working well. First, they process the food that we eat, digest the food, convert the vitamins after the absorption of nutrients, and regulate our metabolisms. The gut houses most of the immune system, and it also prevents toxins and pathogens from entering the body. So it literally keeps the bad stuff out and the good stuff in. It repairs any damage caused by anything foreign in the body, like inflammation and infections. The digestive tract is a key organ in detoxification and removing toxins from the body (among others that are the skin, lungs, liver and kidney). Three fourths of the body's neurotransmitters are found and made in the gut, including 50 percent of the body's dopamine and 90 percent of the body's serotonin.

The body also houses trillions of tiny microscopic organisms that live in and on us, from every inch of our skin, mouth and digestive tract. Human cells are outnumbered 10:1 as there are approximately 360 million microbial genes for every human gene.[3] Science is learning more and more about the microbiome on a daily basis.

From conception, we are exposed to trillions of bacteria daily, and our microbiome continues to grow with us, constantly changing.[4] Our inner garden contains a unique composition of good bugs (mutualists), bad bugs (pathogens), and neutral bugs (commensals) that contain bacteria, yeasts, parasites, viruses and archaea which are involved in most, if not all, biological processes that constitute human health and disease by directly affecting our epigenetics, minds and immune systems. Our keys to optimal health and well-being are determined by this microbial balance and diversity.

The microbiome is a critical player in multiple physiological functions and promotes normal gastrointestinal function, thus digesting multiple nutrients, synthesizing hormones and vitamins, and balancing pH. It also helps extract energy and harvest calories from undigested food particles as they pass through the digestive tract, just as it absorbs food, manufactures neurotransmitters and even controls blood sugar balance. The microbiome is also very important for the production of vitamins and folic acid, thus increasing the absorption of minerals and manufacturing short chain and essential fatty acids. They break down and rebuild hormones, and help maintain a healthy weight and metabolism. The microbiome has a key role in immunity, via the gut associated lymphatic tissue (GALT), and is the first line of defence between the internal and external world. The bacteria interact with the immune system, influence the T cells (a critical part of the immune system), help fight off colds and infections, help to organize the right level of response to an invader; they also have antitumor and anticancer effects and break down bacterial toxins.

O mankind, eat from whatever is on earth [that is] lawful and good and do not follow the footsteps of Satan. Indeed, he is to you a clear enemy. (Qur'an 2:168)

O messengers, eat from pure things and act righteously, for I know what you do. (Qur'an 23:51)

Allah, glorified and exalted is He, linked what we put in our mouths with our brains and the decisions we make. Allah even commanded the Messenger to eat pure foods and do good, thus connecting food to action. Now science has proven the connection between the gut and the brain.

The microbiome helps to shape the brain, behaviour, mood and decision-making. The gut contains the same neurotransmitters found in the brain. Negative changes to the microbiome can lead to cytokine release, thus increasing stress and inflammation and leading to mood disturbances, bad decisions and even bad food cravings, partly via the vagus nerve. Positive changes in the microbiome create a calming response. The microbiome has the power to influence the expression of our genetic code, influence cellular functions and cravings for healthy foods (vegetables, protein, healthy fats and fruit). These bugs also influence the genes. When genes are turned on, they command the body to take action, and it doesn't matter if it's human gene or a bacterial gene. The absence of healthy gut bacteria alters genes, leading to inflammation and the alteration of signaling pathways involved in learning, motor control, memory and craving for the wrong type of foods (artificial, processed, white toxic food).

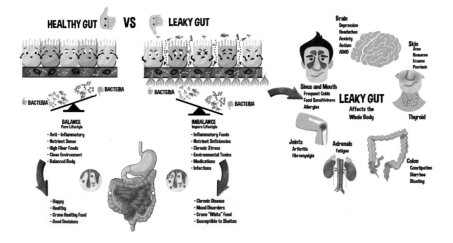

PICTURE 3.3 HEALTHY GUT VS LEAKY GUT

Lowering this bacterial richness of good bugs and increasing the amount of bad bugs can all lead to higher weight, high cholesterol, insulin resistance, increased inflammatory markers, chronic diseases and even bad decisions.[5] The health of our immune system is directly related to a healthy relationship with beneficial microbes that maintain the function of the small intestinal lining protecting us from unwanted foreign toxins/protein and infectious agents seeping into our blood stream.

These amazing tiny organisms play a vital role in the development of the immune system, will lay the foundation for our health for years to come. Changing this balance by adopting an impure lifestyle or through other impurities like infectious triggers can be responsible for inflammation leading to chronic disease[6].

All *Khabīth* Things Disrupt the Gut Microbiome

...He makes lawful to them the goodly pure things and forbids them from harmful impurely things... (Qur'an 7:157)

There are a number of factors that disrupt the gut microbiome, and they are all *khabīth* (impure). Some conditions have a genetic component, but many researchers have determined that less than 10 percent of those with the genes for an autoimmune disease will actually develop it. However, we have control over our genes. *Tayyib* factors help us to maintain good health, by reducing the exposure to triggers that can help put out the fire and leading to optimal health and healing for years to come.

Khabīth/Impure Food. What we eat and drink can directly affect the composition and metabolism of our microbiomes, and can either hurt or help us. The *tayyib* pure foods feed the "good" bugs, while the *khabīth* impure foods feed the "bad" bugs. Eating *khabīth* foods, with limited or no nutritional value, processed foods, an excessive amount of sugars, artificial foods, food additives and genetically modified crops filled with pesticides can create a dangerous toxic load in our bodies, throwing off our bacterial balance and creating an inflammatory response, leading to chronic disease and bad decisions. The pure foods that Allah, glorified and exalted is He, has provided us keep our microbiomes and brains healthy.

Chronic Stress/Khabīth/Impure Thoughts. Chronic stress can increase the level of stress hormones that negatively affect the microbiome, thus affecting the genes and leading to an overgrowth of yeast in the gut and inflammation, and vice versa. A deficiency in Akkermansia (good bacteria), a type of bacteria found in the intestine, can more likely lead to developing obesity and Type-1 diabetes. Stress hormones, like cortisol, and catecholamines, like epinephrine and norepinephrine, reduce the level of Akkermansia.

Khabīth/Impure Environment. The daily exposure to toxic environmental contaminants can put stresses on our immune defences. These toxins kill off many beneficial strains and microbes, strain the body's ability to repair itself and lead to chronic delays of necessary routine repairs.

Medications. Though some medications can save lives, they do come with a side disadvantage, so we need to weigh their risks vs. their benefits when we take any medications. Some medications, especially nonsteroidal anti-inflammatory drugs, other pain killers, birth control pills, steroids, chemotherapy drugs, acid blocking medications, opiates, antibiotics and sleep medications can negatively affect the microbiome.

Other factors include over strenuous exercise which may increase pro-inflammatory cytokines in the bloodstream and harm the lining of the intestinal wall, thus affecting the microbiome, and exposure to infections that were never resolved (bacteria, viruses, fungi or parasites, etc.).

How Impure (*Khabīth*) Substances and Foods Mess Us Up

The gut lining can be destroyed upon eating impure foods or living an impure lifestyle. The intestines are covered by intestinal epithelium, a single layer of cells that separate the body from all the stuff found in the intestines. The gut is naturally permeable in order to allow vital nutrients, like proteins, starches and digested fats to pass through the tight junctions and enter the blood stream.[7] Normally, the cells that line the intestines stick together very tightly to form a protective barrier that is very hard to penetrate, and this keeps bigger particles that can damage the system out. It also acts as a relay switch for the messages coming from the rest of the body to the good bacteria in the gut.

If an imbalanced gut microbiome or dysbiosis goes on for a while, pathogenic microbes or improperly digested proteins may activate the immune system, creating a fire or war in the gut as they trigger the immune cells leading to inflammation, damaging the gut wall epithelial cells and the junctions become leaky and increasingly permeable.[8] Over time, this leads to increased intestinal permeability or leaky gut syndrome.[9] When the gut becomes permeable, weak or compromised, it allows things to pass through the membrane into the blood stream, when normally they should not, such as undigested food particles, gluten, viruses, bad bacteria and toxins that trigger the immune system,[10] and this imbalances the gut microbes further. So biodiversity is key to keeping the immune system healthy and happy.

For short periods of time, acute inflammation isn't bad, but it's bad when the immune system is constantly in the "on" position for months because then it turns into a chronic inflammation. Over time the immune system becomes highly reactive, responding to stimuli that it ignored hitherto, like foreign substances such as zonulin (protein that modulates the permeability of tight junctions between the cells of the wall of the digestive system) which then keeps the gates open. When this continues for months and becomes chronic, it can lead to the translocation of bacteria and bacterial products, like lipopolysaccharides (LPS), also known as an endotoxin, which then penetrate the bloodstream, activating the immune system and releasing cytokines that instigate inflammation through the body and central nervous system (CNS).

Leaky Gut and Leaky Brain – The Gut-Brain Connection

O mankind, eat from whatever is on earth [that is] lawful and pure things and do not follow the footsteps of Satan. Indeed, he is to you a clear enemy. (Qur'an 2:168)

Verily, Allah has commanded the believers as He commanded his messengers. Allah said: O messengers, eat from good things and act righteously, for I know what you

51

do. And indeed this, your religion, is one religion, and I am your Lord, so fear Me. (Qur'an 23:51–52)

Allah, glorified and exalted is He, directly connects what we put in our mouths with the decisions we make. For every message from the brain that goes down to the gut microbiome, there are nine messages from the gut going up to the brain. These messages can influence the brain's response to a stressful situation, the activation of the brain's immune system, the adaptability of these new cells to learn (neuroplasticity), brain hormone production (that controls how the brain works) and the growth of new brain cells (neurogenesis).

An imbalanced microbiome creates an inflammatory environment that creates intestinal permeability. When it comes to the brain, this can also lead to a leaky gut, low grade inflammation and affect brain hormone production. Constant inflammation of the brain and body increases the risk of Alzheimer's, mood disorders, brain fog, mood swings and even memory loss. The microbiome has a direct impact on the breach in the blood brain barrier, which allows macromolecules from the blood to sneak inside the brain tissues. The specialized immune system in the brain (glia cells) are activated to fight the invaders leading to more inflammation. Breaches in the blood brain barrier can also come from head trauma, and a *khabīth* internal and external environment!

According to research published in journals like *Clinical Gastroenterology* and *Hepatology and Gut*, there are a number of health conditions that cause leaky gut or can be caused by it. Increased intestinal permeability can also lead to impaired glucose metabolism, insulin resistance, obesity, metabolic syndrome, Type-2 diabetes, food sensitivities, malnutrition and nutrient deficiencies like that of B12, magnesium and iron, and neurotransmitter deficiencies.

Leaky gut can be implicated in infections and acute inflammation like sepsis.[11] It can also be responsible for food sensitivities,[12] autoimmune diseases[13] celiac disease, non-celiac gluten sensitivity,[14] multiple sclerosis,[15] lupus,[16] Hashimoto's[17] and rheumatoid arthritis.[18] Leaky gut has been implicated in cardiovascular problems like hypertension[19] hyperlipidemia, CVD,[20] dermatological issues (eczema, psoriasis, rosacea, dermatitis, and acne),[21] endocrine issues like metabolic syndrome,[22] diabetes 1[23] and 2,[24] ENT problems like allergies[25] and sinus problems. Other conditions it is directly related to include gastrointestinal problems like gas, bloating, and digestive pain,[26] irritable bowel syndrome,[27] Crohn's disease,[28] ulcerative colitis,[29] ulcers, non-alcoholic steric hepatitis,[30] non-alcoholic fatty liver disease (NAFLD), other liver issues,[31] pancreatic disease[32] and other digestive symptoms like belching, bloating, and bad breath.

Studies have demonstrated leaky gut connection with even gynaecological problems like yeast overgrowth,[33] PCOS (polycystic ovarian syndrome)[34] and other hormonal chaos. Damage to the microbiome can lead to an oestrogen dominance that may lead to painful breasts, lumps, heavy periods, infertility, increased risk of miscarriages and lowered libido; it can even increase the risk of oestrogen dependent cancers (breast, endometrial, and ovarian). Other connections include neurological problems like migraines,[35] Alzheimer's,[36] ALS,[37] and parkinsonism,[38] cancer,[39] anaemia, psychological disturbances like alcoholism,[40] anxiety and depression,[41] ADHD,[42] schizophrenia, bipolar disorder, sleep disturbances, rheumatological complaints like arthritis[43] and other degenerative diseases, chronic fatigue syndrome,[44] fibromyalgia,[45] and RLS,[46] and even interstitial cystitis, pediatric issues like autism,[47] asthma and AIDS.[48]

Thus, increased intestinal permeability/leaky gut can cause a vast number of symptoms and disorders, as it starts off as general inflammation but over time advances to become nutrient malabsorption and then food and other chemical insensitivities. For this reason, healing the intestinal lining is the foundation of *The Qur'anic Prescription*.

Eat Ṭayyib (Pure) Foods, Eat Small Amounts to Heal, Succeed and Thrive

But those who disbelieve enjoy themselves and eat as grazing livestock eat, and the Fire will be a residence for them. (Qur'an 47:12)

But waste not by excess for God loves not the wasters. (Qur'an 7:31)

The Prophet, peace be upon him, said: 'The child of Adam fills no vessel worse than his stomach. Sufficient for the child of Adam are a few morsels to keep his back straight. If he must eat more, then a third should be for his food, a third for his drink, and a third left for air.' (Tirmidhī and *Musnad* Aḥmad)

The Prophet, peace and blessings be upon him, said, "The *believer eats in one intestine (is satisfied with a little food) and the non-believer eats in seven intestines (eats much)."* (Bukhārī)

Islam emphasizes the importance of consuming small quantities of food at any given time. In 7:31, Allah (SWT) has commanded us not to consume above and beyond one's needs. We have been commanded and instructed to eat very little food just to keep our backs straight. The Prophet, peace and blessings be upon him, even says that the believer eats with one stomach, while the non-believer eats with seven. Allah, glorified and exalted is He, describes the characteristics of the people of Hellfire as those who graze like cattle. Why is Allah, glorified and exalted is He, linking over and over again belief/disbelief, or even His worship, to food? According to the Qur'an, and now science, the consumption of small quantities of food matters, as eating less is the biggest factor in maintaining good health and even healthy aging. The body is able to digest better with less food. Recent studies have shown that those who reduce their calories by 30 percent live longer and even avoid some age-related diseases.[49] What is amazing is that this study didn't take into account what is eaten but only the amount of food consumed.

Why Does a Small Quantity of Food Matter? Insulin and Leptin

Why does a small quantity of food intake matter according to science? Large quantities of food can lead to insulin and leptin resistance. Insulin manages the glucose levels and leptin helps with satiation. When there is insulin and leptin resistance, hormone imbalances and overeating happen, which wreaks havoc in almost every system of the body, leading to chronic disease of every stripe. Muslims are supposed to eat one third, but when someone has insulin and leptin resistance, they don't even know when their third of the stomach is full, and so they continue eating.

Fake Food and Increased Quantity Foods → Leptin and Insulin Resistance → Sickness and Overeating

What is Insulin Resistance?

The food that we take is absorbed and then enters into our bloodstream. Glucose in the body is needed in the cells for energy. Glucose enters the cell of organs, like the heart, fat and muscles, but only if it has a key, which is insulin. Insulin is a protein and storage hormone produced by the pancreas, which is responsible for controlling blood sugar levels and determining people's metabolism.

Insulin can actually affect every cell in the body, thus determining the life of the cell. It is an anabolic hormone, meaning that it can make bigger things out of smaller things and its effect is determined through what the cell it binds itself to does. Insulin regulates the production of other hormones, makes fat in the liver, helps the muscle cell make new protein, regulates how a cell uses energy as well as hundreds of other tasks.

Over time, the flood of inflammatory signals starts to wear down this key. As it keeps on using it over and over again, the body stops listening to the insulin, until the key stops working altogether and the cells don't open their doors to the insulin and are unable to absorb glucose adequately, leading to insulin resistance. To keep everything in balance and the glucose at a healthy level, the pancreatic beta cells start producing even more insulin. Over time, the beta cells can't keep up with the body's increased demand for insulin, leading to excess glucose in the bloodstream.

Insulin resistance is the root of many of the common chronic diseases, but symptoms can start long before. Symptoms of insulin resistance are fatigue, irritability, brain fog, memory or concentration issues, weight gain around the midsection, sugar crashes in the middle of the day, inability to lose weight, getting cranky, irritable and tired when a meal is missed, and feeling sluggish and sleepy after meals. Someone with insulin resistance can also be addicted to carbohydrates, have hypoglycaemic attacks, acne, irregular periods, have dark and thick skin around folds and creases (acanthosis nigricans), infertility, cysts, PCOS, poor sex drive, and increased hair growth. Obesity is strongly connected to insulin resistance. The best way to determine if you have insulin resistance is through measuring the waist and hip ratio. Measure the largest part of your belly and the largest part of your hips. Divide the waist number by the hip number and ideally it should be below 0.9 for women and below 0.8 for men.

This is a growing problem that leads to inflammation and needs to be addressed for the healing and prevention of disease. Anything that causes insulin resistance will cause inflammation, and vice versa. Insulin resistance results in rapid and premature aging, along with diseases like metabolic syndrome, inflammation, and can lead to heart disease, stroke, dementia, autoimmune diseases and even cancer. Insulin resistance affects most organ systems.

Insulin resistance leads to excess aldosterone which causes water and salt retention, hypertrophy of the vessel wall and the activation of the sympathetic nervous system leading to a lack of supply of nitric oxide to blood vessels whose the dilation and narrowing, dyslipidemia, causes hypertention. Insulin resistance increases blood pressure and the chances of blood vessel damage; it also increases lipid deposits in the blood vessels and inflammation; it infiltrates the blood vessels with macrophages that become increasingly laden with oxidized lipids which then change into foam cells, contributing to athersclerotic plaques.

Insulin resistant men and women are also more likely to be infertile. Polycystic ovary syndrome, associated with insulin resistance, is the most common cause of female infertility, affecting around 10 million women worldwide. Even if affected women get fertility treatments, they usually respond poorly to drugs and typically need higher doses which increases side effects. When blood insulin level is good, the response to clomiphene is good too. Men with higher body fat usually have less testosterone, and this can result in the production of insufficient healthy sperm.

Insulin resistance is a general occurrence in pregnancy, but the metabolic health of the mom and baby is interconnected. If a mother has stronger insulin resistance, it can affect the baby's weight as the babies' weight can be higher than the normal average, and 40 percent of them would be more likely to be obese with metabolic complications in their teenage years and beyond. What is also very serious is that babies weighing less than the normal weight at birth can also be insulin resistant, and they are under a greater risk of becoming obese later in childhood than overweight babies. Insulin resistance can also affect the mother's milk supply, as mothers with insulin resistance had the lowest milk supply.

Insulin resistance makes cancer grow faster, thus doubling the likelihood of dying from cancer. Breast, prostate and colorectal cancers are strongly correlated with insulin resistance. Insulin resistance affects the skin, leading to acanthosis nigricans, skin tags and psoriasis, which can lead to muscle loss, associated with reduced bone mass, osteoarthritis, fibromyalgia, gout, and it can also lead to gastrointestinal issues like gallstones, non-alcoholic fatty liver disease and kidney problems, because too much insulin can lead to an excess of calcium as insulin increases the level of parathyroid hormone. Asthma is also highly linked to insulin resistance.

Sadly, this problem is now present in very young children and is constantly overlooked. A study on insulin resistance in early teenage children showed that, children with at least one parent with insulin resistance, were more insulin resistant with fasting insulin levels, and had around 20 percent higher levels than in children who had no parents with insulin resistance. Insulin resistant children are more likely to experience alterations in puberty. Studies have shown that children with the highest levels of insulin were 36 times more likely to become obese as adults.

An impure lifestyle can lead to prediabetes/insulin resistance and diabetes leading to more chronic illnesses, as genetics have only accounted for 5 percent of all cases of type two diabetes, and even fewer cases of insulin resistance. We are living in a more *khabīth* environment and eating more *khabīth* foods and they are creating imbalances. Diets full of *khabīth*/impure foods are causing the rise of insulin in the body now more than ever before. Cereals made with corn raise blood sugar level more than sugar. The lack of fibre can lead to increased visceral fat while artificial sweeteners have been linked to weight gain and diabetes. Stress increases cortisol and insulin levels, and this makes insulin resistance worse. Leaky gut or dysbiosis increases inflammation, worsening obesity and belly weight. Toxins in the environment, like air pollution, cigarette smoke, BPA exposure, pesticides and even MSG, are now making the cells numb to insulin. Sleep deprivation, a sedentary lifestyle and stress can influence hormones, which can then alter insulin sensitivity. One week of sedentary life can increase insulin resistance by seven folds.

Having less thyroid hormone is associated with reduced insulin sensitivity. Deficiencies due to food and lifestyle (especially vitamin D and magnesium deficiency) are leading to insulin resistance. Insulin sensitivity also reduces with age as the older we get the more insulin resistant we become. Medications like steroids and hydrochlorothiazide (first line medication for blood pressure) can increase blood sugar level, leading to insulin resistance.

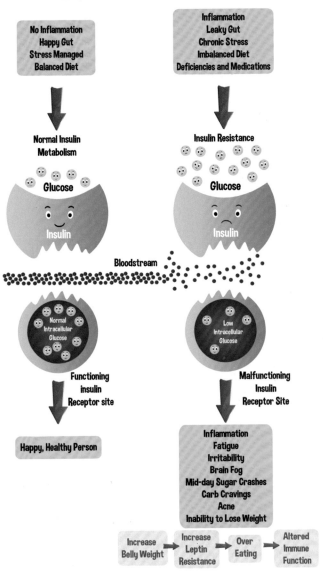

PICTURE 3.4   INSULIN RESISTANCE

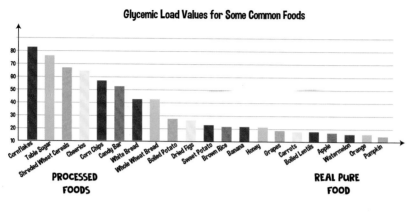

Glycemic Load Values for Some Common Foods

PROCESSED FOODS

REAL PURE FOOD

PICTURE 3.5   GLYCAEMIC LOAD

Let's Talk About Leptin

Leptin is the hormone of hunger produced by fat cells that inform us when we are satiated so that we stop eating. It is the gatekeeper of fat metabolism, monitoring how much energy an organism takes in. When the stomach starts to fill up, fat cells release leptin to tell the brain to stop eating. When the body is constantly overloaded, it can

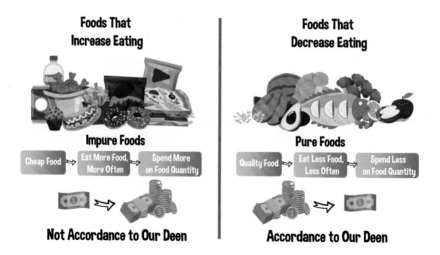

Foods That Increase Eating

Impure Foods

Cheap Food ▸ Eat More Food, More Often ▸ Spend More on Food Quantity

Not Accordance to Our Deen

Foods That Decrease Eating

Pure Foods

Quality Food ▸ Eat Less Food, Less Often ▸ Spend Less on Food Quantity

Accordance to Our Deen

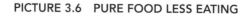

PICTURE 3.6   PURE FOOD LESS EATING

overwhelm the system because of the constant surges of leptin. Like insulin, overtime the body's receptors start to turn off and become leptin resistant, which means that the body stops listening to the leptin signal. Just as all hormone issues, leptin resistance is a complex issue. Overeating, weight gain and obesity ensue with too much leptin and the unresponsiveness of the body to it. The majority of overweight individuals who have difficulty losing weight have leptin resistance.

Pure foods which are high in fibre heal the gut and a small intake of food balances out insulin and leptin levels. Most diseases that lead to suffering and disability are lifestyle diseases, and a *tayyib* lifestyle can prevent and treat chronic diseases. *Tayyib* foods are very nutrient-dense and more powerful than any drug when it comes to reversing disease, as most drugs only manage diseases and don't prevent them. If you are insulin resistant, fasting and reducing carbohydrate intake activate the liver glycogen and atophagia, and inhibit fat stores.

The Qur'anic/ Prophetic Diet – Eat to Live, Not Live to Eat

He sends down water from the sky, and with it we bring forth the plant of everything. From these we bring forth green foliage and composite grain, palm trees laden with clusters of dates within reach, vineyards and olive groves and pomegranates alike and unlike. Behold their fruits when they bear fruit and ripen. Surely here are signs for a nation who believe. (Qur'an 6:99).

The Qur'anic/Prophetic lifestyle is ideal for us. The Qur'anic/Prophetic diet is a rich diet of whole foods that are rich in phytonutrients, good fats, fibre and low glycaemic foods rich in nutrients.[50]

In summary, if you are very hungry, at the most you must fill one third of the stomach, so it is important to focus on the foods you *can* have - the *tayyib* foods. If you eat processed carbs first, you deprive the body of nutrient-dense foods. Each meal should have a balance of vegetables, fats, protein source with adequate hydration and fruit. Such meals help with satiation, optimize gut health and decrease insulin resistance[51] by improving the immune system, improving metabolism, healing and preventing chronic disease.

The Qur'anic/Prophetic superfoods are antidiabetic, anticancer, immune modulator, anti-inflammatory, protect the liver and are even analgesic and have healing properties. The foods that have been recommended by Prophet Muhammad, peace and blessings be upon him, have now become superfoods with powerful healing properties.[52]

Quranic/Prophetic (S) Foods
Nutrient Dense, Balance Gut Bacteria and Hormone Levels and Optimize Immune System

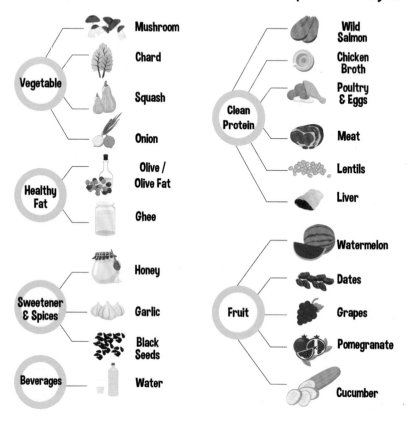

PICTURE 3.7   THE QUR'ANIC/PROPHETIC FOODS

Vegetables

The diet of the Prophet Muhammad, peace and blessings be upon him, was plant-based for a good reason. Few vegetables were common in the Arabian Peninsula at the time of the Prophet, peace and blessings be upon him. To the best of our knowledge, he ate truffles/mushrooms, lemongrass, chard, squashes and pumpkins.

Allah, glorified and exalted is He, has created vegetables in so many colours and each colour has a specific nutritional benefit. They are a rich source of minerals, vitamins and disease fighting phytonutrients (phyto means plants), a group of chemicals essential for vibrant health that protect from inflammation and chronic disease.[53] There are about 250,000 to 300,000 known edible plant species, but humans only consume between 150–200 of them.[54] Sadly, during 2007–2010, half of the total of the U.S. population consumed less than 1 cup of fruit and less than 1.5 cups of vegetables daily; 76 percent did not meet fruit intake recommendations, and 87 percent did not meet vegetable intake recommendations.[55] Seventy-eight percent of the world's population doesn't eat the minimum of five servings of fruits and vegetables a day, as about three-quarters of the world generally only eat twelve plant and five animal species.

This needs to change, as long ago our hunter ancestors ate more than 800 varieties of plants, including medicine in the forms of plants; indeed, vegetables are critical for health. They help to keep the body alkaline, optimize detoxification, reduce inflammation,[56] and also contain fibre that acts as a fertilizer for the good bacteria in the gut. They also help to lose weight, and prevent cancer and heart disease.[57] Veggies can turn on and off genes, as some studies have shown that plants genetics may regulate our genetics.[58]

Half of your plate ought to be vegetables, and clean protein and healthy fats should only be in small portions. This dynamic combination speeds up your metabolism and reduces the risk of chronic illness.

Try to eat local, whole, organic vegetables whenever possible (heirloom varieties are the best) as the whole plant is full of vital nutrients. They can be eaten raw, juiced, cooked (some are great cooked and cooled, as that process creates resistant starch),

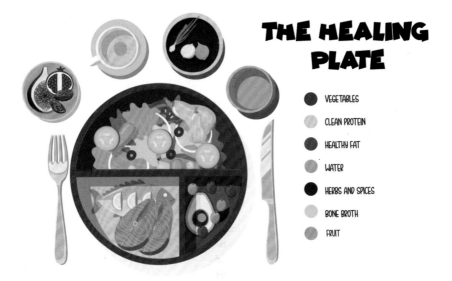

THE HEALING PLATE

- VEGETABLES
- CLEAN PROTEIN
- HEALTHY FAT
- WATER
- HERBS AND SPICES
- BONE BROTH
- FRUIT

and cultured. You must avoid microwaving food as it can create AGE's molecules that create inflammation. Deep frying veggies can destroy their beneficial compounds. You should also avoid power washing veggies, for it is fine to rinse them because a bit of soil is good for the body as this adds diversity to our microbiome, lowering inflammation. Try to keep the skin and peels of fruits and vegetables on, as they are highly nutritious, regulate appetite and affect fat storage, control blood sugar, insulin release, optimize detoxification, and improve overall inflammation.[59]

Eat Allah's Rainbow. The more diverse food we have in our diet, the better our health will be. Each colour has a specific health benefit for the human body. Some will actually have a more powerful effect when eaten together. Eat lots of different varieties of coloured veggies. The colour has so many more nutrients (phytonutrients) that give the plants their rich colour, scent and taste and they are more detoxifying and anti-inflammatory.

Red veggies (like tomatoes, red onions, bell peppers, beets and carrots) contain lycopene which can protect against heart disease and genetic damage from free radicals (antioxidant) that can cause cancer. Beets contain phytonutrients called betalains which are antioxidants, anti-inflammatory and are important for detoxification support. Red cabbage contains antioxidants like anthocyanins that can help the heart by blocking blood clot formation and they help with cellular aging.

Orange veggies (carrots, pumpkins, sweet potatoes, orange bell peppers and squash varieties) have alpha carotene and beta carotene which protect the skin, sight help fighting against cancer and optimize the immune system.

Yellow-green, which may not look yellow to the eye, include greens, spinach, mustard, turnip greens, yellow corn and even avocado which signals the carotenoids lutein and zeaxanthin and are beneficial for the eyes and protect against atherosclerosis (hardening of the arteries). Yellow summer squash is also a good source of fibre.

Green veggies (greens, collards, broccoli, bok choy, cabbage, kale, arugula, watercress, mustard, fennel, broccoli rabe and sprouts, etc.) indicate phytochemicals, isocyanates, indoles and sulforaphane, which raise glutathione, boost detoxification and inhibit carcinogens. Cruciferous vegetables are packed with fibre and have glucosinolate that can reduce inflammation and fight cancer. They also have nutrients like A, C and K while sea vegetables, like seaweed or edible algae, are a rich source of iodine, contain important antioxidants and nutrients to fight inflammation and even cancer and strengthen the immune system.

Vegetables that are pale green-white (such as garlic, leeks, onions, cauliflower etc.) get their colour from allicins. The latter has powerful antimicrobial properties and helps in boosting the immune system, improving the health of the heart, immune function and are also anti-cancer and anti-tumor. Cauliflower is rich in glucosinolates and sulphur which contains phytonutrients that have an antioxidant, anticancer and detoxifying activity. Sulforaphane is a phytochemical found in cruciferous veggies which may help to prevent cancer by improving antioxidant activity in the body and also contributes to detoxification. Other foods in this group can also contain antioxidant flavonoids like kaempferol and quercetin.

The colour in blue purple veggies is caused by anthocyanins (found in purple potatoes, red cabbage, eggplants) and flavonoids that prevent cell aging, improve vascular/cognitive function, blood flow, reduce inflammation, inhibit DNA damage in the brain, and improve bone, urinary and immune health. Purple potatoes are antiangiogenic and can kill cancer stem cells, and those properties can be preserved when a potato is cooked, baked or boiled.

Brown foods (mushrooms) see below

Most of these veggies have fibre, with different types of fibre (like soluble and insoluble fibre) offering different immune and biological effects. Fibre is important as it suppresses appetite, helps us feel full, controls craving, and stabilizes the rise of blood sugar insulin levels after a meal; it also decreases inflammation and lowers blood pressure, improves cholesterol and memory, helps fight chronic disease like cancer, and removes toxins from our system, feeding the healthy bacteria.

Soluble fibres like beta-glucans regulate the function of several types of immune cells, lower cholesterol, LDL levels, combat cancer and optimize heart and gut health. This type of fibre is found in mushrooms, algae and seeweed. Other soluble fibres include inulin which is an important prebiotic for certain strands of bacteria in the gut that lowers inflammation and helps with blood sugar regulation. Sources of inulin are onions, garlic, asparagus and bananas. Pectin, a soluble fibre (though some can be insoluble), is also great as a prebiotic for gut bacteria, as it improves cholesterol and blood sugar and is found in apples, strawberries, citrus, potatoes and carrots.

Insoluble fibre, like psyllium husk, is a prebiotic that softens stool making them easier to pass, lignin comes from nuts, flax seeds, cauliflower, zucchini, fruits, avocado, ripe bananas.

Fibre should be part of every meal and can be found in broccoli, asparagus, kale, green beans, artichoke, sweet potato, okra, tomatoes, and butternut squash. Other foods with fibre are nuts, seeds, and fresh produce like avocados. Fruit sources include apples, pears, blueberries, oranges, raspberries, strawberries, peaches, and pineapple. Beans and lentils are also great sources, if tolerated. Men should aim for about 25-30 grams of fibre per day and women should aim for 30-38 grams as studies have shown that different fibres feed different strains of bacteria and build the immune system.

Some vegetables also have resistant starches (i.e. they are not digested in the small intestine) that improve digestion, regulate blood sugar, improve weight loss and fat burning, influence metabolism, reduce appetite, improve lipids and optimize gut flora; examples include psyllium husk, inulin from chicory, parsnips, turnips, sweet potatoes, yams, green plantains, cassava, tiger nuts, jicama, taro root, cold potatoes, green mangos, chestnuts, rutabagas, persimmons, yucca or Jerusalem artichokes. Low glycaemic index resistant starches are jicama, cashews, uncooked green bananas and plantains.

Qur'anic/Prophetic Veggies Spotlight

Squashes and Pumpkins

And We caused a plant of gourd to grow over him. (Qur'an 37: 146)

Pumpkins or a similar vegetable are mentioned in the Qur'an, in connection with the Prophet Yūnus (Jonah) (peace be upon him) and the Prophet, peace and blessings be upon him, is also reported to have loved squash.

> Anas ibn Mālik said: 'The Prophet loved gourd. A tailor once invited the Prophet over some food he had made. Anas went with the Prophet and the tailor brought him some bread made from barley and some soup with gourd and dried meat in it. Anas said, "I saw the Messenger of Allah follow the traces of the gourd all around the edge of the pot (with a piece of bread), which made me love gourd ever since."' (Bukhārī and Muslim)

Though it is not clear what exact type of squash was meant by the Prophet's advice, we know now in science that squashes are high in antioxidants, reduce inflammation, boost the immune system and even prevent and fight cancer. Squashes are filled with vitamin A, vitamin C, vitamin E, B vitamins and minerals like magnesium, potassium, copper, phosphorus, calcium and iron. Pumpkins are high in vitamin A, lutein and zeaxanthin contents may protect the eyes and contain compounds that help the skin, heart, stabilize blood sugar levels and weight. Pumpkin seed oil is effective in preventing sperm abnormalities and in increasing sperm count.[60]

Truffles and Mushrooms

Sa'īd ibn Zayd reported that Allah's Messenger (peace and blessings of Allah be to him) said: 'The *Kama'* (mushroom-truffle) is like the *mann* (in that it is obtained without effort) and its water is a cure (medicine) for eye troubles.' (Bukhārī).

Truffles (a treat of the forest) are a fungus that grow in forested areas, usually in the shade near trees. They can be found mainly in Europe and the Middle East. Truffles, one of the most expensive foods on the planet, are considered a delicacy due to their intense aroma and are also loaded with antioxidants and flavonoids that can fight disease and boost overall health.[61] You can treat yourself by shaving some over your food. These contain immune boosters called anandamide that also work as a neurotransmitter, protect the DNA, improve muscle function and energy metabolism.

Mushrooms are prebiotic foods that have great benefits as they are rich in vitamin B and also contain beta-glucans that keep the immune cells alert and lower inflammation. As they grow in rich soils, they can also help increase the diversity of the microbiome. They also contain glutathione and another powerful anxtioxidant called ergothioneine, which are particularly high in porcini mushrooms. The part of the mushroom which helps a great deal in healing is called the mycelia (part below the ground) and has been shown to balance the microbiome, help detoxification, destroy cancer cells, protect the heart, lower blood sugar, optimize brain health, provide antifungal and antiviral benefits, and it has liver-protecting properties that also balance cortisol and other stress hormones.[62] They also have bioactive compounds that may help protect against Alzheimer's disease. Types of mushrooms include cordyceps, reishi, shiitake, lion's mane, and turkey tail.

Beets

> Umm Mundhir said: 'The Prophet, peace and blessings be upon him, visited me and 'Alī was with him. We had bunches of dates hanging and the Prophet, peace and blessings be upon him, began eating from them. 'Alī also began eating with him. Then the Prophet, peace and blessings be upon him, stopped him. saying, "You have just recovered from illness and should not eat this." He therefore stopped and the Prophet, peace and blessings be upon him, continued eating. Umm Mundhir said: I then cooked some barley and beetroot and the Prophet, peace and blessings be upon him, said to 'Alī: "Eat this, it is suitable for you."' (Tirmidhī)

Beets are packed with phytonutrients, antioxidants and fibre that lower inflammation. They contain betalains that give the beet its bright red colour. A 2019 review of studies found that certain compounds in beets, like these betalains, can disrupt cancerous mutations.[63] A study in the *British Journal of Nutrition* showed that beetroot juice helped to significantly lower both systolic and diastolic blood pressure after 24 hours of its intake.[64] Beets have also been shown to lower cholesterol. They are packed with nitrates that help to lower blood pressure, improve blood flow, help enhance exercise capacity and boost brain function. Nitric oxide acts as a vasodilator which helps to decrease blood pressure and improve blood flow. As they are rich in fibre, beets help to support bowel movements, digestive health and weight loss because they help in feeling full. Beets also support liver function so by extension, they help in detoxification. In a 2019 review of studies which looked at the effects of alpha lipoic acid on symptoms of diabetic neuropathy, it was discovered that alpha lipoic acid supplement led to a decrease in symptoms of diabetic neuropathy, and beets contain alpha lipoic acid (though the dose of the ALA used in the study was more than what is found in beetroot). Beetroots and their tops are also rich in carotenoids that improve eye health. However, those prone to developing oxalate type kidney stones should avoid consuming too much of beet tops.

Chard

Chard, or Swiss chard, is one of the most nutrient-dense vegetables out there and is packed with vitamin C and glutathione (which boosts detoxification). It can come in the form of polyphenol, carotenoid phytonutrients and betalain that are all very powerful in fighting free radical damage (because they are high in antioxidants), and they also protect the heart, fight cancer,[65] help with skin and eye health,[66] prevent diabetes,[67] protect bones,[68] reduce fractures,[69] and maintain healthy brain function.[70] Chard is full of magnesium, potassium, calcium and other minerals that are important for the nervous system and muscle health[71] as well as in lowering inflammation. There are a variety of colours in chard, including red, yellow and purples. Other types of Swiss chard include rhubarb, burgundy, Geneva, Lucullus, winter king and when different colours are bunched together it is known as "rainbow chard". A 2018 study published in *Neurology* concluded that the 'consumption of approximately one serving per day of green leafy vegetables and foods rich in phyllopquinone, lutein, nitrate, folate, a-tocopherol and kaempferol may help to slow cognitive decline with aging.'[72]

Garlic and Onions

...And [recall] when you said, "O Moses, we can never endure one [kind of] food. So call upon your Lord to bring forth for us from the earth its green herbs and its cucumbers and its garlic and its lentils and its onions." [Moses] said, "Would you exchange what is better for what is less? Go into [any] settlement and indeed, you will have what you have asked... (Qur'an 2:61)

Garlic has antioxidant, anti-inflammatory, liver-protecting and detoxification properties. The active component of garlic is allicin which is a rich source of organosulphur compounds that can help upregulate genes and enzymes that are important for detoxification. There are over 6000 peer reviewed articles that demonstrate the benefits of garlic.[73] Garlic and onions and their bioactive sulphur compounds are believed to have effects at each stage of cancer formation and are super antiangiogenic foods which heal and prevent cancer,[74] help treat diabetes,[75] improve inflammation, protect against colds and infections,[76] lower blood pressure,[77] improve health,[78] and even improve brain health.[79] Aged garlic can strengthen the immune defence against everyday infection and potentially even cancer.

Onions are rich in antioxidants, flavonoids like quercetin and anthrocyanins, which are the same type of protective compounds found in cherries and berries, along with organosulfides and nutrients like vitamin C, so they enhance immunity and have cancer protection properties.[80] Onions also protect the heart,[81] strengthen bones,[82] protect against diabetes[83] as well as against respiratory infections.[84] Because onions are antioxidants, they may also improve fertility.[85]

Garlic and onions are all prebiotic foods. Other prebiotic foods include chicory root, dandelion greens, eggplant, garlic, Jerusalem artichokes, jicama, kefir, leeks, onions, peas, asparagus and burdock root. Prebiotic foods help heal the gut lining by providing food for the probiotics, thus optimizing detoxification, soothing inflamed tissues and protecting against further inflammation.

> Prophet Muhammad, peace and blessings be upon him, said: 'Anyone who eats garlic and onions or leeks should not come near our Mosque. The angels are harmed by what harms the sons of Adam.' (Bukhārī, Muslim)

Garlic breath is a real thing. When garlic cloves are cut, crushed, or even chewed, they release a sulphur bearing compound called allicin which gives garlic a pungent taste. Hence, try not to overdo it. You should not eat garlic on an empty stomach to avoid GI irritation, just as you should always talk to your doctor first before starting on garlic. Garlic in any form can increase bleeding risk because it acts as a natural blood thinner. Therefore try to avoid taking raw garlic in big amounts. Crushing or chopping garlic and letting it sit a few minutes, before adding it to your cooked recipes, releases anti-platelet enzymes that help prevent coronary artery blockages. Muslims are advised to cook onions thoroughly, and not to approach the mosques with 'onion/garlic breath'. The Prophet, peace and blessings be upon him, advised us to "cook it thoroughly" for it to lose its strong odour. (Muslim, Ibn Mājah, Nasā'ī and Aḥmad.) To get rid of the strong smell of garlic and onion, you could try to eat raw parsley.

Clean Protein – Quality over Quantity

The body needs protein to heal and the latter is crucial for the immune system, muscle synthesis and appetite control. Protein ensures that the gut lining is appropriately constructed and that there is enough building material for enzymes, neurotransmitters and building lean muscle. But quality is more important than quantity. Prophet Muhammad, peace and blessings be upon him, called meat the king of foods, but it should be eaten occasionally and in small amounts.

When meat is mentioned in the Qur'an, fruits are often mentioned first. Allah, glorified and exalted is He, says,

And we shall provide them with fruit and meat, such they desire. (Qur'an 52:22)

And fruit, that they may chose, and the flesh of fowls that they desire. (Qur'an 56:20–21)

Note: Science has now shown that fruits are rich in digestive enzymes that might help with food absorption. Fruits, like pineapple, contain digestive enzymes called bromelain which break down proteins into building blocks, including amino acids. Papayas contain papain which breaks down protein into building blocks, including amino acids while mango contains the digestive enzymes amylase which breaks down carbs from starch into sugars like glucose and maltose. Bananas contain amylases and glucosidases, two enzymes that digest complex starches into easily absorbed sugars while kiwi contains digestive enzymes actinidain which help digest protein. So adding these foods can promote digestion and better gut health.

Allah, glorified and exalted is He, also discusses how meat should be prepared and eaten:

So eat of (meats) on which Allah's name hath been pronounced, if you have faith in His signs. (Qur'an 6:118)

Eat not of (meats) on which Allah's name hath not been pronounced: That would be impiety. But the evil ones ever inspire their friends to contend with you if you were to obey them, ye would indeed be polytheists. (Qur'an 6:121)

They ask them what is lawful to them (as food). Say: lawful unto you are (all) things good and pure: and what you have taught your trained hunting animals (to catch) in the manner directed to you by Allah. Eat what they catch for you, but pronounce the name of Allah over it, and fear Allah. For Allah is swift in taking account. (Qur'an 5:4)

Forbidden to you (for food) are: dead meat, blood, the flesh of swine, and that on which hath been invoked the name of other than Allah, that which hath been killed by strangling, or by a violent blow, or by a headlong fall, or by being gored to death; that which hath been (partly) eaten by a wild animal; unless you are able to slaughter it (in due form); that which is sacrificed on stone (altars); (forbidden) also is the division (of meat) by raffling with arrows: that is impiety. (Qur'an 5:3)

Furthermore Allah, glorified and exalted, tells us how Prophet Ibrāhīm (peace be upon him) honoured his guests with a roasted calf as a gesture of generosity:

... And he hastened to entertain them with a roasted calf. (Qur'an 11: 69)

Eating protein increases metabolic fire and the ability to burn calories while reducing appetite which helps us to feel full. Studies show that inflammation went down when people added to their diets lean meats instead of carbohydrates.[86]

When eating protein you need to take into consideration the source of the meat and its impact on the environment. Industrial farming is one of the largest factors in climate change, while regenerative agriculture is important to restore the planet's biodiversity and reverse climate change. The Intergovernmental Panel on Climate Change (IPCC) estimates that livestock production on factory farms produces about 14.5 percent of greenhouse gasses, and 9.5 percent of that is from the production, transportation and processing that occurs in the feeding of feedlots, and 5 percent from methane produced by livestock. Landfills full of rotting vegetables produce three times more methane (a more potent green house gas than carbon dioxide) than livestock.

In the US, modern Animal Feeding Operations (AFOs) are agricultural enterprises in which animals are kept and raised in a confined situation. They congregate animals, feed, urine, dead animals and manure on a small area of land where feed is brought to the animals. The modern Concentrated Animal Feeding Operations (CAFO) is where animals are fed unnatural diets of soy, animal parts and excrements, candy, antibiotics, corn, and hormones and it is destroying our planet. In these CAFOs, there are more than 1000 animal units (an animal unit is defined as an animal equivalent of a 1000 pounds live weight that is equal to 700 dairy cows, 125,000 broiler chicken and 1000 head of beef cattle) confined on site for more than 45 days a year. Unfortunately, a reported 24 million antibiotics are used every year in the US, mostly given to animals, and 70 percent of the antibiotics given are for the sake of speeding up the growth of animals. Every country is different and so, it is important as Muslims that we educate ourselves about the harms of industrial farming and stop eating factory farmed meat. Fortunately, the European Union has banned the use of growth hormone and feeding animals antibiotics or drugs.

Unfortunately, our massive multibillion dollar "halal" industry is only focussed on the few moments before the animal's death, and overlooks the other 99.9 percent of the animal's life, so the halal certification doesn't account for how the animal was treated. The Prophet, peace and blessings be upon him, condemned the beating of animals and cruelty towards them while he praised those who showed compassion to them.

May God curse anyone who maims animals. (Muslim)

As Muslims, we need to take another look at the halal industry and create a change. It is sad that in the United States, it is difficult to find grass-fed, organic halal meat. It is easier to find kosher organic than it is to find organic halal meat. This needs to change. Muslims need to choose the meat of animals that are grass-fed, pastured, organic, and that have not had any antibiotics and GMO feed. It is best to mix up your diet with high quality plant and animal sources of protein.

If you can't eat clean, then you should eat lean protein like beef sirloin, turkey or chicken breast, avoiding the cuts of meat that have a lot of fat and ground beef. Integrating these animals into a regenerative farm can help to build the ecosystem, reducing net greenhouse gas emissions by 86 percent. Regenerative agriculture is the number one solution to get carbon out of the atmosphere and reverse climate change.

Qur'anic/Prophetic Protein Spotlight

The quality of the protein we have is more important than the quantity. Hence, you must choose clean protein.

Fish

> And He it is Who has subjected the sea [to you], that you eat from it fresh tender meat [fish] ... (Qur'an 16: 14)

> ... And from them both you eat fresh tender meat [fish]... (Qur'an 35: 12)

People who eat seafood live longer[87] because such a diet lowers the risk of Type-2 diabetes, autoimmune diseases[88] and even cancer.[89] Many seafoods contain healthy sources of EPA and DHA. They are great sources of dietary protein, vitamin D, B12, iodine and selenium. Our oceans are polluted and many fish are full of contaminants. Small wild fish are best because they have less toxins, as farmed fish contains higher levels of toxins like polycholorinated piphenyls (PCBs) and persistent organic pollutants (POPs).[90] Tuna, swordfish, shark, king mackerel and tilefish are the fish with the biggest mercury problem.

Small wild fish are highly nutrient-dense. The best fish to consume, due to the high amount of antiangiogenic omega-3s they contain, are hake, sea bass, Bluefin tuna, cockles, bottarga, caviar, fish roe (salmon), manila clam and sea cucumber. Try to consume smaller and wild fish or sustainably cold-water raised fish including wild salmon, mackerel, sardines, herring, small halibut, anchovies and sable (black cod).

But if you opt to buy farmed fish, then aim to look for sustainable organic fisheries with high environmental welfare standards; organic standards are best in closed systems. If you choose to consume canned fish, then sardines, clams, oysters and salmons are great options as long as they are in a non BPA can and packed in olive oil. You can also eat the bones of fish, for they are a great source of calcium. Pregnant women should consume 8 oz of fish per week, but these should be low in mercury, like sardines, herring, anchovies, wild salmon and mackerel. Fish oil supplementation maybe better.

Poultry and Eggs

... And We sent down on you Manna and quails, [saying], 'Eat of the good lawful things We have provided for you ... (Qur'an 2: 57)

Poultry is also an excellent source of protein. Allah, glorified and exalted is He, mentions quails in particular as a gift to the children of Israel. Poultry is a good source of some crucial nutrients: protein, B vitamins, choline, and minerals like selenium, sulphur, iron and phosphorus. Dark chicken meat contains vitamin K2, or menaquinone, naturally occurring fat-soluble vitamins which have anti-cancer properties, just like fish.[91] Pastured poultry have more EFAs, but today's chickens have a lot less nutrients and can have more inflammatory Omega-6 fatty acids.

Eggs are an excellent source of choline that is needed for brain health and detoxification. They are also full of lutein and zeaxanthin that support eye health and other antioxidants, minerals, and vitamins, especially vitamin D. Eggs also protect against heart disease.[92] If you are not sensitive, aim to buy pastured organic eggs and have them in so many ways: soft boiled, poached or cooked on low temperature, whenever possible. You should also make sure to use a healthy oil when you scramble or fry eggs.

Meat

It is reported in Bukhārī and Muslim that the Prophet, peace and blessings be upon him, liked eating the shoulder of muttons. One of his favourite dishes was the *tharīd*, which is a meat and bread dish. He said:

The merit of ʿĀʾishah when compared to other women is like the merit of the *tharīd* when compared to all other dishes. (Bukhārī, Muslim, Tirmidhī, Nasāʾī, Ibn Mājah and Aḥmad)

Meat has always been a grey area, with different research proving both its benefit and harm. But the one thing that is certain is that we need to focus on the quality of meat consumed and not on its quantity. In a 2019 review of sixty one studies of 4 million people, researchers found no link between meat and death or disease.[93]

Quality is important because grain-fed animals are more inflammatory to humans. Studies have shown that there has been no link between heart disease and dietary fats.[94] Meat from grass-fed animals is full of micronutrients.[95] It is also full of beneficial fats and Omega-3s with an optimal ratio between Omega-6 and Omega-3, just as it lowers overall fat content, increases absorbable form of vitamin E content and conjugated linolenic acid and vaccenic acid and also lowers inflammation and rebuilds healthy cells.[96] Switching from grain-fed to grass-fed meat and dairy products has lowered women's risk of breast cancer by 60 percent compared to those with the lowest levels of CLA. Grass-fed meat has been found to have a rich array of phytonutrients, and goats that are raised on pastures have the same amount of phenolic compounds as green tea and can contain anti-inflammatory substances like quercetin and caffeic acid that all lower inflammation. Organ meat from grass-fed or pastured animals is also very beneficial. Liver contains vitamins (B12, vitamin C, A and folate), nutrients and minerals (copper, iron, zinc, magnesium and phosphorus) and even CoQ10.[97]

Meat wasn't regularly eaten by the Prophet, peace and blessings be upon him (as he ate very little) so a little goes a long way. Look for animal products that are pasture-raised, organic, grass-fed and grass-finished; animals which have been fed-GMO feeds, antibiotic, hormones or grass sprayed with pesticide. Avoid factory farmed meat whenever possible. The latter may be cheaper, but it is pumped full of hormones, antibiotics, GMOs, pesticides[98] and even sugar and candy[99] to fatten up the animals faster for mass production.

As the Prophet, peace and blessings be upon him, demonstrated, meat shouldn't be the main part of our plate. Some research indicates that we should eat more plant protein as we get older, but you should determine what works best for you. The way you prepare meat and what it is prepared with are important, as grilling can produce toxic chemicals that can lead to cancer. Cook meat slowly with lots of spices as this can be protective. You should avoid processed, charred and burnt meats and make sure that the meat is marinated. Some spices have been shown to reduce toxins.[100]

Vegetarian Options

Because of food shortage, the Prophet, peace and blessings be upon him, didn't have meat regularly.

> 'Ā'ishah states: 'We (the family of Muhammad, peace and blessings be upon him) used to spend weeks on end without kindling a fire as (we had nothing to cook), confining ourselves to just dates and water.' (Muslim)

There are a lot of other sources of protein, like hemp seed protein powder, chia protein powder, and pea protein powder; lentils and beans are also great if you can tolerate them. We can't get all the protein the body needs from plants, and as people age, many among them need more.[1] Plant protein contains low levels of leucine, compared to animal protein.[101] Examples of plant protein include tempeh (20 grams

---

[1] Earlier in the page, the author says that some research indicates that we should eat more plant protein as we get older. Here, she says we can't get all the protein we need from plants especially as we age. It can sound a little confusing to readers.

of protein), pea protein (15 grams), hemp protein powder (15 grams), nut butter, lentils, beans (all around 8 grams of protein) and nuts and seeds (5 grams).

Beans are packed with fibre, zinc, iron, folate, potassium and magnesium. Observational studies have shown that fruits, veggies and beans were associated with less risk of death and heart disease.[102] Though beans may not be a great source of protein, they do feed the good bacteria because of the resistant starches which keep the colons healthy and feed the gut bacteria.[103] However, some people may not be able to tolerate them because they contain lectins and phytates (see part 3).

Some types of soy can be good for people, but because most soy is genetically modified, we should try to avoid it. They also contain elevated levels of an enzyme inhibitor that prevents from absorbing nutrients, but fermentation can solve this. Peanuts are another source of protein, and legumes may have fungus, aflatoxins, a carcinogen that can grow on it depending on how they were stored. So these two should be kept to a minimum.

The Prophet, peace and blessings be upon him was not a vegan or vegetarian, yet most of his diet consisted of plants, but a plant-based diet can cause deficiencies in vitamin K, Omega-3 fats, B12, vitamin A, iron and even calcium.[104]

Protein Powders

There are numerous protein powders on the market, so look for those with the least ingredients. Egg protein, beef collagen or gelatin are good sources that may even heal the gut lining. Rotate protein sources in order to avoid developing sensitivities.

The Forbidden Protein

> *Forbidden to you (for food) are: dead meat, blood, the flesh of swine, and that on which hath been invoked the name of other than Allah.*(Qur'an 5:3)

Pork has been forbidden, as now science has proven that it is infested with viruses and parasites while processed meat like ham, bacon and sausage can lead to an increased risk of cancer.

Healthy Fats

The body and every cell in it need fat. Eating fat will not make us fat or sick unless we eat it with lots of carbohydrates. Strange as it may sound, healthy fats are important in weight loss[105] (especially compared to low-fat diets) as well as in lowering inflammation.[106]

Healthy fats are essential to life and cellular function because they are essential for absorbing fat soluble nutrients, which is required to make cholesterol, and also aid in the body's hormonal, metabolic functions and immune system functioning. They are also needed for cell structure and are vital for brain and nerve function, as more than half of the brain is made of fat and is also needed for developing the brains of babies.[107] They also balance mood, aid in dementia prevention, optimize bone and digestive health, and are also required to make hormones like testosterone and oestrogen and metabolizing vitamin D 25. Fat makes us satiated by turning on leptin, the hormone that regulates the feeling of fullness, which is often disrupted by eating too many processed and refined carbohydrates as well as bad fat.

There are different types of fats: saturated (butter and coconut oil), monounsaturated (olives, avocado, and many nuts), polyunsaturated (Omega-3 and 6), and trans-fats. Monounsaturated fatty acids (MUFA), which come from animals and plants can protect from heart disease, improve insulin sensitivity and reduce the cholesterol that is responsible for accelerating the hardening of arteries[108] (the small dense LDL particles), improve HDL, improve hormone health and brain neurotransmitters and lubricate the body's joints. Examples of this type of fat include beef tallow, butter, duck fat, egg yolks from pastured chickens, but also olives, nuts and avocados (key in the Mediterranean diet of the Prophet, peace and blessings be upon him). This type of fat is filled with antioxidants and nutrients. It can also be found in canola oil, but the latter has been altered with strong chemicals and high heat, which can damage the oil and make it harmful.[109]

There are also polyunsaturated fatty acids (PUFA), linoleic acid and Omega-3 fats (EPA and DHA), found mostly in fish and grass-fed meat. Omega-3 fatty acids reduce inflammation, protect the brain, and are important in preventing and healing chronic conditions.[110] What is sad is that about 90 percent of Americans are deficient in Omega-3 fatty acids. Plants, such as flax seeds and walnuts, contain ALA that the body can convert to EPA/DHA, but it only access less than 10 percent of its which isn't enough for the body's needs. Unfortunately, Americans are eating too much Omega-6 fats and too little Omega-3s, which sets the stage for chronic inflammation.

Some studies have now shown that there is no link between saturated fat, cholesterol and heart disease.[111] Healthy fats, including Omega-3s, are actually protective and important in reversing every single indicator of heart disease risk, including cholesterol, hypertension, diabetes and inflammation, just as they protect against autoimmune diseases and depression.[112] Studies have shown that the fats in the blood that can lead to heart attacks are the ones that come from eating bad carbs and sugar.[113] Eating carbohydrates can increase the amount of saturated fats in the blood which is linked to disease.[114] It is actually a low cholesterol diet that forces the body to work extra hard to make more of it leading to higher cholesterol levels.

Saturated fat is essential for fat-soluble vitamins and nutrients, and is beneficial because it can lower triglycerides, raise HDL and the less harmful (fluffy) type of

LDL. It also causes less hardening,[115] lowers inflammation by turning off the genes that produce cytokines, and prevents leaky gut. Saturated fats reduce inflammation and chronic diseases, like heart disease, cancer, diabetes, depression, and others. Adding fats to our diet can also reduce overall calorie intake.[116] Be careful with saturated fats if you follow a high refined carbohydrate diet[117] and low Omega-3 intake as this may lead to inflammation. Fats like coconut oil and butter don't raise saturated fats,[118] but it is the carbohydrates we eat that forces the liver to make fat, leading to high cholesterol, especially the bad type of LDL, triglycerides and lowering HDL.[119]

Healthy fats satiate us, keep the blood sugar balanced and increase our metabolism. Focus on eating *tayyib*/pure oils that our ancestors ate, and avoid processed *khabīth* oils and fats. A typical serving of fat is about a tablespoon of oil, a handful of nuts, or 4 oz. of fish or other animal protein. Aim not to eat fats with carbohydrates, sugar and starches because it can lead to weight gain.

Examples of good fats: olives, olive oil, avocado, nuts, seeds, coconut oil, medium chain triglycerides (MCT oil), butter (organic pasteurized and raw), ghee (clarified butter, free of A1-beta casein), flaxseed oil (full of essential fatty acids) and fatty fish and fish oils all improve constipation, reduce the risk of heart disease, and optimize cellular function.

Qur'anic/Prophetic Fat Spotlight

Olive/Olive Oil

> *By the fig, and the olive, by Mount Sinai, and by this city of security [Makkah], verily, We created the human of the best stature.* (Qur'an 95: 1–4)

> *With it He causes to grow for you the crops, the olives, the date palms, the grapes, and every kind of fruit. In this is indeed an evident proof and a manifest sign for people who give thought.* (Qur'an 16: 11)

Olives have been mentioned six times in the Qur'an. Olives also contain oleic acid that prevents colon, breast, prostate, pancreas and endometrial cancers. It also contains olecanthal that lowers inflammation, enhances the immune system and has analgesic properties, and oleurpein that lowers blood sugar levels.

Olive oil is one of the healthiest foods on this earth,[120] as it is full of antioxidants and polyphenols. It is good for the brain and reduces inflammation,[121] hsCRP and even cancers.[122] It is also great for optimizing gut health because it helps in reducing bad bugs like H pylori,[123] thus reducing the risk of heart disease, lowering blood pressure,[124] preventing heart attacks[125] and cholesterol panels.[126] You should use extra virgin olive oil because it possesses more anti-inflammatory properties[127] (in dark tinted glass bottles to prevent oxidation). Olive oil can oxidize quickly when exposed to heat because it has a low smoke point, and can release free radicals and other toxic substances, so it not recommended for cooking.

Butter and Ghee

> The two children of Busr said: 'The Messenger of Allah (peace be upon him) came by us and we offered him some butter and dried dates, as he liked eating butter and dried dates.' (Abū Dāwūd)

Science has now concluded that butter is instrumental in heart disease prevention;[128] it is also a factor in reducing inflammation and in diabetes prevention. Science has also established that there is no link between butter and heart disease.[129] You should choose the butter of grass-fed animals because it is richer in fat soluble vitamins and nutrients and has three to five times more CLA than the butter of grain-fed animals[130] which is full of choline and vitamin A.[131] Ghee has the same anti-inflammatory properties as butter, so you can also look for the ghee of grass-fed animals. The ghee of grass-fed animals is full of vitamin D, A, E, K Omega-3s, CLA, and butyrate, which promotes intestinal health, healthy skin and vision. In ghee, the milk solids are removed, and so it is casein and lactose free and can easily be tolerated by those with lactose intolerance or those with dairy allergies.

Other Sources of Fats

Nuts and seeds: Nuts are a great source of proteins, minerals, fibre, and essential fatty acids. They also contain potent antiangiogenic Omega-3 PUFAs. Studies[132] have proven that nuts lower the incidence of cardiovascular disease and cancer,[133] improve brain function,[134] and are good for weight loss.[135] They also improve cholesterol,[136] prevent blood glucose from spiking,[137] lower the risk of Type-2 diabetes[138] and even the risk of death.[139]

The nuts that you purchase should ideally be organic (because they can absorb pesticides easily), raw, soaked (overnight for up to twenty-four hours), sprouted then roasted and then stored in closed, tight and dark containers in a cool location. This helps to reduce their lectins and phytates content. The skins of nuts are highly nutritious.[140] You can freeze nuts and seeds for up to three months. A handful or two of nuts a day (such as almonds, pecans, walnuts, hazel, macadamia, pistachio and seeds like chia, flax, and pumpkin) are enough to gain all the benefits. If you want to drink nut milk, it is best to make it yourself, as the ones bought in stores have additives like carrageenan and different gums that can alter the gut flora.

Seeds are also packed with healthy protein, fats, fibre, minerals, antioxidants and Omega-3's (eg. flax seeds) that can reduce inflammation, improve gut function, and prevent autoimmunity and heart disease.

Avocado: It is full of good fat, and helps to build lean muscle mass, detoxify, and build healthy skin, hair and sight, and also helps the function of the brain and digestion. It also protects against insulin resistance and helps burn fat. Being full of nutrients, fibre, antioxidants and minerals, it helps reduce inflammation, prevent cancer, heart disease, strokes[141] and makes us feel satiated.

Coconut oil: Coconut oil can be a healthy addition to your diet for it is anti-inflammatory, antifungal and antimicrobial. It contains anti-inflammatory fats like lauric acid, combats viral infections, increases metabolism and promotes weight loss. It also increases conjugated linolic acid which strengthens the immune system and helps cells communicate better, thus protecting from cancer, just as it increases caprillic acid that has antifungal properties, and keeps the gut and urinary tract working properly.

Coconut oil can reduce inflammation, raise HDL, improve cholesterol and heart health,[142] and it is not associated with an increased risk of heart attack and stroke.[143] Coconut oil also fights off fungus[144] and bad bacteria,[145] and improves digestion, brain health and metabolism,[146] just as it lowers insulin levels,[147] and acts as an antioxidant, improves memory for those with Alzheimer's disease, and improves thyroid function and sport performance. Coconut oil remains stable with heating up to 350 degrees F, so it can be used for cooking. You should look for virgin, organic, expeller cold pressed, unrefined, and unbleached coconut oil.

Medium chain triglycerides: Coconut oil is about two-thirds MCT oil. MCT oil is a great source of fat, as it also boosts metabolism and promotes weight loss. It also improves cognitive function, thus supporting the immune system, and helps to heal obesity-related fatty liver, and reduces the ratio of total cholesterol to HDL.[148]

Respect the oil: If not treated properly, even good oils can go bad. Oils that contain strong double bonds, like saturated fats, are more stable during cooking and have less chance of releasing toxins, while others can get damaged at certain temperatures. When damaged, they can destroy valuable nutrients (smoke point).

I have listed the oils that can be used and at what temperatures, and added their smoke points.

High heat/medium heat: coconut oil (350F/176C), butter (350F/176C), ghee (450F/204C), avocado oil (520F/271C), beef tallow (400F/204C) or duck/chicken fat

Low heat/no heat: extra virgin olive oil (320F/160C), flaxseed oil (225F/107C), walnut oil, macadamia oil, sesame oil, walnut oil, almond oil, tahini, hemp oil raw.

Water/Drinks

Optimal hydration is key in delivering nutrients to cells, decreasing inflammation, and optimizing cell function. It also improves mood and cognition and regulates the temperature of the body, flushes out toxins through the kidneys, prevents infections, promotes weight loss, increases energy, improves sleep and promotes healthy bowel movements. However, it should be the right, *tayyib* kind.

Sugary drinks have invaded our everyday lives. The commercials have brainwashed us to believe that the only thing that will quench our thirst is sugary drinks. Unfortunately, sugary drinks are responsible for about 184,000 deaths a year worldwide via diabetes, cancer and heart diseases.[149] Sugar sweetened beverages lead to kidney failure,[150] high blood pressure,[151] diabetes,[152] fatty liver[153] and heart disease.[154] You should also avoid fruit juices because they contain a lot of sugar.

Qur'anic/Prophetic Spotlight

Water

> *.. And We have made from water every living thing ..* (Qur'an 21: 30)

> *.. And We have given you to drink sweet water.* (Qur'an 77: 27)

To optimize healing, you must stay hydrated.

> He (the Prophet, peace and blessings be upon him) used to drink in three sips, not exhaling into the cup, and he said of this method: 'This is more healthy and better in quenching thirst.' (Muslim)

Filtered water is the best. Aim to drink water in a separate, clean glass or container, as it is not permissible to drink water straight from a pitcher, container, or other water receptacles (Bukhārī). You should then recite the name of Allah, glorified and exalted is He, before drinking (Tirmidhī), and never eat and drink with the left hand (Muslim). You should also remember to sit and drink water (Muslim) and not to drink after a meal, as it may hamper digestion. When you finish drinking, don't forget to say *Alḥamdulillāh*.

Zamzam water

> Prophet Muhammad, peace and blessings be upon him, said: 'It (Zamzam) is a nutritious food and a cure from ailments.' (Muslim)

The water of Zamzam is drawn from the well of Zamzam which is located in the masjid al-Haram in Makkah, Saudi Arabia. The alkalinity of Zamzam water and the presence of trace elements may be the cause of its healing power (but more studies are needed on this).[155] Some studies have also found that Zamzam could reduce clastogenic and cytotoxic effects of gamma irradiation.[156]

Nabeez (Nabīdh)

Ibn 'Abbās reported that some *nabīdh* was prepared for Allah's Messenger, peace and blessings be upon him, at the beginning of the night and he drank it in the morning and the following night and the following day and the night after that up to the afternoon. If anything was left out of that, he gave it to his servant or gave orders for it to be poured out. (Muslim)

Nabeez (*nabīdh*) was one of the drinks consumed by the Prophet, peace and blessings be upon him. In his time, it was typically made from dates or raisins and water, which was then left to soak overnight.

Broth

The Messenger of Allah, peace and blessings be upon him, commanded me thus, 'O Abū Dharr! Whenever you prepare a broth, put plenty of water in it, and give some of it to your neighbours.' (Muslim)

Bone broth contains nutrients that can easily be absorbed, like calcium, magnesium, phosphorus and sulphur which help heal and seal the gut lining. It also promotes the growth of good bacteria, and reduces inflammation and food sensitivities. It also contains collagen and glutathione (a super antioxidant, key in the regulation of cell death and proliferation of nutrient metabolism). You should drink about a minimum of a cup of bone broth per day.

Other drinks

A lot of people drink coffee, but research on it can be confusing. Depending on your genetics, it could be either good or bad. Coffee contains nutrients like magnesium, antioxidants, flavonoids, polyphenols and vitamin C.[157] And its benefits include lowering the risk of heart disease, colon cancer, depression, cirrhosis of the liver, Alzheimer's and even premature death.[158] But it should be avoided by those who have diabetes, prediabetes, highly stressed lives, mood disorders or difficulty sleeping, because it can increase insulin production[159] and cortisol and, as a stimulant, it can stress the adrenal out more.[160] Some people can tolerate coffee (black or with coconut milk).

Other options that you can drink include fresh veggie juice, fresh raw veggie juice and smoothies, which are also a great option when you want fast meals.

Organic teas (black, white, green, herbal, or yerba mate) are a great drink to enjoy with lots of benefits. Chamomile tea is rich in bioactives that have antiangiogenic properties and can inhibit angiogenesis by interfering with the signals needed to activate vascular cells to start developing blood vessels. Green tea is anti-inflammatory and has antioxidants, phytonutrients and detoxifying properties. The bioactives and flavour of tea are generally stable for two years.

Vinegar/Fermented Foods

The Prophet, peace be upon him, once said to his wife when she told him that they had only vinegar for dinner: 'What an excellent condiment is vinegar!' (Muslim)

Fermented foods, like vinegar will optimize health and healing because they support digestion, detoxify the liver, and strengthen the immune system. Vinegar consumption was found to regulate blood sugar levels and increase insulin sensitivity[161] and satiety, just as it helps people lose weight.[162] Vinegar is also antibacterial,[163] while apple cider vinegar promotes heart health by decreasing cholesterol.[164]

Other fermented foods, like sauerkraut and kimchi, are rich in glutamine, improve inflammation and can decrease total cholesterol and LDL,[165] and they also help regulate the glucose level. Natto is made from fermented soybeans (if you can tolerate soy); it has been shown to enhance vitamin K2, boost the immune system, support cardiovascular health, and contain bacillus subtilis.[166] Other fermented foods you can try are miso, kombucha, kvass, pickles, pickled ginger, and homemade ketchup.

Allah's Candy – Fruit!

Verily, the pious shall be amidst shades and springs, and fruits, such as they desire. [It will be said to them,] Eat and drink comfortably for that which you used to do. (Qur'an 77: 41–43)

Then let humankind look at their food: that We pour forth water in abundance, and We split the earth in clefts, and We cause therein the grain to grow, and grapes and clover plants [green fodder for the cattle], and olives and date-palms, and gardens, dense with many trees, and fruits and herbage [greens], [to be] a provision and benefit for you and your cattle. (Qur'an 80: 24–32)

Humans naturally have a sweet tooth, and Allah provided them with the perfect food not only to satisfy that craving but also to nourish and heal their bodies. Different types of fruit have been mentioned in the Qur'an and Sunnah, and now science is proving their health benefits. The colour of every fruit and veggie represents a different family of healing compounds (see above in vegetable section).

Eating the rainbow of fruit prevents cancer, diabetes, heart disease,[167] stroke,[168] and improves blood pressure, insulin levels, cholesterol and triglycerides, just as it lowers cognitive decline[169] and overall mortality risk.[170]

Fructose can increase triglycerides. Fructose with fibre, like in fruit, does cause any problem, as the fibre can slow its absorption and feeds the good bugs in the gut, thus cleaning the intestine.

Aim to eat local, organic and seasonal fruits in moderation, and if you are diabetic, overweight or insulin resistant, then you should choose low glycaemic fruits like oranges, pears, plums, peaches, watermelon, cantaloupe, apples and nectarine, to be taken in less than a cup per day. You can also combine fruit with protein, which is a fat source that keeps inflammation at bay.

There are so many fruits specifically mentioned in the Qur'an and Sunnah, and now science considers these foods as superfoods.[171] Let's examine these in a little bit more detail.

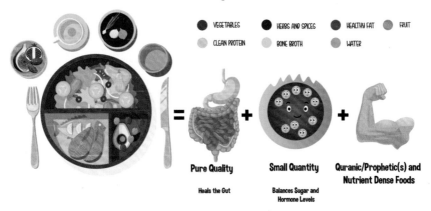

The Quranic Perspective on Food

● VEGETABLES   ● HERBS AND SPICES   ● HEALTHY FAT   ● FRUIT
● CLEAN PROTEIN   ● BONE BROTH   ● WATER

Pure Quality + **Small Quantity** + **Quranic/Prophetic(s) and Nutrient Dense Foods**

Heals the Gut   Balances Sugar and Hormone Levels

Qur'anic/Prophetic Fruits Spotlight

Dates

And shake the trunk of date-palm towards you; it will let fall fresh, ripe dates upon you. So eat and drink and be glad... (Qur'an 19: 25–26)

And We have made therein gardens of date-palms and grapes, and We have caused springs of water to gush forth therein. (Qur'an 36: 34)

And the earth He has put for the creatures. Therein are fruits, date palms producing sheathed fruit-stalks [enclosing dates]. (Qur'an 55: 10–11)

Dates were the most favoured food of Prophet Muhammad, peace and blessings be upon him, and are a great alternative natural sweetener with a lot of benefits.

Prophet Muhammad, peace and blessings be upon him, once told his wife 'Ā'ishah: 'A house with no dates - its people are hungry.' (Muslim)

If someone eats seven dates from the vicinity of Madinah, no poison will harm him until the evening. (Muslim)

Dates contain polyphenol that inhibit colon cancer, carbohydrate (1->3)B D glucan that inhibits sarcomas and proantocyanidin that protects against chemically induced hepatorenal toxicity. Dates also lower cholesterol and triglycerides naturally, relieve constipation and boost energy. They are rich in calcium and phosphorus that help with bone health. Prophet, peace and blessings be upon him, also liked to eat his dates with other foods; he ate ripe dates with cucumber (Bukhārī) and also recommended the breaking of fast with dates whenever possible.

If anyone of you is fasting, let him break his fast with dates. In case he does not have them, then with water. Verily water is a purifier. (Bukhārī)

Figs

There is a chapter in the Qur'an called *The Fig*. The fact that Allah, glorified and exalted is He, swears by this tree indicates its fruit's tremendous benefits and great value:

By the fig, and the olive, by Mount Sinai, and by this city of security [Makkah]. (Qur'an 95: 1–3)

Figs are powerful antioxidants,[172] a property which applies to the whole plant;[173] they also have anticancer properties,[174] treat common illnesses,[175] and are antibacterial and antifungal,[176] just as they contain compounds that are cytotoxic and fight against human cancer.[177] Dates have also antilipidemic and antidiabetic effects.[178] Drying figs makes them an even better source of phenolic compounds and increases their antioxidant properties.[179]

Grapes

Grapes are mentioned many times in the Qur'an in connection with Paradise (and the rewards of the Hereafter) as well as with the countless blessings of Allah, glorified and exalted is He, to His creatures on earth:

Would any of you wish to have a garden with date-palms and grapevines?... (Qur'an 2: 266)

With it He causes to grow for you the crops, the olives, the datepalms, the grapes, and every kind of fruit. Verily, in this is indeed an evident proof and a manifest sign for people who give thought. (Qur'an 16: 11)

Then let humans look at their food, that We pour forth water in abundance, and We split the earth in clefts, and We cause therein the grain to grow, and grapes and clover plants [green fodder for the cattle]. (Qur'an 80: 24–28)

Verily, for those who are pious [ever conscious of Allah], there will be success [Paradise]; gardens and grapevines. (Qur'an 78: 31–32)

Prophet Muhammad, peace and blessings be upon him, liked eating soaked raisins, though he forbade soaking both raisins and dates in the same bowl. (Bukhārī, Muslim)

Prophet Muhammad, peace and blessings be upon him, loved grapes. Grapes are rich in antioxidants, including flavonoids and polyphenols that reduce systolic blood pressure and cardiovascular diseases.[180] They also have antimicrobial properties,[181] along with proanthocyanidins that protect against skin, breast,[182] prostate, lung, neck and head cancers. Grapes also contain resveratrol, which has been shown to increase the expression of all three genes that are related to living longer.[183]These delicious fruits have also been shown to reduce obesity, lower inflammation,[184] and improve memory function. You have to make sure to purchase organic grapes to limit your exposure to pesticides.

Pomegranates

In them [both] will be fruits, and date-palms and pomegranates. (Qur'an 55: 68)

Pomegranates are powerful fruits, and research has now shown that they can help prevent and treat lots of chronic conditions such as high blood pressure, oxidative stress and even cancer through lowering overall inflammation.[185] They contain fibre, iron and ellagic acid that helps to boost energy and antagonize the effect of mutagens. They also contain gallic acid that suppress the accumulation of advanced glycation end products and lower down cholesterol levels.

Pomegranate seeds, as antioxidant, heal from the inside out, by altering the microbiome. They are also anitcarcinogenic,[186] They also reduce arthritis and joint pain,[187] are cardioprotective and lower blood pressure.[188] There is a bacteria in the gut called Akkermansia Muciniphila which makes up 1–3 percent of all bacteria in the gut and has a huge impact on it, as it can help improve glucose metabolism, decrease inflammation and combat obesity.[189] Patients with this gut bacteria are more likely to respond to cancer treatment and are able to call their immune system to fight cancer. When we lack this gut bacteria, our immune system does not respond to cancer treatment. Pomegranates and cranberries can increase this gut bacteria, because they are loaded with ellagitannins, a specific group of bioactives in about 70 percent of people which can metabolize into urolithin-A, another bio active. Urolithin-A has an antioxidant, anti-inflammatory and anti-cancer activity.

Bananas

Among Talh, [banana plants] with fruits piled one above another, in shade long-extended, by water flowing constantly. (Qur'an 56: 29–31)

Bananas are a great source of magnesium, potassium, fibre, pectin (which decreases as bananas ripen), resistant starch (found in unripe bananas), vitamin C and antioxidants. They help to boost energy and improve digestive health (resistant starch is food for the beneficial bacteria in the gut). They also contain tryptophans that are used to produce serotonin which enhances the mood, improves kidney function[190] and even supports heart health because of the minerals they contain (such as potassium[191] and magnesium).[192] Bananas can also help in modulating blood sugar levels after meals and may reduce the appetite by slowing the emptying of the stomach.[193] However, bananas should be enjoyed in moderation due to its relatively higher sugar content.

Watermelons

Prophet Muhammad, peace and blessings be upon him, used to eat watermelons with ripe dates, commenting that the heat of one (dates) is overcome by the coolness of the other (watermelon). (Tirmidhī and Abū Dāwūd)

Watermelon is great for hydration, as it is 92 percent water; it keeps us full, acts as a natural diuretic, protects the kidney, aids in detoxification, and supports weight loss.[194] Watermelon contains antioxidants like vitamin C, carotenoids and lycopene[195] that improve cancers of the digestive system, boosts immunity, and may have anticancer effects as it appears to reduce the risk of cancer by lowering the insulin like growth factor (IGF).[196] Watermelon also improves heart health by reducing inflammation, relieves arterial stiffness,[197] thus improving lipid levels,[198] just as it improves sore muscles after exercise[199] and contains nutrients for the skin (vitamin C and vitamin A) and eyes (lutein, zeaxanthin, vitamin C, vitamin A and beta carotene).

Citrons

It is reported in Bukhārī that the Prophet, peace and blessings be upon him, once said: 'The simile of the believer who recites the Qur'an (well, and acts upon its commandments) is like the citron. It tastes sweet and its smell is sweet.' (Bukhārī, Muslim, Nasā'ī, Abū Dāwūd, Tirmidhī, Ibn Mājah and Aḥmad)

Citron fruit is one of the original four citrus fruits, with a bumpy skin and colour like a lemon. This fruit is rich in antioxidants, especially in vitamin C, and so it helps to promote immunity,[200] decrease inflammation,[201] improve heart health,[202] and reduce hypertension[203] and cancer risk.[204]

Jujube

Jujube (or *nabaq* in Arabic) is the fruit produced by the lote tree, a green spiny tree belonging to the buckthorn family, Rhamnaceae, which is very similar to a small date, but has a crisp texture.

Prophet Muhammad, peace and blessings be upon him, said:

On the night that I was taken on the Night Journey, I was shown *Sidrat al-Muntahā* (a tree in the seventh heaven) and I saw its *nabaq* fruits which resembled the clay jugs of Hajr (a town in Arabia). (Bukhārī)

And indeed he [Muhammad] saw him [Jibrīl or Gabriel] at a second descent [another time], near Sidrat al-Muntahā [the lote tree of the utmost boundary (beyond which none can pass)], near it is the Paradise of Abode. When that covered the lote tree which did cover it! (Qur'an 53: 13–16)

And those on the Right Hand, who will be those on the Right Hand? [They will be] among thornless lote trees, among 'Talh, [banana plants] with fruits piled one above another. (Qur'an 56: 27–29)

These tiny fruits have so many benefits and have several biological compounds which hold therapeutic potentials for disease prevention[205] as they are rich in antioxidants, are anti-inflammatory,[206] improve sleep and brain function,[207] may fight cancer cells,[208] are antimicrobial, improve metabolic disorders via its hypoglycaemic and anti-diabetic actions, and help to treat gastrointestinal disorders,[209] as some studies show, because its fibre serves as food for the beneficial gut bacteria.[210]

Cucumber

> 'Ā'ishah reported that the Messenger of Allah often ate cucumber mixed with wet dates. (Bukhārī, Tirmidhī).

Cucumber, which is a fruit and not a vegetable, is well known for lowering lipid as well as for its antioxidant and antidiabetic activity. Cucumbers are naturally cooling and contain few calories which supply powerful polyphenol compounds that help naturally slow aging, fight cancer and alkalize the body. They also improve heart health[211] and blood pressure levels.

Others Fruits

Berries are rich in antioxidants, which prevent toxins from damaging the body, as well as cancer, dementia, diabetes and inflammation; they are also rich in pranthocyanidins, which have been shown to reverse inflammation, and they have gallic acid, which protects the brain from inflammation, oxidative stress, and cancer.[212] They are also antimicrobial, support heart health by reducing harmful enzymes called NADPH,[213] and support digestion, help to control appetite and promote weight loss.[214] Amla or indian gooseberry are rich in antioxidants, and others are goji berries, raspberries, cranberries and blueberries.

Stone fruits like peaches, plums, nectarines, apricots, cherries, lychee and mango are antiangiogenic, regenerative and DNA protective while apples contain a number of antiangiogenic polyphenols like caffeic and ferulic acid.

Sweeteners

Most people have a sweet tooth, and so did the Prophet, peace and blessings be upon him, and as an occasional treat, we can still enjoy sweet things.

> *There comes forth from their bellies, a drink of varying colour wherein is healing for people. Verily, in this is indeed a sign for people who think.* (Qur'an 16: 69)

It was reported by his wife 'Ā'ishah that Prophet Muhammad, peace and blessings be upon him, loved sweets and honey. (Bukhārī, Muslim, Abū Dāwūd, Tirmidhī and Ibn Mājah)

A man came to the Prophet, peace and blessings be upon him, and said: "My brother is complaining about his stomach (he has diarrhoea)." The Prophet said, "Give him some honey to drink." The man left and came back later saying, "I have given him some honey but it did not help (or in other words, 'it made his diarrhoea worse)." The Prophet, peace and blessings be upon him, told him again, "Give him some honey to drink." The man repeated this twice or three times and each time the Prophet, peace and blessings be upon him, gave the same answer. The third or fourth time, the Prophet, peace and blessings be upon him, said, "Allah has spoken the truth while your brother's stomach has lied." It was reported that the man's brother was finally cured. (Bukhārī and Muslim.)

Honey is a natural and least-processed sweetener which is full of antioxidants, vitamins and minerals. It helps to lower inflammation, aids the gut to digest through acting as a natural digestive enzyme and a prebiotic and neutralizing free radicals. It also helps in improving conditions like allergies, coughs and asthma.[215] It is best to choose cold expressed raw organic honey, or manuka honey, but you should use it sparingly to keep glucose levels under control. Honey has both antimicrobial and antifungal properties as well.

Maple syrup also contains many beneficial antioxidants,[216] decreases the plasma glucose,[217] protects the microbiome and also fights against cancer.[218] Other sweeteners that are full of antioxidants are molasses from raw cane sugar[218] and date sugar which have the same level of antioxidants as a serving of blueberries.[219] You must avoid sugar at all cost (discussed in detail below).

Organic stevia whole plant extract can also be used, as it doesn't raise the glucose levels. It is a plant that is grown in areas like China, Brazil and Japan. Stevia is 200-300 times more intense than table sugar, so a little of it goes a long way. However, you should look for pure sources. Dark chocolate which contains more than 70 percent cocoa is best, for it has numerous health benefits because it contains cocoa flavanols which is a highly unique blend of phytonutrients found only in cacao beans, and can also be enjoyed as cocoa powder or cacao nibs. Studies have shown that they can improve cognitive function and blood vessel function, lower blood pressure and improve metabolic health. You should look for the sources of cocoa flavanols that have low sugar, low lead and cadmium levels, as the latter can affect many cocoa products because of man-made pollution. Cadmium and lead levels are usually the least concentrated in chocolate and the highest in cocoa powder.

Herbs and Spices

Herbs and spices are powerful antioxidants, anti-inflammatories and detoxifiers.

Qur'anic/Prophetic Spotlights

Garlic detoxifiers decreases blood pressure, prevents clots and improves cholesterol (crush and chop to release its secret power, allicin, (discussed above).

Lemongrass

It was narrated that the Prophet, peace and blessings be upon him, said (about Makkah when the Muslims were about to enter it after they had reclaimed it in battle against the pagans): "Do not cut its plants," to which al-'Abbās pleaded, "Except for the lemongrass, O Messenger of Allah, for the people of Makkah use it in their houses and graves." So the Prophet, peace and blessings be upon him, said, "Except for the lemongrass." (Bukhārī, Muslim, Abū Dāwūd and Nasā'ī)

Lemongrass is a herb that belongs to the grass family of Poaceae, and grows in clumps. It has been used as a medicinal herb, and popularly for making teas and essential oils. Lemongrass essential oil is rich in vitamin A, B1, B2, B3, B5, B6, folate, vitamin C, magnesium, phosphorus, manganese, copper, potassium, calcium, zinc and iron. It can be used for headache relief; it can also kills bacteria,[220] reduce fever, support the immune system,[221] treat digestive disorders, reduce inflammation,[222] just as it has an antioxidant effect,[223] lowers cholesterol[224] and even helps to detoxify because it is a natural diuretic.[225]

Basil

Basil is an antioxidant[226] which protects DNA. It is also anti-inflammatory and fights against cancer,[227] and bacteria[228] and virus infections. It also relieves stress,[229] boosts heart and brain health, supports the health of the liver[230] and digestive system, and reduces the amount of blood glucose levels, just as it protects against diabetes.[231]and is an anti-aging herb.

Also grain, with [its] leaves and stalk for fodder and sweet-smelling plants. (Qur'an 55: 12)

Basil was also recommended by the Prophet, peace and blessings be upon him, in this following hadith:

Whoever is offered basil let him not refuse it, as it is from heaven. (Nasā'ī and Abū Dāwūd)

Eucalyptus

As to the Righteous, they shall drink of a Cup [of Wine] mixed with Kafoor [eucalyptus]. (Qur'an 76: 5)

Eucalyptus boosts the immune system and has great immune modulating and antimicrobial/antiviral effects.[232] It can also help with respiratory illnesses and pain.[233]

Nigella (Black Seeds)

Prophet Muhammad, peace and blessings be upon him, said: 'Use this black seed, for it cures every disease, except death.' (Bukhārī, Muslim, Tirmidhī, Ibn Mājah and Aḥmad)

Black seeds are also known as roman coriander, black cumin, black caraway and black sesame. Black seeds (made from the seeds of the back cumin) are full of antioxidant, antimicrobial[234] and anticancer properties,[235] which prevent insulin resistance,[236] and obesity,[237] just as they optimize hair, skin,[238] and liver functions.[239] Black seeds have been shown to kill MRSA, relieve joint pain, and they also stimulate the regeneration of beta cells in Type 1 diabetics. Two grams of black seeds each day can significantly reduce the formation of blood glycation, blood sugar levels and insulin resistance. Black seed oil is often composed of single chemicals or simple combinations of single chemicals. An Iranian study in which volunteers were asked to use the oil of black seeds for three weeks noticed that it leads to controlling pain. Black cumin seed oil rebalances an out of control immune system and lowers inflammation by increasing T regulatory cells.

Ginger

Ginger lowers inflammation,[240] fights fungal infections,[241] cancer,[242] regulates blood sugar,[243] lipid levels[244] and atherosclerosis and improves digestion.[245] Ginger root has been used as a medicinal herb in Asia for thousands of years. Ginger is mentioned in the Qur'an as a drink for the pious ones in paradise:

And there they will be given to drink a cup [of wine) mixed with Zanjabīl [ginger]. (Qur'an 76: 17)

Other powerful herbs and spices include cardamom which stimulates bile and optimizes liver health and fat metabolism. Cinnamon helps to stabilize blood sugar and blood pressure. It also improves circulation and has antimicrobial effects and also lowers bad cholesterol. Turmeric is a powerful anti-inflammatory which optimizes detoxification. Black pepper helps with nutrient absorption. Hot chilli and cayenne increase

89

circulation, lower inflammation and boost metabolism. Green herbs, like oregano, have antifungal, antibacterial, antiparasitic, and antioxidant properties; and others like mint, dill, chives, paprika, rosemary and parsley are also beneficial. Thyme has powerful antiseptic, antioxidant and anti-inflammatory properties which help in digestion and are good for lung function. Sage lowers blood sugar and is good for the brain. It is also an antioxidant, anti-inflammatory and can improve blood pressure. Cumin is anticancer and helps the immune system. Organic spices in glass bottles are the best option. Adding these nutritious herbs and spices is the best way to fight inflammation.

Salt

Salt is fundamental for healthy brain and body functions. Low sodium levels have been linked to cognitive decline and other metabolic problems. A study of 94,000 people showed that those who had the lowest intake of sodium had the highest risk of heart disease, with no increased risks seen at intakes of up to 5g per day.[246]

Modern table salt is different from sea salt. Table salt has been overly processed and its chemical composition is altered and toxic. It is a natural distillation of pure sodium chloride, usually combined with iodine and a small amount of sugar to stabilize the iodine and anti-caking agents, stripping it of its nutritional benefit, leading to fluid retention. Now sea salt, Celtic salt, and Himalayan salt are the best salt we can use. Pink Himalayan salt contains 84 minerals and traces of elements like potassium, magnesium, copper, iron and calcium, which are needed for the body to function optimally. You have to make sure to get adequate iodine in your diet from sea vegetables, shrimp and turkey.

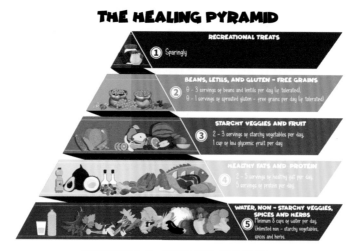

PICTURE 3.8   HEALING PYRAMID

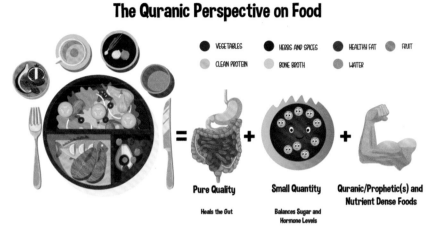

PICTURE 3.9   HEALING PLATE WITH LOGOS

Which Are More *Ṭayyib*, Organic or Non-Organic Products?

The above question crosses our mind every time we step into a grocery store: Is the price increase worth the benefits? The short answer is yes; organic food is sustainable, nutritious and better for human beings and the planet. In the past, most agriculture was pesticide free, but this changed after World War II. Agriculture now relies on pesticides to kill insects, control weeds and stave off fungi. More than 5.6 billion pounds of pesticides are used in farming every year, with 1 billion pounds of pesticides being used in the United States alone.

The difference between organic and non-organic foods lies in the way crops are grown. For organic foods, with a USDA label, the guidelines prohibit the use of pesticides or herbicides, hormones, genetic engineering or antibiotics. Conventional produces do not abide by any of these restrictions. So what is wrong with pesticide? Industrial agriculture relies on two main types of chemicals, pesticides and fertilizers. Pesticides are any substances or mixture of substances that are meant for destroying, repelling or mitigating any pests. For farmers, pesticides can provide a higher yield and save labour

In a study published in the *Journal of Applied Nutrition*, organically and conventionally grown apples, pears, potatoes, wheat and sweet corn were compared and analyzed for their mineral content over a two-year period and organic produce was found to be more nutrient dense.[247] Every year, the US Department of Agriculture tests more than 6900 kinds of produce and pesticides residue is found in 75 percent of the samples; 146 different pesticides are found in these samples.[248] Studies have shown that pesticides are carcinogenic,[249] neurotoxic,[250] and lead to depression[251] and respiratory issues.

Now which one sounds more *tayyib* (pure)? The answer is obviously organic produce, so choosing organic foods is best. You can consult the information provided by the Environmental Working Group on this issue. They have a list of the "dirty dozen" and the "clean fifteen" (foods with and without pesticides). Apart from being more *tayyib*, organic foods have much higher mineral content.[252] Studies have shown that participants who ate more organic foods had less insecticide in their urine, despite eating 70 percent more produce than other participants who ate conventional produce.[253] Eating *tayyib* and organic foods creates richer soils that are more resilient to climate change and capable of absorbing and retaining more carbon monoxide from the atmosphere.

In order to eliminate any pesticide residues from your fruits and vegetables, rub them, because rubbing them can eliminate the contaminants on the surface or wash them in a diluted solution of water mixed with 3 percent hydrogen peroxide.

Some Qur'anic/Prophetic Foods that One Should Limit

The Qur'anic/Prophetic diet is perfect. There is no question about that. But when people start to manipulate foods or eat the wrong types of food, the body suffers.

The foods we eat always influence our health. Some foods can help us while others can hurt. Certain foods can worsen symptoms and/or contribute to leaky gut syndrome, which in turn increases the risk of developing food sensitivities or make existing ones even worse. For instance, in a leaky gut, food is improperly digested and particles of it then leak through a weak intestinal barrier. The immune cells read the "name tags" on the food particles, telling the body how it should respond. If the immune cells label the particles as invaders, they can make antibodies against the specific food, thus causing or exacerbating chronic disease or chronic symptoms. If we are sensitive to certain foods, the effects can be either dramatic and immediate, i.e. food allergy, or subtle and gradual, food sensitivity.

If we have developed IgE antibodies to a certain food, when we eat it or are exposed to it, we will experience an immediate response, such as hives, swelling or difficulty in breathing, and we become allergic to the exposure. With repeated exposure to the foods that bother us, and if the food creates IgG antibodies, this can lead to leaky gut, IBS, depression, headaches, heart palpitations, fatigue, brain fog, post nasal drip, sinus issues and other symptoms of inflammation, also known as developing a food sensitivity or intolerance to those specific foods. Although the symptoms are usually less severe, food sensitivities play an integral part in causing immune-mediated conditions. Because the reactions can be outside the realm of the digestive tract and are often delayed, it can be hard to connect a particular food to how we feel. The following foods are the major common culprits in allergies or sensitivities, inflammation, and chronic disease.

If you are dealing with a chronic issue, it is highly recommend to remove these foods from your diet, as removing them can greatly improve your health. Most people do really well and their symptoms improve immediately once they remove from their diets all *khabīth* foods (sugar, processed/artificial foods, soy) as well as some of the *ṭayyib* foods like dairy and grains, specifically wheat/gluten. It is true that the latter foods are Qur'anic/Prophetic but it remains that they are highly processed and people have overindulged on these foods. A process of elimination of certain foods from your diet or even a blood test can help you determine which foods you are sensitive to.

Dairy

And verily, in the cattle there is a lesson for you. We give you to drink of that which is in their bellies, from between excretions and blood, pure milk; palatable to the drinkers. (Qur'an 16: 66)

The description of Paradise which the God-fearing [pious] have been promised is that in it are rivers of water the taste and smell of which are not changed; rivers of milk of which the taste never changes ... (Qur'an 47: 15)

It is narrated that on the night of the *Isrā'*, the Messenger of Allah, peace and blessings be upon him, was given two cups: one containing milk and the other wine. The Prophet looked at them, then chose the milk. Gabriel said, "Thank Allah Who has led you to what is natural, if you had taken the wine, your followers would have gone astray." (Bukhārī and Muslim)

Prophet Muhammad, peace and blessings be upon him, taught us: 'Whoever Allah gives food let him supplicate, "O Allah! Bless it for us and grant us what is better." And whoever Allah grants some milk let him say, "O Allah! Bless it for us and grant us more of it," for I do not know of a more complete food or drink than milk.' (Tirmidhī and Abū Dāwūd)

The Prophet, peace and blessings be upon him, also used to eat cheese. He brought some cheese in Tabook and asked for a knife, saying, 'In the Name of Allah,' and then he cut it. (Muslim and Abū Dāwūd.)

Dairy products are packed with magnesium, calcium, vitamin A, B6, B12, added vitamin D, zinc, selenium and A2 milk boosts glutathione. But unfortunately,

93

the cows of yesterday are no longer the cows of today, as about 70 percent of the world's population is lactose intolerant and this leads to milk related digestive issues[254] which affects up to 90 percent of East Asians. The reason for this is that people have been drinking the processed, more toxic form of dairy for too long, milk from these genetically improved cows (high level of A1 casein) triggers an inflammatory response capable of attacking the body's own tissues, with any form of dairy. Originally, all mammals produced a type of milk called A2, but then a mutation occurred in Europe, leading to a new type of cow's milk called A1. Overtime, the vast majority of cow's milk in the Western world became A1. Studies have shown that this newer A1 milk is linked to many inflammatory diseases. After the age of five, the body stops producing the enzymes that break down the macromolecules found in milk (lactose and milk proteins). The milk of commercial cows contains cancer causing growth factors, insulin like growth factor (IGF-1),[255] reproductive hormones, antibiotics, and milk allergens.[256]

Normally, milk should separate easily for easy digestion, but because it's been modified by pasteurization and homogenization to kill the bad bacteria,[257] healthy probiotics, vitamins, minerals, enzymes, nutritious proteins and lactose are also getting destroyed in the process, making milk difficult to digest, and this creates free radicals, alters the casein protein, and creates a molecule that resembles the gliadin protein in gluten which confuses the immune system. The undigested molecules lead to leaky gut syndrome, causing an inflammatory response and creating more problems for those with IBS.[258] This has also been linked to prostate cancer.[259] Most notably the casein proteins, which induce inflammation, lead to eczema.[260]

In children, cow's milk is a common cause of food sensitivity/allergy[261] which can also be associated with recurrent ear infections during childhood, congestion and sinus problems,[262] an opioid that can create a shortage of antioxidants in the brain and has been linked to schizophrenia,[263] ADHD, autism,[264] and can also trigger autoimmunity and diabetes.[265]

Another concern pertains to the natural oestrogens from pregnant cows that can increase the risk of hormonal sensitive cancers and early puberty. For someone with sensitivity to dairy, even cultured products like yoghurt can cause problems

But once you have healed from such allergies and sensitivities, you can gradually introduce in your diet raw grassfed A2 whole milk. You should start with raw, organic, pastured goat, sheep, camel yak or even buffalo milk. You can also make goat's milk kefir to boost healthy fats and improve the gut flora. Raw milk (best from Jersey or Guernsey cows or from source-certified cows) modulates epigenetics, thus increasing microbial diversity and lowering allergies. Grass-fed dairy also contains the ideal ratio of Omega-6 and Omega-3 needed to optimize health and healing.[266] Low-heat boiling preserves the milk benefits better than high-heat boiling.

Alternatives include: coconut milk kefir, with its wonderful antifungal and antiviral properties, which help heal leaky guts, and almond milk. Most people can tolerate grass-fed butter and ghee. Keep in mind that milk can weaken the bones, and there are far better calcium sources than milk that are necessary for optimal bone health and good general health such as flax seeds, spinach, sardines, walnuts, Brazil nuts, greens (e.g., mustard and collard), sesame seeds, wild salmon, broccoli and kale.

Gluten and Grains

And We send down blessed water [rain] from the sky, then We produce therewith gardens and grains [every kind of harvest] that are reaped. (Qur'an 50: 9)

And also grain, with [its] husks, leaves and stalk for fodder, and sweet-scented plants. (Qur'an 55: 12)

And have sent down from the rain-laden clouds abundant water, that We may produce therewith corn and vegetation, and gardens of thick growth. (Qur'an 78: 14–16)

Then let human beings look at their food, that We pour forth water in abundance, and We split the earth in clefts, and We cause therein the grain to grow, and grapes and clover plants [green fodder for the cattle], and olives and date-palms, and gardens, dense with many trees, and fruits and herbage [greens], [to be] a provision and benefit for you and your cattle. (Qur'an 80: 24–32)

At the time of the Prophet, peace and blessings be upon him, flour was prepared by grinding whole grains and the Prophet Muhammad, peace and blessings be upon him, forbade his Companions from eating bread made from refined flour.

Sahl said he was asked: 'During the Prophet's lifetime did you have white flour?' Sahl answered, 'No' then he was asked, 'Did you sift barley flour?' He replied, 'No, but we used to blow on it (to remove the chaff).' (Bukhārī)

Bread made from barley flour was the preferred bread in the Prophet's house and he also liked barley porridge.
Another preparation made from barley is *talbīnah*. (Tirmidhī and Aḥmad).

'Ā'ishah said that when any of her relatives died, she would order the preparation of *talbīnah*, then, *tharīd* (a traditional Arabic dish made from meat and bread) would be made, and she would pour the *talbīnah* on it. 'Ā'ishah would then ask the women to eat, saying, 'I heard the Messenger of Allah, peace and blessings be upon him, say: '*Talbīnah* brings relief to the heart of the sick and takes away some of the anguish.' (Bukhārī, Muslim and Aḥmad).

Barley is great for some people but can cause disease for some. This is because people have been eating the wrong type for so long, and this type has gluten. Likewise, the grains that people are eating now are not the same grains which were eaten at the time of the Prophet, peace and blessings be upon him. The Prophet, peace and blessings be upon him, ate more barley than any other grain and he didn't eat grains all the time. Barley is rich in selenium and has a prebiotic fibre called beta-glucan that promotes the growth of healthy microbes, it lowers total and LDL cholesterol and even helps to regulate blood sugar.

Unfortunately, we are eating more starches and carbs then every before with limited amounts of vegetables: about 50 percent carbs, 34 percent fats and 16 percent protein.[267] Grains can be a great source of fibre, minerals and vitamins but only if they are in their natural state and organic. Once they have been turned into flour, eating just raises the blood sugar and insulin levels, as two slices of whole wheat bread raise the blood sugar more than two tablespoons of table sugar.

So for those with chronic conditions, it is recommend to limit/eliminate processed grains, including all forms of gluten (including barley) from their diets, in order to lower inflammation, stabilize blood sugar levels and optimize/expedite healing.

Once you let the body heal, you can introduce some less processed grains, including gluten foods, back in your diet in moderate amounts, depending on what your body can tolerate.[268] Surprisingly, it is not documented anywhere that the Prophet, peace and blessings be upon him, ate wheat, and some Qur'an commentators believe that the first sin humans made via Adam and Eve was picking the wheat plant/agriculture.

The Problem with Today's Wheat

We have all heard of this new fad called gluten. But what is it? And why are people trying to avoid it if they don't have celiac disease? Gluten (the word comes from the latin word for "glue") is a protein found in grains such as wheat, barley, rye, kamut, and spelt, i.e. all the delicious stuff that we crave for.

Unfortunately, the average human body reacts badly to today's gluten, prompting an immune response, leading to inflammation, including mental illnesses[269] like depression and schizophrenia,[270] autism,[271] dementia,[272] obesity, heart disease, and even cancer.[273] About twenty-one million Americans are thought to have non-celiac gluten sensitivity. Simply removing wheat from the diet can help improve symptoms drastically. Why does today's wheat cause such problems?

People all over the world eat wheat and so, in the last fifty years, and in order to increase its production, modern wheat has been hybridized and manipulated to contain a "super starch", amylopectin A, that raises blood sugar higher than any other starches, leading to insulin resistance.[274] Wheat is also sprayed nowadays with massive amounts of chemical fertilizer and pesticides.[275] This high-yielding dwarf wheat has a much higher amount of gluten, more phytic acid and amylopectin, but fewer nutrients. So this new gluten protein molecule is large, and humans lack the specific enzymes to fully break it down. When the partially digested molecules come in contact with the small intestine, they spark the immune system and create inflammation.

The body undergoes an inflammatory response specifically when gluten is consumed. In 2000, Dr. Alessio Fasano at the University of Maryland isolated a physiological substance that directly controls the tight junctions in the gut wall, a substance he called "zonulin" that leads to leaky gut.[276] Two things can trigger the release of zonulin in the small intestine: exposure to bacteria and exposure to gluten.[277] People are now more exposed to zonulin than ever before, leaving their immune systems in the "on" position and their bodies vulnerable to becoming chronically inflamed.

Gluten can cause the gut cells to release zonulin, the protein that can loosen tight junctions in the intestinal lining, creating a permeable barrier and leading to leaky gut syndrome or increased intestinal permeability. Gluten does not just lead to leaky gut syndrome and food sensitivities, it can also cause large spikes in blood sugar, contributing to blood sugar dysregulation, insulin resistance, obesity and further inflammation. Gluten binds to opioid receptors in the gut, the same receptors that morphine and heroin bind to. This makes the body crave it, thus creating a withdrawal effect when we stop eating gluten. Wheat has been modified in such a way that people are more exposed to gluten than at any other time before, making non-celiac gluten sensitivity a widespread problem. One study reported that an inflammatory gut response was noted in the intestinal cells of healthy volunteers, suggesting that gluten may cause reactions in almost everyone.[278]

Examples of foods with gluten include barley, rye, wheat, durum, graham, kamut, semolina, spelt, oats, and soy sauce and its presence can also be undeclared in other products such as ketchup. Avoid foods that are packaged, processed and canned with "natural flavours."

Other Grains

Science has proven that grains offer very little nutritional value compared to other categories discussed above and are, furthermore, not needed to sustain a healthy existence free of disease. Grains are the edible part of the plant: the seed with the embryo. The plant produces natural insecticide to help it pass undigested through the animal system. The truth is that all grains are anti-nutrients (as they contain phytates), preventing the body from absorbing nutrients and minerals (like calcium, magnesium, iron, zinc, and potassium) and decreasing the digestion of fats, protein, and starches, which leads to deficiencies of key nutrients in the. Grains can promote leaky gut, feed unfriendly bacteria and damage the intestinal cells. Grains can be problematic for most people because they contain amylopectin which causes blood sugar spikes that lead to insulin resistance, and it also increases belly fat and inflammation,[279] and lectins (like agglutinins, a natural insecticide, and prolamines), specifically oats, corn and quinoa, which can cause leaky gut and dysbiosis by stimulating the immune system, and thus interfering with cell function, and making it hard to digest. Some may even contain toxins from moulds, called mycotoxins, which increase weight gain and irritability.

Seeds and seed-bearing plants, like grains and legumes, contain amylase inhibitors which block the enzymes used by the body to break down carbohydrates. They also contain protease inhibitors which block the enzymes used by the body to break down proteins. These enzyme inhibitors survive even after cooking these seeds, thus providing nourishment for unhealthy bacteria and promoting SIBO and yeast overgrowth. Seeds and seed-bearing plants also contain saponins, which is found in legumes, pseudo grains and nightshades and which potentially destroy red blood cells and lead to leaky gut.

Once you have healed, and depending on your toleration of them, you can add some occasional grains to your diet. But when doing this, you should sprout the grains because this makes them easier to digest and the nutrients easier to absorb and, at the same time, sprouting deactivates the phytic acid and increases dietary fibre by 50 percent.[280] Examples that can be added include organic sprouted grain flours, such as buckwheat, sorghum, quinoa, millet, amaranth, corn, oats, rice and even sourdough.

Corn

Corn can be as dangerous as gluten, for it contains a lot of starch and can also contribute to leaky guts.[281] Corn is also one of the most common genetically engineered foods, with about 90 percent of corn being genetically modified.[282] Corn is present in many products – such as high-fructose corn syrup, corn oil, and cornstarch – and is even being fed to livestock and poultry, leading to inflammation caused by saturated fats.

> *The likeness of those who spend their wealth in the Way of Allah is as the likeness of a grain [of corn]; it grows seven ears, and each ear has a hundred grains. Allah gives manifold increase to whom He pleases. And Allah is All-Sufficient for His creatures' needs, All Knower.* (Qur'an 2: 261)

Rice

When we say grains, rice and bread come to mind first, but unfortunately people are eating the highly processed versions. Brown rice contains more phytonutrients than white rice, which is associated with an increased risk of diabetes Type-2.[283] The other problem with rice is that it contains arsenic that may cause cancer.[284] Brown rice has the most arsenic in it while basmati rice has the least arsenic in it.

Oatmeal

Oatmeal has been shown to spike blood sugar, and elevate insulin levels, sugar, adrenaline, cortisol,[285] and to make us hungrier. People have been told that it is "heart healthy" (you have to remember that the American Heart Association makes a lot of money when the AHA seal is put on the labels of products), and that maybe due to the oatbran (not oatmeal) which reduces cholesterol. Oatmeal is loaded with sugar and its negative impact on heart health has been demonstrated.[286]

Once you are able to tolerate it, you can add less processed and sprouted grains can be added to your diet. Please do remember that you do not need grains to survive and that vegetables are carbohydrates. Other great carbs are nuts and seeds, lentils and even fruit.

Once your gut has healed, you can occasionally add to your diet black rice, quinoa, amaranth, millet or other forms of gluten-free grains and even sourdough bread and barley, depending on your toleration of them. So you must listen to your body. Sprouting the grains can increase the content of some nutrients and fibre content that improve digestion, the immune system and metabolism. Sprouting can help break down lectins, phytates and other anti-nutrients found in grains and legumes. Try to avoid high-glycaemic carbohydrates as best as you can and stick to the pure and *tayyib* versions (ancient grains) that you can get, as they are better for people and the planet.

Prohibited Food from the Qur'an and Sunnah – The *Khabīth* That Destroys Our Health Is Prohibited in Islam

As discussed above, Allah, glorified and exalted is He, has clearly stated that the *tayyib* is halal for us and if something is not *tayyib*, it is *khabīth*.

Khabīth means impure, artificial, processed foods and GMO foods, i.e. foods not provided by which have been manipulated. *Khabīth* food is anything that harms us, and now science has proven how these foods can hurt people more than they can help them. Anything artificial or *khabīth* causes inflammation. So, if a certain food was not known to our ancestors or didn't exist in their time, we should not eat it.

Artificial/Processed/Fake Food

We should stay away from *khabīth* processed/junk/fast foods. This includes all the white stuff, such as white flour, white bread, cakes, cookies and other baked goods. The latter contain lots of ingredients, have a very high glycaemic index, are full of partially hydrogenated oil (canola, soybean, corn, and other vegetable oils), food additives, artificial preservatives and artificial colours, flavours, etc., i.e. everything that damages the gut flora, leading to leaky gut, intestinal inflammation and chronic illnesses, including cancer.

So if you can't pronounce it or don't know what it is, then refrain from putting it in your mouth. This chart below will help you understand why this is so. All around the world, there are different names for these compounds. In Europe for example, they are known as E numbers, which are codes for substances used as food additives.

E100–E199 (colour additives)
E200–E299 (preservatives)
E300–E399 (antioxidants, acidity regulators)
E400–E499 (thickeners, stabilizers, emulsifiers)
E500–E599 (acidity regulators, anti-caking agents)
E600–E699 (flavour enhancers)
E700–E799 (antibiotics)
E900–E999 (miscellaneous)
E1000–E1599 (additional chemicals)

Artificial colourings	Associated with everything from cancer to hyperactivity in children.
	Blue #1, Brilliant Blue, FCF, E133-worst artificial colour, linked to hyperactivity and risk of kidney tumours, some research suggests it is a potential neurotoxin.[287]
	Blue #2, Indigotine, E132 damages chromosomes and leads to cancer.
	Red #2, linked to asthma and cancer.
	Red #3, Erythosine, E127 animal carcinogen, panned from cosmetics, but still allowed in food.
	Red #40-hyperactivity in children[288], accelerated the appearance of tumours.[289]
	Yellow #5 (Tartrazine, E102) and Yellow #6 (Sunset Yellow FCF, E110)- hyperactivity in children[289] and found to be contaminated by carcinogens like bensidine.[290]
	Green #3, Alurra Red AC, E129 causes bladder cancers.
	Brown HT or E155 causes asthma, cancer and hyperactivity in children.
	Caramel colour- brown food colouring linked to cancer.[291]
Additives	Cause uncontrollable hunger and binge eating.

Aluminum additives	Linked to neurotoxicity.
Azodicarbonamide (dough conditioner)	When baked it can lead to cancer and tumours, because it leads to semicarbazide (a carcinogen) and urethane (suspected carcinogen).[292] The WHO has linked it to respiratory issues, asthma and allergies.
Butane	A known carcinogen.
Butylated hydroxytoluene (BHT)	Affects the signaling from the gut to the brain that tells people to stop eating[293] and has been proven to cause cancer in animal tests.
(preservative)	Butylated hydroxyanisole (BHA) listed by California as a carcinogen.[294]
Calcium propionate	Produces a neurotoxin which affects the microbiome and causes autism and ADHD (found in all commercial bread)[295] and also causes sleep disturbances in children.
Calcium and sodium caseinate	Toxic dairy extract.
Carnauba Wax	Can cause tumours and cancers.
Canola oil	Damages hearts in lab animals.[296]
Carrageenan	Causes leaky gut, inflammation and possible human carcinogen.[297]
Citric acid (additive)	Derived from mould made with GMO corn not from fruit.
Dextrose (heavily processed form of sugar)	Usually made from corn; it has no nutritional value, typically made from GMO corn that produces its own insecticide.
Microwave popcorn	Contains PFOA, a synthetic chemical linked to cancer and hormone disruption.[298]
Monosodium glutamate (MSG)	Directly damages neurological tissue and kills brain cells, causes headaches, allergies, worsens asthma and damages the gut. It also increases food cravings and irresistibility.[299] It was used in one of the earliest methods of getting lab animals to become obese. MSG induces body-wide generalized endocrine disruption which increases the risk of developing insulin resistance, metabolic syndrome hypertension, belly fat, elevated blood lipids and blood sugar. MSG can be disguised as autolyzed protein, yeast extract, calcium caseinate,

gelatin, glutamate, glutamic acid, hydrolyzed plant protein, maltodextrin, modified corn starch, modified food starch, monopotassium glutamate, natural flavour, protein isolate, seasonings, soy sauce, sodium caseinate, textured protein, yeast extract, yeast food and yeast nutrient.

Natural flavors	Flavours derived from a proprietary mixture of chemicals derived from anything in nature. Many flavours may have up to 100 ingredients, including synthetic chemicals, propylene glycol as a solvent, and the preservative BHA, as well as GMO derived ingredients, and MSG.
Nitrates and nitrites	Found in processed meats, "probable" carcinogenic according to the WHO.[300]
Phosphates	Increased link to CVD and osteoporosis
	Sodium phosphate- preservative, accumulation leads to increased risk of heart disease, accelerated aging, kidney disease and mortality.
Polysorbate-80 or lecithin	Commonly found in vitamins, chewing gum and ice cream and linked to autoimmunity.[301]
Potassium bromate	Linked to various cancers (not allowed in the UK, Canada or the EU).
Propyl gallate	Used in food with animal fats, believed to be an endocrine disruptor, may be carcinogenic.
Propylparaben (E216) or Methylparaben	Synthetic preservative which is linked to breast cancer and reproductive problems.[302]
Propyl gallate	It increases the risk of tumours and endocrine disruption, and it is on the list of EWG's additives which should be avoided.[303]
Sodium benzoate (E211) or potassium benzoate (E212)	Synthetic preservatives when combined with vitamin C produce benzene, which is a known carcinogen.
Soy protein isolate	GMO, hormone disruptions, inhibits absorption of calcium and other vital minerals in the diet.
Sulfites	Can cause inflammation leading to problems like asthma, dermatitis and diarrhoea.

Tert-Butylhydroquinone (TBHQ)	Synthetic preservative found in packaged fried foods and commercial seed oils linked to stimulating the immune system, behavioural problems, stomach cancer, liver enlargement, vision issues, and negatively affects T cells and promotes allergies.
Theobromate	In animal testing it had possible effects on reproduction and development.
Titanium dioxide (E171)	Food colour that leads to inflammation.
These are just a few examples	There are so many more.

Khabīth Oils

Most processed foods contain vegetable oils. Canola, corn and soybean oils are tasteless, multi-purpose and industrially processed, including using caustic chemical solvents in their processing, which harms the fat. These oils also contain pro-inflammatory omega-6 fats and lead to gut dysfunction/leaky gut, interference with normal cell metabolism, and are hazardous to health and increase the risk of heart disease. Omega-3 should be consumed in an amount that is proportionate to the amount of Omega-6 that you consume; ideally, the Omega-6 to Omega-3 ratio should be from 4:1 to 1:1 in order to optimize health, fight disease, and stop premature aging.[304] The imbalance between Omega-6 and Omega-3 has been shown to depress the immune system function, contribute to weight gain and lead to inflammation.[305] Ninety percent of canola oil is from genetically modified plants. Avoid vegetable oils, especially those that are partially hydrogenated, such as corn, soybean, canola, safflower, and sunflower. Try to also avoid trans fats which are found in shortening, margarine, spreads, and anything that is hydrogenated including refined baked goods. These are chemically altered so that they can stay solid at room temperature. These fats lead to inflammation and immune dysfunction and they also increase bad cholesterol and lower good cholesterol, raising the risk of heart attack. They also promote obesity,[306] insulin resistance, prediabetes and diabetes Type-2,[307] cancer,[308] and dementia. These processed oils are cheap, so you will find them in most processed foods, restaurant foods and everything in between.

Khabīth Sweeteners

Artificial sweeteners are synthetic chemicals which cause hunger (leading to leptin resistance, which prevents from knowing when we are full),[309] gas and bloating.

Aspartame, which is 200 times sweeter than sugar and used in more than 6000 products, triggers the release of leptin and insulin in the blood; it also lowers neurotransmitters like serotonin and reduces the feeling of satiation which can lead to over-eating. A study that followed people for 25 years found that all those who drank diet soda were 65 percent more likely to become overweight and 41 percent more likely to become obese. Sweeteners act as an excitotoxin, which damages neurons in the brain,[310] leading to some neurological effects like headaches and migraines. They can also contribute to CVD and Type-2 DM, thus causing allergic reactions and various physical ailments such as gut irritation, altering the gut microbiome,[311] insulin resistance, inflammation[312] and even cancer.[313] Sucralose, more specifically, has a detrimental effect on gut bacteria,[314] reducing the latter by up to 50 percent because it is not broken down during the digestion process which makes them arrive in the large intestine fully intact, thus destroying the gut bacteria. Researchers at Duke University Medical Centre also discovered that Splenda significantly reduces beneficial bacteria in the gut and increases fecal pH which decreases the amount of nutrients that are absorbed.[315] It is also linked to liver and kidney damage in rats. Saccharine causes weight gain more than sugar and has been proven to damage the DNA and cells.

Studies have found that people who use artificial sweeteners have an increased appetite which leads to weight gain as we end up eating more because our craving for sugar is not satisfied. Consequently, our waist size increases, thus increasing the chance of developing Type-2 diabetes (by 67 percent),[316] as well as insulin resistance and metabolic syndrome which worsens the obesity epidemic.[317] Artificial sweeteners are also very bad for metabolic health and the brain.[318]

Genetically Modified Organisms (GMOs)

'And I will mislead them, and I will arouse in them [sinful] desires, and I will command them so they will slit the ears of cattle, and I will command them so they will change the creation of Allah.' And whoever takes Satan as an ally instead of Allah has certainly sustained a clear loss. (Qur'an 4:119)

As for the pure land, vegetation comes out by its Lord's will, but poor land produces in agony. We explain Our messages in various ways to those people who are grateful. (Qur'an 7:58)

When human hands change what Allah has provided for human beings, it ceases to be *tayyib*. The *Shaytan* has even promised that this is exactly what he will command humans to do. The verse above can be seen in a new light in today's world, a world filled with genetically engineered plants. GMOs (genetically modified organisms) are created through biotechnology, also called genetic engineering. The DNA of plants, animals, viruses or bacteria are artificially altered in the lab to produce foreign compounds that cannot occur in nature. What is at stake here is natural hybridization, but something which is not natural.

What is GMO? And the Chemical Companies In Charge of Our Food

Genetically modified organisms (GMO) are organisms that have been artificially manipulated in a lab.[319] These organisms' genetic material is manipulated to create combinations of plant, bacteria, virus or animal genes that don't naturally occur. GMOs were engineered to withstand exposure to herbicide and/or to produce an insecticide, but new technologies are now being developed to create new organisms via synthetic biology which artificially develop other plant traits. The biggest GMO companies are Monsanto, Bayer, Syngena, Dow and Du Pont, but all these are also chemical companies. They are engineering plants with which they can spray their chemical herbicide without killing the plants. They are making plants that tolerate poison so that they can use even more poison on them.

Glyphosate, the active herbicide in Roundup, was originally used as an industrial cleaner, but one day it spilled out onto the land and killed all the plants. Monsanto bought glyphosate and patented it as a herbicide. Then they genetically engineered the seeds and plants to be "Roundup ready" such that these plants can survive when sprayed with glyphosate. Unfortunately, 80 percent of GMO seeds are "Roundup ready" varieties and most packaged and processed foods contain ingredients derived from GMO like soy, canola, corn, sugar beets, etc., just as more than 750 different products sold in the US contain high levels of glyphosate. Since its introduction in 1996, the amount of glyphosate used around the world has increased by five folds and Roundup is the most heavily used weedkiller in global agriculture, and the second most popular one at home. In conventional farming, they use Roundup as a desiccant on non-GMO crops like with most wheat, oats, canola and corn, which means that glyphosate is sprayed on these crops just before their harvest so that the stalks are dry and easy to harvest and then processed, leaving those non-GMO foods also covered in chemicals.

In addition to engineering crops to withstand Roundup, they also engineered crops, such as cotton and corn plants, to produce their own toxic insecticide/pesticide called Bt toxin, which create tiny holes in the gut walls of the insects, thus destroying their digestive lining and then killing them.

The Effects of GMO

And when it is said to them, 'Do not cause corruption on the earth,' they say, 'We are but reformers.' Unquestionably, it is they who are the corrupters, but they perceive [it] not. (Qur'an 2:11)

When GMO's were first introduced, what was promised was the plants' resistance to insects, decreasing people's dependence on pesticides, and increasing crops worldwide. However, GMO agriculture has failed to fulfil all these promises: crops have not increased, and instead the USA has been using 21 percent more pesticides. GMO agriculture is definitely not the solution to all the world's problems; in fact, it's causing more disruption.

People were told that GMO agriculture wouldn't affect humans, because humans don't have the pathway through which glyphosate works in plants (the shikimate pathway present in all bacteria, fungi and plants, that synthesizes amino acids into proteins). Unfortunately, the microbes in human guts do have this pathway. This chemical is very active in disrupting beneficial bacteria,[320] leading to leaky gut and imbalanced gut bacteria, because it doesn't kill the bad bacteria, which leads to its overgrowth and damage to the intestinal wall. As a chelator, glyphosate can take out metals and minerals from the body, specifically amino acids like tryptophan and tyrosine that the bacteria in the gut need to make dopamine and serotonin. Scientists are just beginning to understand what kind of effects this will cause, as Bt toxin and Roundup can create leaky gut, and glyphosate has also been patented as an antibiotic. Glyphosate may negatively affect vitamin D3 activation in the liver, potentially explaining the epidemic levels of vitamin D deficiency. Glyphosate exposure has been linked to an increase in the rate of different cancers.[321]

The pesticide (Bt toxin) disrupts the microbiome, compromises the ability to detoxify toxins, depletes vitamin D and other key nutrients and can mimic hormones like oestrogen, which can lead to cancers. The pesticide can be linked to a fourfold increase in celiac disease and other autoimmune conditions, according to 270 studies compiled by MIT in 2013. There is a marked rise in many other diseases since the introduction of GMOs and Roundup, which has increased toxins, allergens and nutritional problems in the foods consumed by humans. For example, GMO soy has up to 7x more allergens than regular soy.[322] Removing these foods can eliminate the dysfunction of the human body.

In the US, GMO foods are soy, corn, sugar, alfalfa, cotton seed oil and fabric, papaya, canola, zucchini and yellow squash. In some areas, apples, potatoes and salmon are also being genetically engineered. A new law in the United States, will make it mandatory to label products that contain GMO by 2022. Fortunately, 19 out of the 27 member state countries of the European Union have voted to either partially or fully ban GMOs. The EU has specific regulation requiring the labelling of GMOs in consumer food. Most nations that prohibit GMO cultivation still allow GMO products to be imported. Countries growing GMO crops currently are Argentina, Australia, Bangladesh, Bolivia, Brazil, Canada, Chile, China, Colombia, Costa Rica, Czech Republic, Honduras, India (but cotton only), Malawi, Mexico, Myanmar, Nigeria, Pakistan, Paraguay, Philippines, Portugal, South Africa, Slovakia, Spain, Sudan, Eswatini (Swaziland), United States, Uruguay, Vietnam, and Zambia.

So why is a chemical company in charge of our food? We know that such food is *khabīth*, and while the rest of the world is still figuring it out, let's get back to the Qur'an and Sunnah and avoid all *khabīth* foods, including GMO. This is an area about which we need to start educating Muslim families. We have talked earlier about corn, let's now talk about soy and sugar.

Soy

Soy is not recognized by the digestive system, as most soy is genetically modified. Soy contains inhibitors that shut down the digestion of proteins, causing gastric discomfort and reducing the absorption of amino acids and minerals such as calcium, iron, magnesium, and zinc. It disrupts the endocrine system, especially dysregulating thyroid and oestrogen, and interferes with leptin, which leads to leptin resistance and making us overeat. It also leads to leaky gut syndrome (when it remains undigested) as it stimulates the immune system to produce antibodies, and leads to food sensitivities and inflammation.[323] Soy is found in tempeh, tofu, edamame, soy sauce and tamari and can be found in meat substitutes and protein shakes, bars and powders. If you decide to eat soy, make sure it's fermented, as in tempeh. The fermentation process breaks down indigestible carbohydrates and dissolves the protein digestion inhibitors.

Sugar

Worldwide intake of free sugars varies according to age, setting and country, but people today are eating more sugar than ever! Americans went from eating 10 pounds of sugar per person in 1800 to 152 pounds of sugar and 146 of flour per person per year today, thus eating a minimum of a pound of sugar daily!

The World Health Organization recommends less than 5 percent of the daily caloric intake, i.e. around 6 teaspoons a day. You might think that you are not consuming too much sugar, but a strawberry yoghurt has 4.75 teaspoons of sugar, Hershey's Milk Chocolate bar has 4.87 teaspoons of sugar, M&Ms have 5.68 teaspoons of sugar, honey nut cereal has 6.67 teaspoons of sugar, 100g of granola has 6 teaspoons of sugar, soda has 7 teaspoons of sugar, and a flavoured coffee has up to 25 teaspoons of sugar! Don't forget that sugar is found in 74 percent of packaged foods.

Most people can't stop at just one cookie because sugar stimulates the brain reward centres, the same parts of the brain that are stimulated by addictive drugs like heroin or cocaine,[324] and when we stop eating sugar, especially suddenly, we experience withdrawal symptoms, just like when people have withdrawal symptoms from dopamine and other addictive drugs.[325] Our willpower has no role here because sugar is biologically addictive. Sugar changes our brain chemistry and turns to glucose in the blood, thus releasing insulin and stimulating the dopamine receptors which give us the feeling of pleasure. This makes sugar eight times more addictive than cocaine.

When the brain senses it is running out of glucose, it goes into a panic mode because it has forgotten how to burn fat, and releases cortisol, making us reach for more sugar. Insulin resistance in the brain cells is associated with brain fog, ADHD/ADD, difficulty focusing and Alzheimer's. The byproduct of sugar metabolism is lactic acid which is acidic, and this leads to neuroinflammation which can manifest as aggression, brain fog, behavioural issues, dementia, ADHD and Parkinsonism.

Sugar breaks down lactic acid which, along with inflammation, contributes to leaky gut, and an increase in toxins in the blood which then lead to systemic inflammation. Bad bacteria thrive on sugar, which then leads to bad bacterial overgrowth of pathogenic bacteria and yeast species like fungi. Oxidative stress damages the gut lining and increases the toxins which then causes more systemic inflammation as well as the increase of fungi which then increases more craving for sugar, creating a vicious cycle. Sugar interferes with the ability of the white blood cells to destroy toxins and fight infection, making us sick – all of this within minutes after eating sugar, and it can last for several hours.

Sugar disrupts the blood sugar balance, with insulin spikes that can be dangerous, leading to fatigue and brain fog, anxiety, and mood swings; sugar also speeds up cell aging,[326] reduces HDL ("good" cholesterol), raises LDL ("bad" cholesterol) and high triglyceride levels, blood pressure and heart disease, just as it causes weight gain and accumulation of belly fat, cancer, diabetes,[327] dementia,[328] insulin resistance, and increases appetite and sugar cravings. It also damages the liver, just like alcohol, and leads to fatty liver.[329] The liver pulls the excess glucose out of the bloodstream, and this leads to non-alcoholic fatty liver disease which can progress into non-alcoholic steatohepatitis which adds inflammation and scaring to the list of liver issues. These liver issues have doubled since the 1980s. Around 25 percent of people with NASH will go on to develop non-alcoholic liver cirrhosis which requires liver transplants.

A major study from the Harvard School of Public Health published in the *Journal of the American Medical Association* found that those who took 25 percent or more of daily calories as sugar were twice more likely to die from heart disease than those who consumed less than 10 percent,[330] and the association was true whether the rest of their diet was fairly healthy or not. Sugar also leads to a rise in fructose which increases the uric acid, leading to inflammation.

Sugar also affects the hormones. Eating sugar leads to more insulin, cueing the fat cells to release more leptin that signals the hypothalamus in the brain that we are full and should stop eating. With leptin resistance, the cells lose the ability to hear leptin signals, and we always feel hungry and constantly crave sweets, needing more and more sugar to satisfy this craving. Sugar's effects on hormones also impacts the thyroid. Insulin resistance has been identified as a risk factor in developing thyroid cancer. Eating sugar leads to fat storage and more production of oestrogen, contributing to oestrogen dominance, progesterone deficiencies and hormonal imbalance which causes symptoms like painful cramps, irregular periods, endometriosis, infertility, PMDD and PMS.

Sugar feeds cancer. Unlike other cells, cancer can't use fat as fuel and relies on sugar. In order for a cancer cell to create the same amount of energy as a normal cell, it must metabolize 18 times more glucose. The higher the HbA1c is, the higher the risk of cancer and heart disease is, even if it just in the pre-diabetic range.

Unfortunately, sugar can be directly related to all the chronic diseases, like heart disease, cancer, stroke, and diabetes, and it has no redeeming nutritional value. So basically, sugar makes us obese, old, and ill. We should avoid sugar and all its other code names: bran sugar, dextrose, glucose, dextran, fructose, agave, barley malt, brown rice syrup, high-fructose corn syrup (HFCS), hydrogenated starch, maltodextrin, maltose, lactose, disaccharides, monosaccharides, sorghum, sucrose and xylose.

Fructose, like in agave and HFCS, has been shown to be associated with insulin resistance, hypertension, and impaired glucose tolerance. A diet full of processed sugar leads to obesity and inflammation and is responsible for the diabetes, heart disease and dementia epidemic, all of which leads to a premature death. Sugars such as refined sugar, corn syrup, and agave nectar (very high in fructose, worsening insulin resistance) should be avoided. We should stick to Qur'anic and Prophetic sources of sweetness, as discussed above.

It is also best to keep sugar alcohols at a minimum, because they don't absorb well and cause bacterial overgrowth, unbalancing the gut bacteria leading to GI upset type symptoms. If you need a sugar alcohol, then erythritol is better because it is absorbed, but can lead to weight gain.[331]

Try to avoid drinks such as soda, diet soda, sports drinks, fruit juice, and other sweetened beverages like iced tea and lemonade which are full of sugar and have limited nutritional value.

If you find it difficult to give up sugar, you should remember to focus on real, whole foods, implement stress management practices, exercise, show gratitude and get good sleep. Supplements that can help are chromium which improves blood sugar control and helps with sugar cravings, along with apple cider vinegar that can improve insulin function and insulin resistance. Cinnamon also regulates blood sugar levels.

Alcohol

O you who believe! Intoxicants [all kinds of alcoholic drinks], gambling, stone altars [used for sacrificing to idols] and arrows [for seeking luck or decision] are an abomination of Satan's handiwork. So avoid [strictly all] that [abomination] in order that you may be successful. Satan wants only to excite enmity and hatred between you with intoxicants [alcoholic drinks] and gambling, and to hinder you from the

remembrance of Allah and from ~alat [the prayer]. So, will you not then abstain?
(Qur'an 5: 90–91)

... And do not throw yourselves into destruction ... (Qur'an 2: 195)

They ask you [O Muhammad] concerning alcoholic drink and gambling. Say, 'In them is a great sin and [some] benefit for men, but the sin of them is greater than their benefit.'... (Qur'an 2: 219)

Alcohol is prohibited in Islam, and now science has shown why this should be the case. Alcohol provokes a leaky gut, increases intestinal permeability, opens up junctions between enterocytes and inflames the liver.[332] It impairs our impulse control, so that we are more likely to eat more – and mindlessly at that. In addition, it is simply sugar in another form, meaning that it causes spikes in blood sugar levels, contributing to insulin resistance and increased anxiety, fatigue and brain fog.

How to Eat Food

We need to eat just to live, not live in order to eat. We should eat pure foods, clean, non-GMO and organic (whenever possible). The body has a right over us, and each morsel we take has a purpose, which is to take care of the gift that Allah gave us, our body.

1. Always start with *'Bismillāh'*, a dua and eat with the right hand.

Umar ibn Abi Salamah narrated: "When I was a boy I was under the care of the Messenger of Allah, peace and blessings be upon him, and I used to eat with him and my hand used to move around the dish while eating. The Prophet told me, 'Child, pronounce the Name of Allah (say *bismillāh*), eat with your right hand, and eat from what is nearer to you in the dish.'" (Bukhārī and Muslim).

The Prophet, peace and blessings be upon him, also said: "The Devil eats from the food on which Allah's Name was not mentioned." (Muslim)

When one of you eats let him mention Allah's Name before starting, and if he forgets, let him say, "In the Name of Allah at its beginning and at its end (*Bismillāh awwaluhu wa ākhiruh*)." (Tirmidhī and Abū Dāwūd)

Prophet Muhammad, peace and blessings be upon him, said: "When one of you eats, let him use his right hand and when he drinks let him drink with his right hand, because the Devil eats and drinks with his left hand." (Muslim and Abū Dāwūd)

2. Eat mindfully and simply. Each time you eat, take a couple of seconds to actually think about what you are eating. Your food contains bioactives, so make sure you get them to keep you healthy. That signal of what we want to eat is coming from our microbiome, so eat with the intent that you are feeding and taking care of your gut "bugs". Don't eat reclining (Bukhārī).

3. Don't criticize the food (Bukhari and Muslim) or just say, "I don't feel like eating this." (Bukhari and Muslim), and compliment the food (Muslim), and make dua for those you ate with (Muslim).

4. Eat with people that you enjoy. Humans are social animals, and that love can enhance the healing power of your foods and lifestyle.

5. End every meal with showing gratitude and making a prayer.

When the Prophet, peace and blessings be upon him, completed his meals, he used to say: "All praise be to Allah, blessed is He! Allah, we cannot reject Your Bounty, nor leave it nor suffice ourselves without it." (Bukhārī and Tirmidhī)

Now What Do I Eat?!

If we have to fill no more than 1/3 of our stomach with food, then we need to fill it with the most nutrient dense foods that will heal our body and lower inflammation.

Example of healthy meals include:

Breakfast: veggies, clean protein, healthy fat and some fruits. Examples include foods made with coconut, nut and seed flours like pancakes, waffles, muffins, banana bread/zucchini bread, eggs, quiche, no-nitrate sausages (chicken, beef, and turkey) or kabobs, no-grain cereal in almond milk with fresh or frozen berries, smoothies, greens, fruit or nut or seed butter, fresh fruit, chia pudding, etc..

Snacks: veggies, clean protein, and healthy fat and fruit. Examples include sugar snap peas and guacamole, nuts with blueberries, veggie and protein rollups.

Lunch and dinner: veggies, clean protein and healthy fat. Examples include soups, egg/chicken/tuna salad, veggie and protein rollups, zucchini pasta with meat sauce, lettuce wrap, stir fry, no-grain tortilla/naan, cauliflower rice. The ideas are endless! You can apply these same techniques for *suḥūr*, *iftār*, when you eat out and even how you shop!

Fasting

O you who believe! Fasting is prescribed for you as it was prescribed for those before you, that you may attain piety [God consciousness]. (Qur'an 2: 183)

Fasting is an integral part of Islam, and now science has shed some light on its importance for healing, slowing down aging, optimal health and optimizing the immune system.

Spiritual Benefits

> All the deeds of the Children of Adam are theirs except for fasting: it is Mine and I will reward for it. (Bukhārī)

The spiritual benefits of fasting are countless: denying oneself the basic human necessity of eating, drinking and intimate relations only for the love of Allah; learning self-control, feeling compassion for the less fortunate; building the community and family; learning patience; remembering Allah's blessings and being grateful.

> Abū Hurayrah related that Prophet Muhammad, peace and blessings be upon him, said: "If one does not give up giving false testimony and acting according to it, Allah has no need for him to give up his food and drink." (Bukhārī)

Ramadan is about more than just not eating or drinking; it percolates within every aspect of our daily life. We are taught to work on ourselves such that our whole body fasts, including our mouth, ears, hands, and deportment. Fasting is prescribed so that we may gain *taqwā* and the key to *taqwā* is eating halal and *ṭayyib* foods.

> Zayd ibn Khālid al-Juhnī related that Prophet Muhammad, peace and blessings be upon him, said: "He who provides for the breaking of the fast (*iftār*) of another will acquire the same reward as the fasting person without diminishing in any way the latter's reward." (Tirmidhī)

> Ibn 'Abbās related that the Prophet, peace and blessings be upon him, was the most generous of people, and he was even more generous during Ramadan when Gabriel visited him every night and recited the Qur'an with him. During this period the open-handedness of the Prophet became faster than the rain-bearing wind." (Bukhārī)

> Prophet Muhammad, peace and blessings be upon him, also taught us: "Satan flows through the human being like blood flows in his veins, so restrain his pathways with hunger." (Bukhārī)

The Physical Benefits of Fasting

> ... *And if you fast, it is better for you, if only you knew.* (Qur'an 2: 184)

The body can have two states: an insulin high state and an insulin low state due to fasting.

Modern science has now proven so many physical benefits for fasting. Simply going without food is anti-inflammatory, anti-tumour and anti-aging. Fasting activates the Nrf2 gene pathway that improves detoxification and stem cell activation, triggering new cell formation, increasing mitochondrial function, autophagy (body's natural cleaning process, removing damaged proteins and clears damaged cellular parts that may lead to cancer, eliminates pathogens, helps in cellular repair and regeneration), increases antioxidant function, increases the production of beta-HBA, a super-fuel for the brain and body, stimulates the production of BDNF, the brain's growth hormone that can support function of brain cells, accelerates weight loss,[1] increases fat burning, lowers blood insulin and sugar levels, possibly reverses Type-2 diabetes,[2] possibly improves mental clarity and concentration, increases energy possibly growth hormone, blood cholesterol profile[3] and possibly longer life.[4]

Fasting improves the immune system, reduces immunosenescence (the gradual deterioration of the immune system over time), lowers white blood cell numbers and inflammation, protects against inflammatory related conditions, lowers cortisol at night, supports the healing of the gut lining, increases weight loss, improves heart health, prevents neurological and metabolic diseases and improves cancer treatments.

When a person fasts, the body begins using glycogen (the most easily accessible energy source) which is broken down into glucose molecules to provide energy to other cells and the body as a whole for 24–36 hours. After that, the body primarily breaks down fat from the liver and the muscles for energy and when that runs out, the body starts to move fat and use it to create ketones (a source of energy that powers the brain more effectively). Beta-HBA, the main ketone, has been shown to be a super fuel that produces ATP energy more effectively than glucose; it also protects the brain cells from toxins, increases the number of mitochondria and stimulates the growth of new brain cells and improves antioxidant function.

Fasting has also been shown to supercharge the brain, stimulating BDNF (known as the brain's "growth hormone", a protein that plays a huge role in stimulating new brain cells and in the performance of existing neurons). Studies have also shown that fasting can increase the production of regenerative protein SDF1 and its receptor CXCR4 which together recruit and attract stem cells from the bone marrow into the blood stream.[5] Fasting has lots of benefits, but the problem is that a lot of Muslims gain weight during fasting because they fast the wrong way. Some Muslims eat too much food and the wrong types at that when they break their fast.

One should Always remember the hadith of the Prophet, peace and blessings be upon him:

By Him in whose Hands is the life of Muhammad, the odour of the breath of the one who is fasting is more pleasant to Allah than the fragrance of musk. (Muslim)

Suḥūr and *Ifṭār* Tips

The pre-dawn meal is a *sunnah*; the Prophet, peace and blessings be upon him, said:

> There is a blessing in having the *suḥūr*, so do not skip it. At least drink a sip of water, for Allah and his angels give their blessings to the people who eat their meal before the break of dawn. (Aḥmad)

With *suḥūr* and *ifṭār*, veggies, protein and healthy focus on *tayyib* foods that will help in healing the gut, balance glucose and insulin levels and those that are also packed with nutrients. Focus on fruit, veggies, protein and healthy fats. Smoothies and skillets with eggs, veggies and avocados with fruit/dates work best for *suḥūr*. For *ifṭār*, the simpler the better: a normal meal with veggies, protein and healthy fats with fruit.

Good nutrition is all about avoiding disease and thriving for the sake of Allah, so you can take care of the gift that Allah, glorified and exalted is He, has given. People see immediate results when they switch to a *tayyib* lifestyle and eat real food. Patients with "incurable diseases" are "healed" with a *tayyib* lifestyle and diet.

People can change the world through eating *tayyib*, real food. Eating *tayyib* foods and living a *tayyib* lifestyle can also address issues relating to social justice, poverty, violence and educational gaps in learning. *Tayyib* food can help with restoring the soil, plant and animal species, and even fight against climate change. People can take charge of their lives using food as a major part of transforming their health and the planet.

Detoxing the Body with a *Tayyib* Environment

The Qur'an and Sunnah emphasize the importance of taking care of ourselves and the external world. Through a *khabīth*/impure environment, we create an inward imbalance. Problems happen when humans disrupt Allah's balance.

> *Evil has appeared on land and sea because of what the hands of people have earned [by oppression and evil deeds], that Allah may make them taste a part of that which they have done, in order that they may return.* (Qur'an 30: 41)

> *And when he turns away [from you O Muhammad], his effort in the land is to make mischief therein and to destroy the crops and the cattle, and Allah does not like mischief.* (Qur'an 2: 205)

People are exposed to more and more chemicals, pesticides, pharmaceutical drugs and radiation than ever before. More than one hundred thousand new chemicals in the past few years have slowly penetrated people's lives, forcing their livers to work harder to remove them. Currently, the US imports about 45 million pounds of synthetic chemicals daily and about 1000 new chemicals are put into use every year, only 5 chemicals have ever been banned in the US. It is projected that, over the next 25 years, global chemical production is expected to double, reaching more than a trillion pounds per year! Approximately 90,000 compounds are approved for commercial use right now, but only a handful have been tested for toxicity!

With the existence of toxins everywhere, everything passes through the liver (the body's main detoxifying organ). A toxin or *khabīth* element in our environment can lead to an inflammatory response.

The accumulation of toxins over time overburdens the liver, thus disrupting its ability to detoxify and forcing it to hold on to the toxic stuff (which should be removed). This damages the mitochondria and metabolism, makes the body numb to insulin and leptin, thus increasing blood sugar issues and insulin resistance. Toxins also affect the epigenetics, inflame the gut,[1] lower the immunity, and worsen inflammation, thus leading to autoimmunity, heart disease, stroke, diabetes and even cancer. The cumulative effect of all of this weakens the immune system, causing more inflammation.

The body is not meant to handle enormous amounts of artificial pollutants on a daily basis. In order to deal with the toxic/*khabīth* overload, you must avoid exposure to toxic/*khabīth* stuff, support your body's natural ability to detoxify, and lower inflammation, all of which will help you to become more resilient to the world around you.

Locate the Toxins

Toxins are all around, and some are beyond our control. So we need to focus on what we can control: our home.

In a typical house, the mattress is likely to have chemicals including flame retardants; the bedding has chemicals left from detergents and softeners; the floors backing may have carcinogens such as 4-phenylcyclohexane (4-PC) or perchloroethylene (PERC); chemicals like benzene may have been sprayed on the furniture; our food and water are full of toxins; and our body products are filled with chemicals like parabens, phthlates that are endocrine disruptors.

Hormone disrupting chemicals, specifically xenoestrogens, once absorbed, can send mixed messages to the endocrine system, thus disrupting the hormones' natural actions. Xenoestrogens are endocrine-disrupting chemicals that mimic the effects of oestrogen, build up in fatty tissues and lead to increased inflammation. They can be linked to early puberty, difficult and early periods, male infertility, low sex drive, obesity and even cancer. Xenoestrogens mimic the effects of human hormones.

Heavy metals are also a common toxin in the environment and can be very toxic in low concentrations. Examples of heavy metals include mercury, arsenic and lead.

Khabith Toxin	Found in	Effects
Phthlates	Found in filler ingredients which are added to self-care products, toys, plastic wraps, vinyl flooring, fake fragrances and plastics.	Disrupt development of the hormone system and impairs fertility. Have been implicated in cancers, endocrine disruption, weight gain, asthma in children, birth defects, infertility, ADHD, diabetes, and obesity.[2]
Parabens	Personal care products like hair, beauty and hygiene products, fast food, food packaging, drinking water and even some fish.	One to five different types of parabens have been found in women's breast tissue with cancer. Parabens disrupt hormonal balance, leading to obesity, insulin resistance, and diabetes.[3] They can also lead to neurological, hormonal and developmental disorders.
Triclosan	An antimicrobial agent often added to antibacterial soaps, toothpastes, body washes, deodorants, hairsprays, some findings in kitchenware, toys, furniture and clothing. The Environmental Protection Agency has labelled this as a pesticide and is no more effective than plain soap.[4]	Increased levels of allergies in children and development of antibiotic-resistant superbugs. It is also being studied as a potential cancer-causing agent.
Fluoride	An industrial waste by-product added to water supplies to attempt to minimize dental decay and is classified as a drug, administered without a specific dose for all to consume.[5] All fluoride toothpastes have a warning to call Poison Control if swallowed. Any cavity prevention can be accomplished via topical fluoride and optimal nutrition.[6] Found in supplements, medications, toothpaste, black tea, red tea, and canned food items.	It is a neurotoxin[7] that damages more than two hundred enzymes and causes developmental neurotoxicity that persists over generations. It disrupts the endocrine system, blocks iodine absorption, increases the likelihood of thyroid issues and cancers, increases oxidative stress, and interferes with cell signaling from neurotransmitters, growth factors, and hormones. As of 2010, 41 percent of kids aged 12–15 had some sort of dental fluorosis, according to the CDC.[8]

BPA/BPS (bisphenol-A/S)	Synthetic oestrogen used in plastics such as containers, coats store receipts, bottles, children's toys, fast food packaging and baby formula cans.	Impairs brain development in newborn babies, stimulates autoantibody production, and causes problems in the small intestine.[9] Leads to problems in hormonal signaling, disrupting oestrogen, thyroid, leptin and androgen functions in the body, promoting weight gain, insulin resistance, and diabetes.
Perfluorooctainoic Acid (PFOA)	A group of man-made chemicals (aka as the forever chemicals as they remain in the soil and water for long periods of time). Found in contaminated fish and food packaging that prevents it from sticking or leaking, cosmetics, water supplies, contaminated soil and cookware. It is a chemical released when nonstick pans that contain Teflon or polytetrafluoroethylene (PTFE) are scratched and/or heated.	They disrupt the hormonal and immune systems, decrease energy, lead to liver damage, decrease mental concentration, lead to developmental problems in animals, and are known carcinogens.
Pesticides	Used in agriculture to kill insects.	Over time, it can disrupt the microbiome and hormones, leading to weight gain, insulin resistance, diabetes, fatigue, forgetfulness, depression, mood issues and even overall inflammation and autoantibody production.
Dioxins and polychlorinated biphenyls (PCBs)	Banned in the 1970s, but they still persist in the environment and in our bodies. Found in meat, dairy, and fish.	PCBs lead to inflammation, autoimmunity, cancer, diabetes and heart problems.

(continued)

Khabith Toxin	Found in	Effects
Bromide (polybrominated diphenylethers [PBDEs])	Found in flame retardants in furniture and upholstery and in mattresses (making the mattress inflammable), baked foods, plastics used in computers/appliances and other electronics, tea, citrus-flavored drinks, and gluten free productions.	It has been shown to increase the risk of autoimmunity, diabetes and ADHD.
Chlorine	Found in industrial products, lubricants, coolants, industrial chemicals, pools, plastics, pesticides, paper products, and cleaning products.	Increases the prevalence of antibiotic resistance and the number of genes of new antibiotic-resistant strains.
DEA (diethanolamine)	Used in foaming agents, shampoos and bubble baths, and toothpastes.	In lab animals, it is linked to esophageal and stomach cancer. It is banned in many countries but still blesses the United States with its presence.
Volatile organic compounds or VOCs	Found in perfumes, air fresheners, household cleaners, and shampoos.	Neurotoxic.
DEHA	Plastic wrap and PVC plastic.	Linked to developmental toxicity and is a probable carcinogen.
Perchloroethylene (PERC)	Dry cleaning fluid and spot removers.	Probable carcinogen.

Heavy Metals		
Mercury	Can be found in silver filings, cosmetics, pesticides, some vaccines and certain fish (highest in tuna and swordfish).	Exposure to it can lead to dementia and developmental problems, like mental retardation, cerebellar ataxia, limb deformities, altered physical growth, sensory impairments, and cerebral palsy.[10]
Lead	Can still be present in older homes, paint, older water pipes, and occasionally in certain cosmetics and pottery from China. In 2020, UNICEF and Pure Earth reported that every third child in the world has too much lead in their body, about 800 million children are still exposed to lead.	Stored in our bones for years,[11] and is a neurotoxin which leads to impaired IQ and heart problems.
Arsenic	Found in drinking water, rice, chicken, some produce, household detergents, coloured chalk, rat poison, and automobile exhaust.	Leads to diabetes, gout, cancer and autoimmunity.

Move Fluids to Detoxify!

O you who believe! When you intend to offer salat [the prayer], wash your faces and your hands [and forearms] up to the elbows, rub [by passing wet hands over] your heads, and [wash] your feet up to the ankles. If you are in a state of janabah [post-sex impurity or had a sexual discharge], purify yourself [bathe your whole body with water] ... (Qur'an 5: 6)

The skin is a major organ for the elimination of toxins. Sweating and cleansing yourself will help to eliminate what is harmful or not needed by the body. Examples of ways of sweating include exercising, spending some time in a sauna and brushing/exfoliating our skin. Taking a bath with Epsom salt, sodium bicarbonate, seaweed, or sea salt (preferably alternating them), may be helpful in eliminating toxins and is great for lowering any die-off reactions. Sweating can get more toxins out of the body than urinating.

Oil-pulling and infrared saunas can also be helpful in expelling toxins from the body, for it can boost circulation, relieve sore muscles, induce relaxation and improve sleep. When you sit in a sauna, your heart rate increases just like when you are exercising because heat stress can induce a similar response from the body. Heat causes blood cells to dilate and increase blood flow all over the body, just as it has mood boosting properties. The use of saunas can improve the immune system, reduce incidence of colds/flus and improve autoimmune and chronic inflammatory conditions. It also detoxes the body through the sweating of chemical toxins and heavy metals, increases energy ATP production by the cells' mitochondria and oxygenation of cells, promotes wound healing, stimulates the production of stem cells and increases melatonin production. The easiest way to increase your exposure to infrared is through exposure to sunlight.

Keep your bodily fluids moving. Drinking more water helps to increase urination, which gets rid of toxic waste, especially with hot lemon water in the morning. Make sure that your bowels are working properly. Enemas and colon cleansers may be helpful with the elimination of toxins and this is especially important for those who do not have regular bowel movements.

Improving your lymphatic flow is important for detoxification. Massage turns the extracellular matrix from a jelly-like substance into a more liquid state, improving elimination through the lymphatic system and helping to relax. You can also alternate between hot and cold showers, as this also boosts circulation and improves detoxification. All you need to do is to stand under a shower, and for one minute use cold water, as tolerated, and then for one minute use hot water, as tolerated, repeating this about five times. This will get the vessels to relax and dilate, helping your skin pump blood. Skin brushing can help to eliminate toxins, by removing all the dead cells from blocked pores. Use a natural soft bristle brush, which helps to scrub your skin from the extremities and the belly towards the heart. Foam rolling and stretching can improve the flow and release of any blockages and swelling.

Eat Ṭayyib/Pure Foods – Eat to Detoxify

Foods that will help you detox:

1. Alkaline the body;
2. Rich in sulphur and fibre;
3. Glutathione.

The ability to create a more alkaline environment in the body with an acidic pH in the stomach may help with the detoxification process. Sulphur and fibre foods also help us detoxify. Glutathione is the most important antioxidant produced by the body and is found in every cell in the body, but its highest concentration is in the liver. Glutathione recycles other antioxidants extending their life spans. It also helps to mop up heavy metals like arsenic, cadmium, mercury, end products and anything that can damage cells by binding to free radicals and carrying them out of the body. Numerous environmental exposures can cause the glutathione to get used up which leads to damaged tissues and inflammation. Glutathione also helps with DNA protection, mitochondrial and immune support and protects against heart disease, cancer, dementia, and other chronic illnesses. N-acetyl cysteine is a precursor to glutathione which helps to remove chemical toxins, radiation, heavy metals, pesticides from the body and it also reduces insulin resistance and inflammation. NAC protects the lungs against disease, reduces gut inflammation and protects against small intestinal bacterial overgrowth. Alpha lipoic acid, a fat-soluble molecule found in every cell of the body which cleans up glutathione and helps it get back to work, is a potent antioxidant that protects the skin and balances blood sugar. It is used for toxin-related illnesses and detoxifying mercury.

As people age, their ability to produce glutathione deminishes. Once people get to their 40s, deficiency symptoms creep up like fatigue, aches and pains, low immunity and poor sleep. Food can help to improve glutathione levels. Sulphur contains cysteine and methionine which are used to make glutathione. Selenium is needed for glutathione activity. Focus on raw fruits, vegetables, herbs and spices because they have the most potent detoxifying effects and try to get as many servings as possible. Each contains a number of compounds that help the body detoxify from even heavy metals. These can prime the body's detoxification system and upregulate chemicals like glutathione.

Choosing a variety of nutrient dense foods helps with deficiencies and gives the body the tools it needs to get rid of toxins. Foods that boost detoxification are asparagus, bok choy, celery, citrus, green apples, kiefer, kimchi, sauerkraut, olives, plums, cruciferous vegetables, such as broccoli, Brussels sprouts, beets, cauliflower, watercress, cabbage, kale, swiss chard and collard greens (raw are more alkaline when cooked). Other foods that are great for liver support are salmon, berries, pumpkin seeds, olive oil, lentils, brazil nuts, wheatgrass, and grapes. All these are full of enzymes that support the liver and gallbladder. Moreover, not only do they help with alkalinity, they are also rich in sulphur and fibre which help in binding toxins and eliminating them through stool. One should Aim for about 30–40g of fibre per day, but this can vary depending on how much more detoxfying your body needs, so you should listen to your body. Acidic foods consist of dairy, processed foods, sugar, flour and meat.

Some patients have handicapped enzymes, but eating the right foods can help give them the raw materials required for making them. Foods rich in cysteine are beef, fish, poultry, eggs, and vegetables like garlic, Brussels sprouts, cauliflower, kale, watercress, mustard greens and broccoli. The body can only produce as much glutathione as its cysteine supplies allow. Sources of alpha lipoic acid include dark green leafy vegetables, animal foods and organ meats. Cruciferous vegetables also contain other compounds that are directly involved in detoxification, including cyanohydroxybutaine and diindolyl-methane (DIM).

Top beverages that help in detoxification include apple cider vinegar, dandelion tea, milk thistle tea, and chamomile tea because they all cleanse the liver and gallbladder. Herbs that can help in detoxification include caraway, dill seeds, curcumin (turmeric), rosemary, thyme, cumin, basil, poppy seeds, oregano, black pepper, and cilantro (a natural chelator). Raw fruits and vegetables are more alkaline when they are cooked.

Swap Out Impure/*Khabīth* for *Ṭayyib*/Pure Foods

Environmental toxins are bad for the body and the planet. Unfortunately, the care products used in our food, water, air, home and body are often the sources of hidden toxins/*khabīth* substances with which we interact daily. So we obviously need to eat and drink *ṭayyib* foods and drinks.

Create a *Ṭayyib* Home

Creating a toxin-free environment starts at home. Here are some strategies:

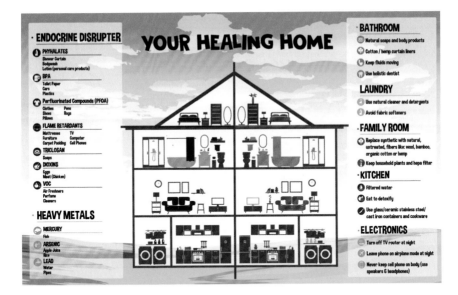

Air

Nine out of ten people in the world breathe polluted air. People breathe the air in their homes more that they breathe the outside air. According to the EWG, the air inside our house is about 2–3 times more polluted than outside air. All the chemicals in our house are still likely off gassing and inhaling chemicals, which are perhaps as dangerous as consuming them. Dirty air can lead to serious effects, including reduction in cognitive performance. About seven million people die every year from exposure to polluted air. Ninety-one percent of the world's population lives in places where air pollution exceeds WHO guidelines. These pollutants can directly affect the brain chemistry in a variety of ways, like carrying particulate matter though small passageways, directly entering the brain. One study showed that in more than 25,000 people living throughout China, exposure to increased levels of air pollution were tied to lower verbal test scores. Pollution also increases the risk of degenerative diseases like dementia, as the study suggests. This should be taken very seriously, especially since some of the most polluted cities in the world are found in Muslim countries, such as Pakistan, Afghanistan, Bahrain and Egypt.

Filtering the air from toxins can optimize your health. More specifically, before you sleep, shut off all the things that you do not need. You can also turn on an air filter, so you can breathe clean air throughout the night, thus lowering the body burden of toxins, optimizing detoxification and healing the body while you sleep.

Do not leave the fire lit in your homes while you are sleeping: this fire is your enemy so put it out before you sleep. (Bukhārī)

According to a 1989 NASA (National Aeronautics and Space Administration) study, several houseplant species are particularly adept at cleaning the air in our homes. Decorate your home with house plants, like spider plants, aloe vera, weeping fig, Chinese evergreen, bamboo, gerber daisies, English ivies, snake plant, peace lily, golden pothos, Janet Craig plant, warneckei, and chrysanthemums. This study suggested putting two large plants per 100 square feet in one's home. Plants can also lift your mood.

One should also Switch chemical cleaners with natural, non-toxic or "green" household cleaners, including soaps and dishwashing detergents. Vinegar, baking soda and hydrogen peroxide can take care of most of what we need done. Use a HEPA vacuum cleaner because they are the best and clean your heating systems and change the filters of AC systems regularly.

Over time, aim to replace synthetic carpets, rugs, window treatments, furniture cloth or bedding (as they can gradually release synthetic materials into the air we breathe) with natural, untreated fibres like wool, organic cotton, hemp or bamboo. Try to avoid flame retardants, paint indoor surfaces with a low or no-VOC and abstain from using air fresheners. Moreover, don't spray pesticides in or around your home.

Water

What we eat and drink can lead to disease. Toxins in water can disrupt the gut microbiome and lead to inflammation. To reduce the amount of toxins or even drugs in tap water, you should use purified water with a reverse osmosis unit, equiped with a triple filtration process. It is important to reduce the amount of toxins/drugs, heavy metals, bacteria/viruses/parasites, nitrates, VOCs, sediments, medications and copper in tap water. One should even Consider buying a purification system for the entire house that also includes a fluoride filtration system. Trace minerals are necessary and provide flavour to the water, and so these can be added back to the water if needed. But until you install a filter, it is easy to purchase filtered water in glass bottles.

Kitchen

Change cookware to pots and pans made of glass, ceramic, non-coated stainless steel, or cast iron. You should avoid cast iron if you have excessive iron stores. If you opt for using ceramic pots, you should look for lead free, unglazed/unvarnished ones. Eliminate all plastic utensils and replace them with glass or ceramic ones.

Try to store food in ceramic or glass containers and avoid cling wrap, use unbleached parchment paper and look for BPA free cans. Try to also minimize the use of the microwave, and never put plastic in it. It is better to cook food at home, as restaurants are a major source of BPAs. Minimize the use of plastic disposables. Plastic containers should be kept away from hot environments like our cars. Avoid cooking food and then placing it in a plastic bag in boiling water (sous vide cooking).

Avoid plastic tea bags, because a Canadian research team has found that steeping a single plastic tea bag releases 12 billion microplastics and 2 billion nano plastic particles, yeilding 16 µg of indigestible plastic per cup. Avoid farmed fish, European and US farmed salmon are high in PBDEs. To avoid arsenic, avoid brown rice grown in southern United States, and instead one should use organic rice from California, India and Pakistan. If you don't know where the rice comes from, make sure to use white rice. Quinoa has a lot less arsenic than any other type of rice. Avoid processed baby foods and fruit juices, because toxic heavy metals were found in these products.

Bathroom

Change vinyl shower curtains to PVC free materials like organic cotton or hemp curtain liners. Natural soaps, like castile soap, and essential oils, like tea tree oil, have a mild antibacterial quality. Avoid hand sanitizers.

Laundry

Change laundry detergent to a non-toxic, green cleaner and avoid fabric softeners. Look for 100 percent organic cotton sheets. Between loads, keep the washer door open to prevent mould formation. Look for clean, organic and eco dry cleaners. Do also make it a habit to look at the labels of clothing because a lot of pajamas have flame retardants.

> The Prophet, peace and blessings be upon him, said: "When one of you goes to bed, he should dust it off with his clothes, as no-one knows what was on it after him." (Bukhārī)

Living Room

Choose flame retardant free furniture and avoid stain-resistant carpets, rugs and furniture. Also, choose brominated flame retardant electronics whenever possible and use a HEPA filter vacuum. Aim to dust regularly with a damp cloth or sponge to trap contaminated dust and check your home for lead based paint, especially if it was built before 1978.

Personal Care Products and Cosmetics

What we put on our skin is as important as what we eat, as the skin is an excellent delivery system for chemicals. Choose organic, gluten-free non-allergenic skin-care, cosmetics and feminine hygiene products, and choose cosmetics with no preservatives. Avoid fragrance products and look for a mineral based sunscreen and shun chemical sunblocks with avobenzone, oxybenzone (endocrine-disrupting potential), octocrylene and ecamsule. One of the dangers of common chemical sunblocks is their mutation into very harmful compounds. This was recently demonstrated with avobenzone which was transformed into a chemical leading to nervous system issues, cancer, liver and kidney disorders. There are also several naturally occurring compounds in foods like lycopene (cabbage, pink grapefruit and asparagus), omega 3 fatty acids, sulforaphane and vitamin C that can offer protective properties from the sun.

Look for a natural brand of deodorant that doesn't contain aluminium, but a light dusting of baking soda can also work. The Prophet, peace and blessings be upon him, loved perfumes, but today most of these perfumes are artificial. Essential oils are a great way to get the perfume without all the chemicals.

The Prophet, peace and blessings be upon him, said: "Whoever is offered some perfume should not refuse it." (Muslim)

Oral Health

The health of our mouth determines the health of our bodies. Brushing with non-fluoride, natural and organic toothpaste and flossing are important for oral health. Avoid antiseptic mouthwash. The Prophet Muhammad, peace and blessings be upon him, used to rinse his mouth with water even after drinking milk, saying:

It has fat. (Bukhārī and Muslim)

Studies have shown that the milk drunk by babies all night long in bottles can lead to cavities. So oral health is important. Prophet Muhammad, peace and blessings be upon him, taught us how to keep the mouth clean. He always commenced his ablution with the use of a tooth-cleansing-stick (*siwāk*).

He, peace and blessings be upon him, also said:

"Had I not thought that I would make it difficult for my followers, I would have ordered them to use the *siwāk* before each prayer." (Bukhārī, Muslim, Abū Dāwūd, Tirmidhī, Nasā'ī, Ibn Mājah and Aḥmad)

The use of the *siwāk* purifies the mouth and pleases Allah. (Bukhārī, Nasā'ī, Ibn Mājah and Aḥmad)

Siwāk is the Arabic name for Salvadore Persica, a plant native to the Arabian Peninsula. The best type of *siwāk* is said to come from the 'Arak' tree.

Science has now proven that chewing these sticks has a therapeutic effect on gingival diseases, and is found to be antibacterial, anti-helminthic, antioxidant. It has also been proven that using the *miswāk* as an adjunct to tooth brushing leads to a significant improvement in the plaque score and gingival health.[12]

Most procedures done by regular dentists can pose a threat to people because of their exposure to toxin, so make sure to see a holistic or biological dentist who will see to it that the biocompatible materials are safe and right for you. Avoid amalgam fillings and replace all metal fillings with white resin (though it is plastic, it better than mercury) or zirconium. Look into what other precautions are used to protect the staff. One should always ask if a rubber dam and amalgam separator are used when removing the mercury filling to keep everyone protected and after the procedure, rinse your mouth with activated charcoal.

Exposure to Electronics and EMF

The Prophet, peace and blessings be upon him, also said: "Turn off the lamps while sleeping." (Bukhārī)

People nowadays are constantly surrounded by electronics, but this doesn't come without its hazards from charged electromagnetic fields. Three to ten percent of the world's population are sensitive to EMFs and can experience symptoms when they are exposed to it. A 2012 independent review, conducted by 29 independent scientists and health experts who examined 1800 studies, found evidence for the damaging effects of EMFs. These EMFs are capable of causing heat production to tissues, cause a level of interference to normal signaling in the body which hurts the mitochondria, leading to tiredness, brain fog and sleepiness. EMFs can also lead to DNA damage, sleep issues, psychological and cell membrane damage and oxidative stress. Electromagnetic radiation of all kinds can change the voltage that regulates how much calcium can get into the cell, leading to a free radical called peroxynitrite release that spikes oxidative damage, hurting cell membranes and mitochondria and damaging gene expression.[13] Matters are getting worse with the new fifth generation telecommunications networks (5G).

Common EMF sources that have low frequency, which are from 1 to 300 Hz, are hair dryers, electrical wiring, kitchen appliances, TV, computers and mobile devices when charging. Intermediate frequency, from 300 Hz to 100 kHz, include TV and computer screen. High frequency, which is from 100 kHz to 300 kHz, is released from smart meters, mobile devices and Wi-Fi. EMFs can be present in electric power lines, cell phone towers, Bluetooth headsets, Wi-Fi routers, radio and television towers, fluorescent and compact fluorescent lighting.

Limiting exposure to EMF sources can optimize health and healing. To reduce exposure to EMF sources, turning off the TV router at night, never carrying a cell phone on our body and using the speaker or headsets at all times is a good start and also switching it to airplane mode anytime we can (especially at night). Unplug all electrical devices that you are not using and keep them far away and also avoid using cordless phones and microwaves. Getting out in nature, getting sufficient sleep, grounding daily, eating a diet packed with antioxidants and lowering stress can help to protect the body against EMFs.

Noise Pollution

One Danish study found that for every 10 dB increase in traffic noise near someone's residence, the risk of the residents developing type two diabetes increased by 14 percent. Noises also lead to a deterioration in mental health. A study published in the journal of PLOS showed that frequent exposure to aircraft noise was associated with a two fold rise in diabetes and anxiety. The WHO reports that children who live in areas of high aircraft noise do not only have higher stress levels, but it also delayed the age of reading and also increased poor attention. If you live in an area with a lot of noise, noise cancelling headphones, air plugs and white noise machine can help.

Detox from Technology

Nowadays, people are addicted to technology. This leads to the stimulation of the neurotransmitter dopamine which leads to such an addiction that compromises our sleep, self-esteem and relationships. The presence of a smart phone while performing a cognitive task can undermine our thinking skills such as problem solving and memory. Scientists are just beginning to understand how these devices affect people, nevertheless, it is better to limit the use of the social media to at least an hour a day, and look for activities that don't require a phone.

A *Ṭayyib* Life Naturally Detoxifies

Detoxifying isn't a separate and isolated task, but rather a combination of different elements which constitute a whole process. Optimizing digestive health by eating anti-inflammatory and nutritious food, reducing stress through meditation, relaxation, improved sleep, and maintaining a good social life are all important keys in healing. Knowledge is power. Knowledge about what is lurking in the environment allows us to take control of our health and our families' health. Try not to spend time worrying about what can't be controlled. Just by eating *ṭayyib* food and living a *ṭayyib* lifestyle, you can help your gut to heal, balance hormones, and detox.

Conclusion

All that has been mentioned can be quite overwhelming, so we should take it one step at a time. However, the upshot is to live purely and eat *ṭayyib* foods. To recap, the following are steps that can be implemented:

1. Confirm your intention. You're doing this to take care of the body that Allah, glorified and exalted is He, has blessed you with. You are trying to live the *dīn* because you love Allah.
2. Know what is *ṭayyib* and what is *khabīth*:

What is Pure and What is Impure?

Pure and Lawful	Impure and Prohibited
Vegetables	Artificial colours, like candy, coloured drinks like Roohafza, coloured frosting, coloured cake, chicken 65, biryani with colouring, etc.
Fruit	Preservatives like in hot dogs, meats, seafood, salt, jams, bread, fast food, chips, junk food, etc.
Clean Protein	Artificial ingredients, sodas, ice creams, candy, doughnuts, cakes, bread, cereals, fast food, MSG, chips, junk food, etc.
Healthy Fat	GMOs like canola oil, soy, corn, papaya, and some types of zucchini, apples and potatoes.
Organics	Anything Artificial and GMO

3. Learn to read the ingredients. Just like you teach your children about gelatin, you need to teach your children to look for artificial, GMO ingredients, preservatives, etc.
4. Make small changes and easy swaps at a time.
   Take it one meal at a time, one day at a time. You've got this. Just ask yourself? Is this *ṭayyib*?

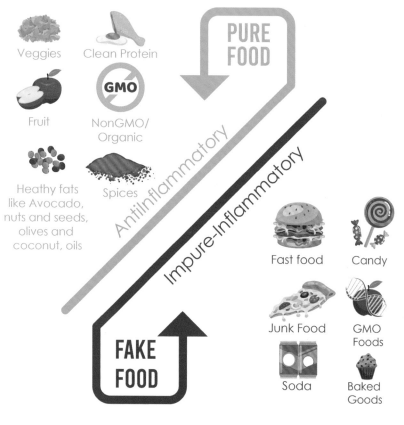

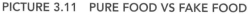

PICTURE 3.11   PURE FOOD VS FAKE FOOD

The Qur'anic Digestive Health and Detoxification Prescription at a Glance:

The Digestive Health and Nutrition Prescription

- Focusing on *tayyib* food;
- Eating less;
- Incorporating Qur'anic/Prophetic foods into the diet;
- Incorporating veggies, clean protein, healthy fat, fruits (based on tolerance) in each meal;
- Fasting.

The Detox Prescription

- Locating the *khabīth* stuff/toxins;
- Keeping the fluids moving (like using Epsom salt baths);
- Eating *tayyib* foods to keep the body alkaline;
- Cleaning up the environment – swaping out what is *khabīth* with what is *tayyib*;
- Detoxifying the body and mind.

The Four S's: Stress, Sleep, Social and Spiritual Health Ṭayyib Mental Health and a Tranquil Mindful Heart

Creating a Ṭayyib/Pure Internal World – Let's Talk About Stress

And whosoever fears Allah and keeps his duty to Him, He will make a way for him to get out [from every difficulty], and He will provide for him from [sources] he never could imagine. And whosoever puts his trust in Allah, then He will suffice for him. Verily, Allah will accomplish His purpose. Indeed Allah has set a measure for all things. (Qur'an 65: 2–3)

Wars, hate crimes and negativity create a world filled with chronic stress, *khabīth*/impure emotions, thoughts and actions. People wake up with negativity, surround themselves with negativity and turn on the news that breeds negativity. People then go to sleep in a state of worry, fear and feeling as if they have failed.

Stress exacerbates almost any chronic illness, causing more than 80 percent of complaints that are presented to the doctors. Our thoughts, feelings and emotions have an effect on our physical and mental health, and the latter affects our emotional, spiritual and psychological well-being. Incorporating daily regular stress management techniques – prayer, breathing techniques, mindfulness, meditation, etc. – can have a powerful impact on our physical and spiritual health, as they are linked to a lower expression of the genes involved in the stress-related pathways and even inflammation.[1] Incorporating these stress management skills can help to keep damaging hormones at bay, teaching the body to be a little calmer and more resilient.

The Stress Response

When the muscles tighten and the heart races – this is a stress response. This occurs when the body feels threatened, also known as the "fight or flight" mechanism. Sensing this threat, the amygdala activates stress pathways thus impairing the prefrontal cortex. To deal with the stressor and protect the body, the latter releases cortisol, which then triggers numerous biological processes in the body, especially when adrenaline and noradrenaline flood the system. This response can be lifesaving in emergency situations, where we need to act immediately, but it wears the body down when there is constant bombardment of stress in our everyday life.

Cortisol continues to be secreted until the cause of stress is resolved, adrenal glands tire out (a state normally referred to as adrenal fatigue), or the stress is managed effectively. In the case of chronic stress, with limited downtime between stressors, the body feels as if it is constantly under stress. In this state of imbalance, the immune system is suppressed and inflammation and chronic illnesses ensue, and every organ of the body can be affected. Elevated levels of cortisol have been shown to inhibit the neurogenesis in the hippocampus, diminishing its functional capacity, leading to the inability to create, store or retrieve memories. Chronic stress can also sabotage the relationship between the prefrontal cortex and the amygdala,[2] which shows that stressful life events weaken this connection and promote new neuronal growth in the amygdala, leading to bad decision making and impulsivity.

Studies have shown that stress can double the chance of becoming obese,[3] just as it can cause diabetes[4] and lead to a five-fold increased risk of dying from heart related problems,[5] a 65 percent increased risk of developing dementia,[6] an increased risk of breast cancer,[7] and a 70 percent increased risk of disabilities in later life.[8] *The Journal of the American Medical Association* found that too much stress can be as bad for our heart as smoking and high cholesterol.[9]

The Effects of Stress

Stress and the Immune System

- Stress suppresses the secretion of IgA, which is an immune molecule.[10]
- Stress causes the release of substances like adrenaline and norepinephrine into the gut which makes the lining of the digestive system more permeable (i.e., leaky gut) and inflammatory.[11]
- Stress makes us susceptible to the re-activation of infections (specifically Epstein Barr virus) that may lead to autoimmunity.

Stress and the Gut

The brain and gut (aka the second brain) are connected via the vagus nerve, which is a thick bundle of nerves that runs along the spinal column,[13] also known as the gut-brain-microbiota axis.[14] The gut contains its own receptors that react to the gut bacteria as well as its metabolites and produces neurotransmitters (brain chemicals that communicate information between the brain and the body).

- Even short bouts of stress can trigger or worsen leaky gut/intestinal permeability.[12]
- Stress can also lower the release of hydrochloric acid and affect the activity of digestive enzymes, thus lowering the absorption of nutrients.[15]
- Stress, even when acute, can also affect good bacteria negatively, lowering the level of probiotics[16]– promoting an overgrowth of the bad bacteria in the small bowel.
- These pathogenic bacteria interfere with the production of vital neurotransmitters. So the more good bacteria we have, the more neurotransmitters and the less pronounced our response to stress is, for at that point we produce an optimal level of neurotransmitters and experiences less depression, anxiety and other mood disorders.
- Stress increases craving for food to allow the bad bacteria to thrive further.

Studies have shown that adding back in good bacteria like B. longum[17] and L. rhamnosis[18], along with the use of prebiotics, can relieve stress and lower cortisol.[19]

Stress and the Hormones

- Stress leads to high cortisol levels which cause a rise in blood sugar levels.
- Stress triggers leptin and insulin resistance.[20]
- Stress promotes weight gain [21]around the waist.
- Stress can also create imbalances in the reproductive hormones, leading to increased polycystic ovarian syndrome, which prevents ovulation and causes infertility.
- Stress may ultimately cause full-blown diabetes and further inflammation.[22]

A daily practice of relaxation techniques can help decrease anxiety, lower blood pressure and heart rate, keep damaging hormones at bay, change gene expression, improve blood circulation and digestion, and enhance the overall immune system.

What is Stressing People Out?

People are bombarded with stress on a daily basis, literally at every corner they turn, and this leads to chronic stress. Listening to the news is easier and more stressful than before, but this disconnects the amygdala from the prefrontal cortex, leading to anxiety and fear. People are addicted to their phones and screens as well as to the dopamine surges that occur every time they check their inboxes or social media accounts for comments and likes. They don't realize that while they are doing this, they are also disconnecting from their prefrontal cortices, and wasting precious time. Let's face it, people are addicted to the internet and no longer know how to quit and devote some time for inner reflexion. But what is putting people out of balance?

Is the stress caused due to a childhood experience or life's traumas? Early childhood trauma can create subtle shifts in our microbiome early in life and can alter our healthy HPA axis, cue the body to produce more cortisol and fewer good bugs, leading to increased stress response later in life, and inflammation. What are your personal challenges? Is the issue relating to emotions, unrealistic expectations, low self-esteem, fear or guilt? And if this is the case, are you taking care of yourself (imbalanced diet, lack of sleep, too many medications, and deficiency of nutrients)? Make a list of any past, present and future external or internal issues.

Calming Stress

... Allah puts no burden on any person beyond what He has given him. Allah will grant after hardship, ease. (Qur'an 65: 7)

Allah burdens no person beyond his scope... (Qur'an 2:286)

Allah, glorified and exalted is He, never tests a person with more than he or she can handle, and He also promises ease after hardships. With this in mind, it is best to help our nervous system to re-establish equilibrium, as this is the key to lowering inflammation and optimizing the mitochondrial function to heal, and prevent chronic diseases at all ages.

Relaxation techniques, like spending time in nature, prayer, *dhikr*, breathing techniques and even mindfulness can restore the balance of our nervous system and create a deep calmness, thus allowing us to be fully present in life despite facing its challenges and stress. These relaxation activities can trigger the vagus nerve and help support the function of the peripheral nervous system,[23] helping us be more physically, emotionally, and spiritually resilient. Research has shown that toning down the fight or flight response can help decrease the inflammatory response in autoimmune conditions like rheumatoid arthritis.[24]

Verily Allah does not change men's condition unless they change their inner selves. (Qur'an 13: 11)

So first, we need to change what is in ourselves for our situation to change.

Steps to Less Stress and True Success:

1. Consigning our stress to Allah - Trust in Him.
2. Healing with Nature.
3. Mindfulness and Meditation.
4. Prayer and *Du'ā'*.
5. *Dhikr.*

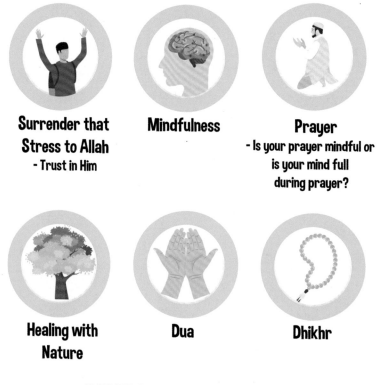

Stress Management in Islam
Steps to Less Stress and True Success

Surrender that Stress to Allah
- Trust in Him

Mindfulness

Prayer
- Is your prayer mindful or is your mind full during prayer?

Healing with Nature

Dua

Dhikhr

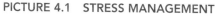

PICTURE 4.1   STRESS MANAGEMENT

Changing Our Mindset – Surrendering Our Stress to Allah and Trusting in Him for He is in Control

Say, "Nothing shall ever happen to us except what Allah has ordained for us. He is our Mawla [Allah, Helper and Protector]. And in Allah let the believers put their trust." (Qur'an 9: 51)

And put your trust in the All-Mighty, the Most Merciful, Who sees you [O Muhammad] when you stand up [alone at night for tahajjud prayers], and your movements among those who fall prostrate [along with you to Allah in the five compulsory congregational prayers). Verily! He, only He, is the All-Hearer, the All-Knower. (Qur'an 26: 217–220)

The Prophet, peace and blessings be upon him, taught a *du'ā'* which helps us surrender our pain to Allah, glorified and exalted is He, and ask for His guidance.

Prophet Muhammad, peace and blessings be upon him, said: "Seek the help of Allah, do not be frustrated and if something befalls you, do not say, 'If I had done this, so and so would have happened,' but say, 'Allah decreed, and what Allah wills, He does.' Indeed, 'if" opens the door of the Devil." (Muslim)

Then, when they had both submitted themselves [to the Will of Allah], and he had laid him prostrate on his forehead [or on the side of his forehead for slaughtering]; We called out to him, 'O lbraheem! You have fulfilled the dream [vision]!' Verily! Thus do We. reward the doers of good. Verily, that indeed was a clear trial. And We ransomed him with a great sacrifice. (Qur'an 37: 103–107)

Challenges shape us; they can change us, but they will never break us if we have Allah, glorified and exalted is He, on our side. Everything has a reason; everything we go through makes us who we are, in order to help those around. Allah has given us mountains to show us how they can be climbed. However, we are not meant to take on all the stress of the worlds on our shoulders alone. We need to change our mindset regarding stress, just as we need to surrender all our stress to Allah, for He alone can help; we just need to trust in Him.

No disaster strikes on the earth or among yourselves except that it is in a register before We bring it into being. Verily, that is easy for Allah. In order that you may not be sad over that which has eluded you, nor rejoice because of that which has been given to you. And Allah does not like prideful boasters. (Qur'an 57: 22–23)

.. And whosoever fears Allah, He will make his matter easy for him. (Qur'an 65: 4)

.. And whosoever fears Allah- He will remove for him his misdeeds and make great for him his reward. (Qur'an 65: 5)

With difficulty comes ease, and if we fear Allah, He has promised to make it easy, and nothing happens except what Allah, glorified and exalted is He, has ordained, so we should continue to put our trust in Allah.

And it may be that you dislike a thing which is good for you and that you like a thing which is bad for you. Allah knows but you do not know. (Qur'an 2: 216)

Say, 'In the Bounty of Allah, and in His Mercy [Islam and the Qur'an]; therein let them rejoice. That is better than what they accumulate. (Qur'an 10: 58)

It was reported that Salmān once said to Abū al-Dardā': "Allah has a right over you, your own self has a right over you and your spouse has a right over you; so give everyone his due right." When the Prophet, peace and blessings be upon him, was informed of what he had said, he replied, "Salmān has spoken the truth." (Bukhārī)

This world is temporary, stress will come and go, but sticking with Allah guarantees success.

And strain not your eyes in longing for the things We have given for enjoyment to various groups of them [polytheists and disbelievers in the Oneness of Allah] – the splendour of the life of this world that We may test them thereby. But the provision [good reward in the Hereafter] of Allah is better and more lasting. (Qur'an 20: 131)

And put forward to them the example of the life of this world, it is like the water [rain] which We send down from the sky, and the vegetation of the earth mingles with it, and becomes fresh and green. But [later] it becomes dry twigs, which the winds scatter. And Allah is Able to do everything. Wealth and children are the adornment of the life of this world. But the good righteous deeds [five compulsory prayers, deeds of obedience to Allah, good speech, remembrance of Allah with glorification, praises and thanks] that last, are better with Allah for rewards and better in terms of hope. (Qur'an 18: 45–46)

Now whatever you have been given is but a passing comfort for the life of this world, and that which Allah has is better and more lasting for those who believe and put their trust in Allah. (Qur'an 42: 36)

Prophet Muhammad, peace and blessings be upon him, said: "No fatigue, disease, sorrow, sadness, hurt or distress befalls a Muslim, even if it be the prick of a thorn, except that Allah expiates some of his sins for it." (Bukhārī and Muslim)

By putting our stress in Allah's hands, we relieve from ourselves so much of it. By trusting in Allah and incorporating daily stress management techniques, we can truly start to heal from the inside out.

Healing by Nature

Allah has provided humans everything they need to stay balanced, including nature.

> *It is Allah who made for you the earth a place of settlement and the sky a ceiling and formed you and perfected your forms and provided you with good things. That is Allah, your Lord; then blessed is Allah , Lord of the worlds.* (Qur'an 40:64)

With the projections that over 70 percent will move to large cities by 2050,[25] moving away from nature is coming with a consequence, even more so with the stay-at-home guidelines. When we lose connection with the environment, we start to lose connection with Allah. Human beings have been entrusted with this world, but how can they take care of it well if they are completely disconnected from it?

> *And [mention, O Muhammad], when your Lord said to the angels, "Indeed, I will make upon the earth a successive authority." They said, "Will You place upon it one who causes corruption therein and sheds blood, while we declare Your praise and sanctify You?" Allah said, "Indeed, I know that which you do not know."* (Qur'an 2:30)

Over and over again, Allah mentions *Jannah* which He describes as:

> *Allah has promised to the believing men and the believing women gardens, beneath which rivers flow, to abide in them, and goodly dwellings in gardens of perpetual abode; and best of all is Allah's goodly pleasure; that is the grand achievement.* (Qur'an 9:72)

Spending some time in nature can actually relieve stress and lower inflammation.[26] Just the sense of smell we get from open nature can help our mood and improve our immune function.[27]

> The (whole) earth has been made a mosque (or a place of prayer) and a means of purification for me, so wherever a man of my ummah may be when the time for prayer comes, let him pray. (Bukhārī)

Being close to Allah's creations can boost the immune system (as it enhances the immune response of Natural Killer cells and activates Natural Killer cells in humans), restore our brain connection and improve overall brain health, as it boosts serotonin leading to better mood and improved ability to focus, improve sleep, and lower blood pressure, pulse and heart rate variability, increase mindfulness and the ability to cope with whatever stress we face, lowering cortisol and even increasing energy. The trees release an essential oil called phytoncide, which helps to protect them. Another reason nature has a positive effect is that negative ions accumulate in places like beaches and waterfalls which boost immune system function, reduce stress, kill microbes and even improve sleep.

Nature heals the body from the inside out. Try to spend at least thirty minutes a week, if not more, in open nature. The human body and the earth are both electric, and this balance of electrical charges plays a critical role in your health. Electrical charges in humans can become imbalanced due to modern living and because the earth is negatively charged, by placing your feet on the ground (known as grounding or earthing), you can discharge and neutralize this build-up of positive electrical charges. Studies have shown that a simple physical connection to nature, through earthing or grounding, can help to reduce free radical damage, improve various immune related health conditions, improve sleep, and lower inflammation and stress cortisol levels, and even regulate immune function.

By escaping to nature, the body is given time to reconnect with its roots, thus increasing your sense of calmness, mindfulness and helping you to reset your life and feel intimately connected to Allah.

Meditation and Mindfulness

People nowadays find it hard to set aside time for reflection and meditation. But Muslims have been "meditating" for centuries. Their prayer is a form of meditation, as are their *du'a*'s and *dhikr* which are all keys in Islam to obtaining true *falāḥ*/success in this life and the Hereafter.

Meditation

Many people are skeptical when they are told that something as simple as meditation could be beneficial to them. After all, the word meditation quite often conjures up the image of someone in the lotus position, eyes closed and looking peaceful, something that likely requires a great deal of practice, patience, time and effort, and so people put it off. There are so many types of meditation, like mindfulness, transcendental meditation, yoga meditation, zen, seated meditation and guided meditation, just to name a few. In Islam, meditation takes the form of the five daily prayers, *du'ā'*, *dhikr* and reflection. Through these meditation techniques, we can improve the connection in the brain between the amygdala and prefrontal cortex, thus strengthening the areas of the brain that can keep us present and focussed. This state acts like a shield to the constant efforts in our everyday life to throw us off balance, thus increasing our overall well-being, helping us to reach advanced spiritual states and enhancing our acts of worship, prayer and remembrance and putting us back in charge of our thoughts.

Meditation improves the overall quality of life[28] and health, through the changes it makes in the body and mind. Not only does the practice of daily meditation and positivity intensify calmness, it also cultivates optimal physical health. When spiritual energy begins to flow, blood circulation improves,[29] blood pressure goes down,[30] cortisol and stress levels go down, digestion improves,[31] the body detoxes, helping us make better decisions because of smaller amydgalas,[32] reduces cortisol and stress and improves CV health, sleep, memory and focus.[33] Moreover, unhealthy genes are switched off, [34] and the overall immune system,[35] and the control of stress and emotions is enhanced.[36] Overall, meditation helps us to empathize with others and take care of our health and the planet.

All forms of Islamic meditation involve some kind of remembrance or awareness of Allah which helps purify the heart and mind of negativity. But now science has proven that prayer has significant biological benefits, as it promotes a parasympathetic response, producing positive changes in brain function and human well-being, thus promoting relaxation.[37] Prayer and *dhikr* both have a positive effect on the neuroimmunological response.[38] But for all of this to be effective, we must bring our bodies back to mindfulness, to help our brains, avoid the hurdles of life and navigate life much better.

Mindfulness

...And know that Allah, glorified and exalted, knows what is within yourselves, so beware of Him. And know that Allah is Forgiving and Forbearing. (Qur'an 2:235)

Say, "My Salat (Contact Prayers), my worship practices, my life and my death, are all devoted absolutely to God alone, the Lord of the universe. He has no partner. This is what I am commanded to believe, and I am the first to submit." (Qur'an 6:162–163)

Prophet Muhammad, peace and blessings be upon him, taught 'Abdullāh ibn 'Umar the following: "When you wake up, do not talk to yourself about the evening, and if you reach the evening, do not talk to yourself about the morning; take from your life for your death and from your health for your sickness, as you never know, 'Abdullah, what your fate will be tomorrow." (Bukhārī)

Allah has informed human beings that their past and future are in His hands. Hence, we must just focus on the now; what they can do right now. But most people, in this day and age, continue to allow their past to haunt them and their everyday lives are consumed with worries about their future – stealing their everyday joys right from under their noses. When we are stuck in the past, we get depressed. When we get stuck in the future, we get anxious. Muslims need to consign both to Allah.

Mindfulness is how we feel in the moment, THIS moment, internally and externally, without judgement. Staying calm and present in the moment will help to bring our nervous system back into balance and decrease stress. Being present helps us not to worry about the past or future, and this limits stress. Mindfulness can be applied to almost any activity we engage in (eating, exercising, walking, meditation, and/or working).

Mindfulness allows us to see our internal and external environment clearly, showing us how best to respond and be fully aware of many different levels of perception at once. As discussed above, mindfulness and meditation have so many benefits, especially their benefit in moving us to make better decisions and decrease emotional reactivity.

> *O you who believe! Bow down, and prostrate yourselves, and worship Allah and do good, that you may be successful.* (Qur'an 22: 77)

In Islam, mindfulness is the equivalent of *murāqabah* (derived from the root meaning "to observe, to watch") and is defined as 'the constant knowledge of the servant and his conviction in the supervision of the Truth, glory be to Him, over one's outward and inward states.'[39] When we are in *murāqabah*, we are in a conscious state of comprehensive awareness of Allah, glorified and exalted is He, and we are aware of what is going on in our heart, mind and body, just as we have knowledge of the enemy of Allah, the soul's capability to suggest evil and the deeds done for the sake of Allah. When practised effectively, *murāqabah* improves our physical health. Mindfulness can reduce the stress response, increase healing from wounds, lower anxiety and increases the level of telomerase which means that the DNA of our immune system is better protected.

By incorporating modern insights (as long as we remain grounded in the Qur'an and Sunnah), surrendering to Allah the pains of our past and future and focusing on the now, we can increase the quality of our everyday actions, prayers, and heal and prevent chronic diseases.

Two Keys to Keep the Body in Balance: Prayer and Du'ā'

> *O you who believe! Seek help in patience and prayer. Truly Allah is with the patient ones.* (Qur'an 2: 153)

Say [O Muhammad], "Verily, I am commanded to worship Allah [Alone] by obeying Him and doing religious deeds sincerely for Allah's sake only and not to show off, and not to set up rivals with Him in worship." (Qur'an 39: 11)

Prayer = Balance is Blue

People have been given a gift: being directly connected with the Maker of the world, the Changer of hearts, the One Who can create something out of nothing, and the One Who can change what is impossible in the eyes of human beings to something possible, at a minimum of five times per day. Allah wants Muslims talk to Him and entreat Him five times a day.

It is You we worship and You we ask for help. (Qur'an 1:5)

And seek help in patience and prayer, and truly it is extremely heavy and hard except for those who have true humility [those who obey Allah with full submission, fear His Punishment, and believe in His Promise (Paradise) and in His Warnings (Hell)]. (Qur'an 2: 45)

Human beings are urged to seek help from Allah. Not only do prayers renew our connection with Allah, glorified and exalted is He, thus supplying the soul with an infinite source of energy, but science has now proven that during the prayer, parasympathetic activity increases and sympathetic activity decreases, which helps to promote relaxation, reduce cardiovascular risk and minimize anxiety.[40] The prayer increases gamma EEG power which participates in various cerebral functions, like memory, consciousness, synaptic plasticity, motor control, attention and memory, all of which is likely related to an increase in cognitive and attentional processing.[41] The prayer has been found to improve balance in healthy individuals as well as stroke patients, decrease the chances of developing knee osteoarthritis, and provide cardiovascular and compositional benefits.[42]

The importance of the middle prayers when people's minds are most active

Guard strictly the [five obligatory] prayers, especially the middle Salat [i.e. the best prayer 'Asr]. And stand before Allah with obedience [and do not speak to others during the prayers]. (Qur'an 2: 238)

Prophet Muhammad, peace and blessings be upon him, said: "The angels descend to you in succession by night and by day, but they all gather together with you at the dawn and afternoon prayers. Those who have passed the night with you ascend to Heaven and Allah asks them, although He is well aware: 'How did you leave my servants?' The angels would reply: 'They were praying when we left them and when we arrived we found them praying.'" (Bukhārī)

The importance of the night prayers

Stand [to pray] all night, except a little, half of it, or a little less than that, or a little more; and recite the Qur'an [aloud] in a slow, pleasant tone and style. Verily, We shall send down to you a weighty Word [obligations and legal laws]. Verily, the rising by night [for tahajjud prayer] is very hard and most potent and good for governing [the soul], and most suitable for [understanding] the Word [of Allah]. (Qur'an 73: 2–6)

The prayer and other spiritual practices can help to put the body back into balance, thus improving mental health and increasing the quality of life. It has also been shown to eventually change the dopamine gene receptor expressions, resulting in the reduction of cell proliferation and leading to better prevention and management in breast cancer patients compared to other forms of treatment.[43]

The act of performing *wuḍū'*, a sign of the purification of the soul, suppressing thoughts, clearing the mind in order to concentrate and reflecting only on the glorification and worship of Allah all help to prepare the mind to optimize our prayers and concentration.

O you who believe! When you intend to offer the prayer, wash your faces and your hands [forearms] up to the elbows, rub [by passing wet hands over] your heads, and [wash] your feet up to the ankles ... (Qur'an 5: 6)

It was related that Abū Hurayrah said: "I heard the Messenger of Allah say, 'If there was a river at the door of anyone of you and you bathed in it five times daily, would you see any dirt on yourselves?' They (his Companions) answered, 'No trace of dirt would remain.' He, peace and blessings be upon him, added, 'That is the similitude of the five prayers with which Allah blots out evil deeds.'" (Bukhārī)

Prophet Muhammad, peace and blessings be upon him, taught that ablution washes away sins, purifying and cleansing the soul:

If the Muslim performs ablution and washes his face, any offence he committed with his eyes will wash away with the water; and when he washes his hands, any assault he committed with his hands will wash away with the water; and when he washes his feet, any misdeeds to which he walked with his feet will wash away with the water, until he concludes (the ablution) and he is free from sins. (Muslim and Tirmidhī)

The Power of Duʿāʾ

Know that Allah, glorified and exalted is He, alone can lift your suffering and solve all problems, *duʿāʾ*/supplication is a direct conversation with Allah. With every difficulty or moment of happiness, you seek Allah's help and guidance and show gratitude towards Him. This helps you relieve any sadness or anxiety you have and strengthens faith.

And when My slaves ask you [O Muhammad] concerning Me, then [answer them], I am indeed near [to them by My Knowledge]. I respond to the invocations of the supplicant when he calls on Me [without any mediator or intercessor]. So let them obey Me and believe in Me, so that they may be led aright. (Qur'an 2: 186)

And your Master and Creator said, "Invoke Me, [i.e. believe in My Oneness and ask Me for anything], I will respond to you. Verily, those who scorn My worship [i.e. do not invoke Me, and do not believe in My Oneness] will surely enter Hell in humiliation!" (Qur'an 40: 60)

O people! It is you who stand in need of Allah, but Allah is Rich [Free of all wants and needs], Worthy of all praise. (Qur'an 35: 15)

There is nothing as dear to Allah as supplication (to Him by His worshippers). (Aḥmad)

You shouldn't be afraid that an invocation might not be granted, for Prophet Muhammad, peace and blessings be upon him said:

No Muslim invokes with a supplication except that Allah answers it in one of the following three ways: He promptly answers his supplication, or delays it for him until the Hereafter, or keeps him away from an equivalent evil. (Tirmidhī)

Allah, glorified and exalted is He, is always there, we just have to be patient.

One's supplication will be granted if one is not impatient. (Bukhārī)

It was narrated by Anas ibn Mālik that the Prophet, peace and blessings be upon him, passed by a women who was weeping beside a grave. He told her to fear Allah and be patient. She did not recognize him and so she said: "Go away, for you have not been afflicted with a calamity like mine!" When she found out later that it was the Prophet that she talked to in that manner, she went to his house and told him, "I did not recognize you." He said, "Verily, patience should be shown when a calamity first hits." (Bukhārī and Muslim)

145

The stress that ensues due to the things we can't control can drive us to the edge. The Prophet, peace and blessings be upon him has taught that we must do our part and ask Allah, glorified and exalted is He, for the rest. We need to pray for those around: our family, relatives and all Muslims around the world.

> The supplication of the Muslim to his brother is granted; there is an assigned angel at his head, each time he prays for his brother, the assigned angel says: *Āmīn* and the same goes for you. (Muslim, Ibn Mājah and Aḥmad)

Allah, glorified and exalted is He, is Self-Sufficient while human beings are weak; Allah, glorified and exalted is He, is Almighty and All-Powerful while human beings are needy; Allah is the Sustainer of life, the Most Generous and the Most Great while human beings need to put their trust in Allah to lift the burden off their shoulders, thereby removing the thoughts that invade their minds and destroy their health.

> *Say [O Muhammad], "O Allah! Possessor of the kingdom, You give the kingdom to whom You will, and You take the kingdom from whom You will, and You endue with honor whom You will, and You humiliate whom You will. In Your Hand is all good. Verily, You are Able to do all things."* (Qur'an 3: 26)

> *Say [O Muhammad], "Who rescues you from the darkness of the land and the sea [dangers like storms], when you call upon Him in humility and in secret [saying], 'If He [Allah] only saves us from this [danger], we shall truly be grateful.'" Say [O Muhammad], "Allah rescues you from it and from all [other] distresses, and yet you worship others besides Allah."* (Qur'an 6: 63–64)

People's Problem with the Prayer - Their Brains Won't Stop

> *Those who offer their Salât (prayers) with all solemnity and full submissiveness.* (Qur'an 23:2)

> If one prays two units of prayer with full concentration, Allah forgives one for whatever sins one may have committed before. (Bukhārī and Muslim)

People's minds are constantly on the go mode due to their busy and rushed lives. Their minds are constantly racing, thinking about the future and the past. Unfortunately, this ends up impacting our prayers and subsequently our lives. This takes away the benefit that we can derive from the prayer, and because of this, people are getting sicker, socially, spiritually and physically.

Ibn 'Ubayd related that the Messenger of Allah heard someone supplicate in his prayer without first glorifying Allah and invoking blessings upon His Prophet and so he observed: "That one was in a hurry" then he called him and said to him (or to someone beside him), "When one of you supplicates, he should begin with the praise and glorification of Allah and then invoke blessings on the Prophet and then supplicate as he may wish." (Abū Dāwūd, Nasā'ī and Tirmidhī)

Prayer, much like meditation, yoga or breathing techniques, causes the mind and body to focus on a singular focal point, thus aligning the mind, soul and body of the praying person. We simply need to focus and be mindful of our prayers to reap all the benefits.

Dhikr – Allah

... And remember the Name of Allah much [both with tongue and mind], so that you may be successful. (Qur'an 8: 45)

... Verily, in the remembrance of Allah do hearts find rest. (Qur'an 13: 28)

O you who believe! Remember Allah often and much. (Qur'an 33: 41)

And when the Prayer is finished, then may you disperse through the land, and seek of the Bounty of Allah: and celebrate the Praises of Allah often (and without stint): that you may prosper. (Qur'an 62:10)

Dhikr is another type of meditation. and remembrance of Allah, glorified and exalted is He.

Therefore remember Me [through prayer and glorification]. I will remember you... (Qur'an 2: 152)

O you who believe! Let neither your property nor your children divert you from the remembrance of Allah. And whosoever does that, then they are the losers. (Qur'an 63: 9)

The Benefits of Remembrance

And remember Allah by your tongue and within yourself, humbly and with fear, without loudness in words, in the mornings and in the afternoons, and do not be of those who are neglectful. (Qur'an 7: 205)

Imam Ibn Taymiyah said: "Remembrance is like water to the fish: imagine how the fish will be if they leave the water?"

147

Prophet Muhammad, peace and blessings be upon him, said: "The example of the one who remembers Allah and the one who does not is like the living and the dead." (Bukhārī)

Prophet Muhammad, peace and blessings be upon him, said: "Do not talk too much without remembering Allah, as too much useless talk without remembrance of the Divine hardens the heart; and those with hard, cruel hearts are the farthest from Allah." (Tirmidhī)

A man once came to Prophet Muhammad, peace and blessings be upon him, asking him to specify an important Islamic ritual for him to cling to and so the Prophet said: "Keep your tongue moist with the remembrance of Allah." (Tirmidhī, Aḥmad and Ibn Mājah)

Remembering Allah, glorified and exalted is He, in every situation, whether it is happy, sad or painful, brings us closer to Allah while showing our gratitude and being mindful of Allah, glorified and exalted is He, can help our situation. We must accept that human beings have no power without Him, and with the help of Allah, glorified and exalted is He, everything is possible. The remembrance of Allah, glorified and exalted is He, increases our love for Him, and this love brings calmness and peace to the heart and mind.

The Power of Your Breath

Focusing on your breath is the easiest, fastest and most powerful way to distress immediately and is also a great help to weight loss.

This is what you should do: Lie on a flat surface with either legs straight or knees bent; or sit up in a comfortable position. Place one hand on the upper chest and the other on the abdomen – this will enable you to feel whether you are using the diaphragm instead of the chest muscles to breathe; the belly should rise more than the chest. Close the eyes and breathe in slowly through the nose counting to 4, letting the stomach expand against the hand. Hold the breath for a count of 7. Exhale though the mouth slowly and steadily to the count of 8. Let the stomach fall back as you exhale all the air from the lungs. Again, the hand on the upper chest should remain as still as possible. Pause for a count of one and then repeat the cycle for ten breaths. Make the breaths as deep and slow as possible. Practising a simple technique like belly breathing for five minutes, two or three times a day, will help establish equilibrium. Even when you are deep breathing, you can still incorporate your favourite *du'ā's* and *dhikr*. As you breathe in and out, you should be conscious and aware that Allah, glorified and exalted is He, is there for you with every breath you take.

Progressive Muscle Relaxation

In this relaxation technique, you should focus on slowly tensing and then relaxing each muscle group. This will help you become aware of your body and counteract the first signs of muscle tension that accompanies stress. When the body relaxes, the mind relaxes too. There are two steps:

1. Deliberately tensing muscle groups.
2. Releasing the tension in muscle groups.

Putting it All Together

It is He who created the heavens and earth in six days and then established Himself above the Throne. He knows what penetrates into the earth and what emerges from it and what descends from the heaven and what ascends therein; and He is with you wherever you are. And Allah, of what you do, is Seeing. (Qur'an 57:4)

I am as My servant thinks of Me, and I am with him when he remembers Me ... (Bukhārī, Muslim)

The Prophet, peace and blessings be upon him, was an example for all of us. He was given more stress then anyone could imagine. He lost his parents, children, family, and some of his wives. He was thrown out of his home into the dessert; he was abused and hurt, and he had the stress of the world on his shoulders. All that stress did not stop him, peace and blessings be upon him, from remembering Allah, glorified and exalted is He, through prayer, *du'ā'*, *dhikr* and meditation. If the busiest and most stressed out man in the world could escape to mount Ḥirā' to meditate, why can't we?

Usually before or after prayer, we make *wuḍū* , then find a comfortable and relaxed place and position, back supported, where you won't fall asleep. Start by saying "*bismillāh*", focus on the breath, practicing abdominal breathing above, then going into mindfulness, meditation/dhikr and ending with gratitude.

Close the eyes. Inhaling in through the nose for 2 seconds and exhaling through the mouth of the 4 seconds. Then increases slowly, in for 3, out for 6, increasing to in for 4 seconds, hold for 7 seconds and then breathe out for 8 seconds. After doing that for a couple times. Then you want to add mindfulness. Ask yourself, what are you hearing, what are you seeing, what are you feeling...and then putting it all together. Develop an observant, noncritical attitude, becoming aware of your physical sensations. While continue to slowly breathing, now turn your attention to meditation or *dhikr*. Chose a word or small phrase of focus that makes you feel peace inside (ie Allah, the names of Allah (SWT), *subḥānallāh*, *alḥamdulillāh*, *allāhu akbar*, seeking forgiveness of Allah, etc), repeating the word (s), concentrating on it or them. As you continue this dhikr, if your mind starts to wonder, slowly guide it back to the remembrance of Allah and *dhikr*. Continue this for 5-10 minutes then move to gratitude. Gratitude to Allah (SWT) for your health, life and all the complex processes involved to allow yourself to breathe.

It is with stillness that we begin to feel the *murāqabah* of Allah, as 'He is with us wherever we are.' He knows what is going on in our heart and mind at all times, so we should develop that closeness with Allah. Every time our mind starts to wonder, slowly guide it back to breathing and to Allah, as we continue our *dhikr*.

The Prophet, peace and blessings be upon him, said: "Verily, at times there is fog over my heart, so I seek the forgiveness of Allah one hundred times a day." (Muslim)

When distracted, the Prophet, peace and blessings be upon him, used to bring himself back to the state of *murāqabah* through *dhikr*. Dhikr is the calming phrase that the mind will come to associate with the state of *murāqabah*. So every time you get distracted, you should quietly use remembrance or supplication to return to the state of *murāqabah*.

Two words are beloved to the Most Merciful and are light on the tongue but heavy on the Scale: Glory and praise to Allah (*subḥān Allāh wa-bi-ḥamdih*), and glory to Allah the Almighty (*subḥānallāh al-ʿAẓīm*). (Bukhārī)

The best form of remembrance is: there is no God but Allah (*lā ilāha illā Allāh*), and the best form of supplication is: all praise is due to Allah (*alḥamdulillāh*). (Tirmidhī)

Start with five minutes daily then increase the duration as fit but find a combination that works for you.

Live a *Ṭayyib* (Pure) Life to Reduce Stress and Restore Balance

Following the pillars of optimal health in its entirety will help to lower stress, as this helps to balance ourselves and our emotions, and allows us to effectively deal with what is at hand.

To recap:

- Eat *tayyib* foods. This will heal the gut, balance out hormones and provide the body with nutrient dense foods it needs to stay balanced and function properly, Add anti-inflammatory foods, hydrate and leave some room for air every time you eat. Add probiotics and probiotic rich foods, as their addition helps balance the peripheral nervous system. Caffeine may interfere with the sleep cycle, so drink some herbal teas instead, like chamomile, nettle leaf, dandelion, and holy basil tea; these will help to ease stress.

- Live in a *tayyib* environment. By lowering the toxic/*khabīth* burden outside the body, you can lower the stress within. For further relaxation, add lavender oil to your detox baths.

And the earth – We spread it out and cast therein firmly set mountains and made grow therein [something] of every beautiful kind, Giving insight and a reminder for every servant who turns [to Allah]. (Qur'an 50: 7–8)

- Give yourself permission to apply self care. It is important to take care of yourself, otherwise you will not be able to take care of other human beings or responsibilities.
- Spending time in nature, observing and contemplating Allah's creations is important in lowering stress. It is also helpful in detoxing your breath and increasing your sense of peace, allowing you even to digitally detox or spend time away from computers and other electronic devices.
- Maintain a *Ṭayyib* Social Life. Cultivate positive relationships, spend time with people who are supportive, encouraging and those who listen to you. Simply smiling and laughing will lower cortisol and boost brain chemicals like endorphins, which will help improve your mood. Laughing increases the level of T cells, natural killer cells and antibodies, all of which helps to improve the immune system. Massaging is also a therapeutic touch that is healing and is a great way to relieve inflammation and stress. Just doing what you love and scheduling fun rest days during the week will allow the liver, body, mind and soul to detox and relieve stress.
- Optimize sleep. Sleep is important in healing as well as in rejuvenating and improving stress levels.
- Remove unnecessary expectations; eschew unrealistic expectations. These simple techniques will empower you to take back control of your health and time.
- Manage and organize time. You are the master of your own time. Plan, prioritize and create daily reminders for tasks and lists, and delegate tasks to others. Declutter your life, which includes the physical and electronic environments like emails and messages. Learn the causes of your stress and what is important to you. Learn to say no and remove guilt from your dealings with others. Moreover, do not overschedule.
- Connect with your soul and find a higher purpose. Allah, glorified and exalted is He, has put humans in this world for a unique purpose, which is different for every person. Praying, *du'ā'*, mindfulness and gratitude will help you to develop a positive attitude and reframe your stress and tackle it better.

When you clear out the clutter in your brain, you can start to think beyond yourself and find a higher purpose.

- Unplug. Limit your exposure to technology; you do not have to be connected 24/7.
- Exercise. One of the biggest stress busters is exercise. This point is discussed in a little more detail below.

Exercise Can Heal

The strong believer is better and more beloved to Allah than the weak believer, while there is good in both; 'Your body has a right over you.' (Muslim, Bukhārī)

Strike the ground with your foot: This is a spring of water to wash in, cool and a [refreshing] drink. (Qur'an 38: 42)

Do not let your own hands throw yourself into ruin. (Qur'an 2:195)

And the servants of the Most Merciful are those who walk upon the earth easily, and when the ignorant address them [harshly], they say [words of] peace. (Qur'an 25:63)

Any action which is performed without the remembrance of God is either a diversion or heedlessness except for four things: Walking from target to target [during archery practice], training a horse, playing with one's family, and learning to swim. (Ṭabarānī)

Regular exercise is crucial for a *tayyib* lifestyle, as it lowers the markers of systemic inflammation and is also good for the brain and body. Some of the tenets of Islam, such as the prayer and *Hajj*, which require physical exertion, are among the overlooked forms of exercise.

Husbands and their wives can exercise, run and play together.

The wife of the Prophet, peace and blessings be upon him, 'Ā'ishah said: "I raced with the Prophet, peace and blessings be upon him, and beat him in the race. Later, when I had put on weight, we raced again and he beat me, upon which he said: 'This cancels that (referring to the first race).'" (Bukhārī)

Prophet Muhammad, peace and blessings be upon him, advised his followers to be energetic and start their day early.

O God! Make the early morning hours blessed for my nation. (Ahmed)

Not only is exercise an amazing stress reliever, it also has great benefits as it can directly manipulate the DNA expression, reduce cravings, regulate appetite, improve insulin sensitivity,[44] keep cortisol in check,[45] improve self-confidence and digestive function by increasing microbial diversity, slow down aging and make neurochemicals that make brain tissue grow. It also stimulates more growth factors, releases endorphins (the brain chemicals that act as a natural pain reliever and lifts mood), improves detoxification, boosts happy chemicals in the brain,[46] rewires and restructures the brain for better thinking because it restores the brain connections, thus sharpening memory, and strengthens the bones and muscles, reducing the risk of fractures and helping build healthy bones. It also increases self-confidence and makes existing blood vessels healthier, keeps chronic diseases at bay and overall inflammation low.[47] Inactivity, regardless of the body's weight is twice as deadly as being obese, as prolonged sitting for more than eight hours a day with zero physical activity can lead to an early death. Studies have shown that light activity like walking for two minutes every hour was associated with a 33 percent lower chance of dying over a three-year period. Research reveals that exercise can help aging people develop a larger brain (both grey and white matter), due to the increase of BGF, the growth of small blood vessel and more interconnections between brain cells. Exercise protects against many of the inflammatory and immune related conditions. Moderate exercise is safe for most, but if you have a chronic illness, you should speak with your doctor before starting a new exercise programme.

Tips on Exercising

The best type of exercise is the one that you can do. Find an exercise that is enjoyable, and exercise for at least thirty minutes every day. Take time to stretch every morning, before and after exercising. Stretching can improve a range of motions, boost circulation, and keep muscles loose and flexible. Remember to breathe while stretching. The key to exercise is its intensity, not its duration. Maintain a mix of aerobic, strength training, core support and fascia work, remember to walk, dance, clean and play with your kids or pets because all these activities are vital for overall health and burning excess energy. You do not need to exercise in one stretch of time, for studies have shown that three 10-minute sessions of exercise throughout the day can offer similar if not more benefits.

Respond to your body and not overdo it. Strenuous exercise itself increases intestinal permeability. You should exercise for as long as you feel good and energized afterward. If you feel exhausted or worse off after exercise or your symptoms worsen, then you are doing too much.

Strength training helps to increase lean muscle mass, which makes the bones stronger, boosts metabolism and burns more fat at rest. The more muscle mass we have, the more likely we are to maintain insulin sensitivity. Strength training stimulates the body to make more growth hormones. The prayer is an excellent form of strength training when done properly. When bowing down in the prayer, the blood is pumped into the upper body, and when done properly this position tones the muscles of the back and abdomen. Prostration in the prayer stimulates the frontal cortex, thus increasing the blood flow into the upper body and head. Yoga reduces anxiety and stress, and improves flexibility, strength, balance, core support and stamina as it involves a series of moving and stationary poses, combined with deep breathing, which strengthens the relaxation response in our daily life. Other forms of strength training are tai chi, lifting weights/tubing which are all great options and should be done two to three times a week. Both yoga and tai chi help to reduce stress by calming the mind and conditioning the body by focusing on the breath and paying attention to the present moment. Incorporate fascia work in your workouts, as it can help to relax the bands that connect your tissues and keep you flexible.

Aerobic exercise or whole body movement that gets the heart pumping (aka cardiovascular exercise), like spinning, interval training, dancing, cycling, running/jogging, walking or swimming are all great stress relievers. Shorter workouts, like high-intensity interval training or burst training with short speed bursts, are also another option. Some studies have shown that all these exercises can boost metabolism, provide a higher level of brain garden fertilizers in less time and burn more calories all day, even after the exercises are completed. The exercises of older people get a greater mitochondrial boost from HIIT than the exercises of younger persons.

Interval training is characterized by a short period of exertion followed by a rest period then back to exertion (getting the heart rate up to 70–80 percent of its maximum). An example of interval training includes doing a five-minute warm up, with a ten-minute interval to bring the heart up for thirty seconds, then down to target heart rate for ninety seconds, and finishing with a five-minute cool down. It is important to give your body rest, so listen to your body. You may want to limit your HIIT workouts to half your weekly workouts. Aerobic exercise is good for mood, brain and cardiovascular health. I recommend starting off with walking. One step in the right direction is better than no steps at all. Wearing a pedometer will help motivate you to try to aim for about ten thousand steps per day. Studies have shown that a daily walk can kick start energy production, lower diabetes, improve mental clarity and even improve metabolism. In a 2016 study, it was found that a 10 minute walk after dinner dramatically lowers blood sugar. Walking is important, it is even better if you can do it outside, while taking deep cleansing breaths, connecting with nature, while remembering Allah. Taking a brisk walk in the woods can lower stress, heart rate, blood pressure and neuroinflammation. It can also lower inflammation, prevent or delay dementia and improve mood. Exercise while fasting can reduce ROS production, improve insulin sensitivity and increase mitogenesis.[48]

Other Relaxation Techniques

• Hypnosis • Biofeedback • Art therapy • Neuro feedback • Tapping/Emotional Freedom Techniques • Float tank • Binaural beats • Relaxation apps

Stress is inevitable, but it doesn't have to ruin our health or negatively affect our everyday decisions. Bad relationships, financial hardship, trauma, work stress or just the stress of every day living are all from Allah. Trusting in Allah, spending more time in nature, optimizing prayer, *du'ā'* and *dhikr* by being mindful can all be incorporated to manage stress properly. The aim should be to not let stress take over our mind, health and life.

Sleep to Optimize Health

And among his signs is your sleep by night and by day and your seeking of His bounty, verily in that are Signs for those who hearken. (Qur'an 30:23)

Sleep is one of Allah's greatest blessings. The Qur'an discusses different types of sleep which correspond with the different stages of sleep in modern medicine. Getting enough sleep normalizes cortisol levels, improves memory and helps to control weight and overall inflammation. Our bodies don't consume much energy while we sleep, so it leaves more energy available over eight or nine hours per night for the body to remove toxins, make hormones, activate cellular repair, boost the secretion of growth hormone, mend injury and fight infections. Sleep cleans up the hippocampus so it can take in new information which it can then process.

The Stages of Sleep in the Qur'an

No slumber (Sinah) can seize Him nor sleep. (Qur'an 2:255)

Sinah/slumber. Dozing off for a short period of time, with prompt arousal following environmental stimulus.

Remember when He covered you with a slumber (Nu'ās) as a security from him. (Qur'an 8:11)

Nu'ās/short nap. Corresponds to Stage 1 and Stage 2 of sleep. Short naps can reduce stress and blood pressure.

And you would have thought them awake, whereas they were asleep (Ruqūd). (Qur'an 18:18)

Ruqūd/sleep for a long period.

And we made your sleep (Subāt) as a thing for rest. (Qur'an 78:9)

Subāt/Deep sleep. This corresponds to the slow wave sleep identified by modern scientists.

Importance of Sleep

Sleep is highly important in the Qur'an and Sunnah.

If anyone of you feels drowsy while praying, he should go to bed (sleep) until his slumber is over. (Bukhārī)

Offer prayers and also sleep at night, as your body has a right over you. (Bukhārī)

Once the Prophet, peace and blessings be upon him, entered the Mosque and saw a rope hanging between its two pillars and so he asked: *"What is this rope?"* The people said: "This rope is for Zaynab who grabs it when she feels tired (to keep standing in prayer)." The Prophet, peace and blessings be upon him, said: "Don't use it. Remove the rope. You should pray as long as you feel active, and when you get tired, sleep." (Bukhārī)

Unfortunately, a third of all Americans are getting less than seven hours of sleep at night.[1]

Lack of sleep affects every organ in the body.[2] Lack of good circadian rhythms is also associated with numerous serious medical illnesses, as it alters the function of 711 genes that we know of,[3] leading to mental and emotional disturbances like depression (those who don't get enough sleep are twice as likely to feel depressed or anxious[4] and encounter other mood issues), a thinner prefrontal cortex,[5] quadrupling the risk of cancer, doubling our chance of obesity and increasing hunger… obesity[6] and increasing hunger,[7] diabetes,[8] and insulin resistance. Trigger production of inflammatory chemicals[9] increases an inflammatory marker called hsCRP (which is a strong predictor of heart disease)[10] and the risk of heart disease and stroke.[11] Not getting good sleep is also related to something known as frontal lobe syndrome, which involves confusion, impulsivity, poor judgment, the inability to perform tasks, and catatonia. A poor night's sleep can make anyone's amygdala about 60 percent more reactive. Our brains are unable to self-clean,[12] leading to emotional reactivity, brain fog, confusion, memory issues, sexual dysfunction, addictions, the inability to make rational decision, susceptibility to infections and even the shortening of our lifespan! Lack of sleep prevents us from processing information in general.

Less than six hours of sleep can (in prediabetics) increase the chances of having a serious cardiac event (if you already have a history of heart issues),[13] and it has a 44 percent increase in the risk of developing full blown diabetes. Less than five hours of sleep is associated with an increased risk of 68 percent the same![14] This has also been shown with acute sleep deprivation (not getting enough sleep for a full 24 hours). As most people in the world suffer from prediabetes, these are very frightening statistics. Just decreasing our sleep by only one and a half hours per night could reduce our daytime alertness by as much as 32 percent! Sleep helps to regulate most hormone production, including leptin and ghrelin. In a well cited study, people who slept for just four hours a night for two consecutive nights experience 24 percent increase in their hunger and ate high calorie treats like salty snacks and starchy foods. If we under-sleep regularly, we can add up to 150,00 extra calories per year, or 42 lbs of extra fat.

Fifteen percent of human DNA is controlled by the circadian rhythm, including the body's repair mechanism.

The body clears its waste and fluid from the tissues through the lymphatic system. The lymph carries the cellular debris and is filtered as it passes through the lymph nodes. The glymphatic system (promotes efficient elimination of soluble proteins and metabolites from the central nervous system) goes into overdrive at night, so sleep helps to clean and wash the brain. When we fail to get enough sleep, our body is unable to put in the effort needed to do all the important tasks like removing toxins, and this leads to hormonal imbalances and inflammation.

Where Does the Problem Lie?

Our impure, disconnected lifestyles are creating problems regarding our sleep. Blue lights (the wavelength of light on the spectrum of visible light that affects us through the eyes) stimulate us and keep us awake, through lowering the sleep hormone, melatonin. This is having detrimental effects on our health, which experts are just beginning to recognize and study. Exposure to blue light at night can also increase breast cancer.[15]

Optimizing Sleep

Islam enjoins how we should wake up, eat, go to the bathroom, etc., and so it basically dictates how we live our life, and also how we need to sleep. Modern sleep medicine currently recommends many of these same practices. Sleep hygiene[16] includes practices that promote better quality sleep.

Bedtime Routines

The Prophet, peace and blessings be upon him, said: *"One should not sleep before the night prayer nor have discussions after it."* (Bukhārī)

A sleep routine is very important. It is best to go to bed the same time every day (this can change but only by about an hour). Prophet Muhammad, peace and blessings be upon him, encouraged his Companions to go to bed early and wake up early. Exposing our eyes to sunlight first thing in the morning is good to help set our body clock. Neuroscience now backs the importance of morning to absorb the sun. The Prophet, peace and blessings be upon him, encouraged his Companions not to be involved in any activity after the *'Ishā'* prayer and he didn't sleep after Fajr. Going to sleep around 9:00 to 11:30 pm helps to promote the best hormonal environment for sleep, fat burning and regeneration.

We used to offer the Jumu'ah *(Friday) prayer with the Prophet and then take the afternoon nap.* (Bukhārī)

If you are short on sleep one day, try to get back on schedule immediately. If you must nap, do so for twenty to thirty minutes before 4:00 pm. Regular exercise can improve sleep. Start winding down about two hours before bedtime by taking time to relax, using either mindful meditation, prayer, *du'ā'*, *dhikr* or other stress relieving strategies. Maybe take a warm bath with Epsom salt and lavender oil and set aside time to write down your worries.

Put out lamps when you go to bed, shut the doors, and cover water and food containers. (Bukhārī)

Turn off all electronic devices at least ninety minutes before bedtime, as this allows our melatonin and cortisol levels to normalize. Try to minimize the use of blue lights from electronics and use amber lights or glasses to filter the blue light. Digital programmes can be used for computer and electric screens which will change the colour of the computer's light from blue to orange as the sun sets. Don't forget to flip switches to turn off the Wi-Fi, put your phone six feet away on airplane mode, and turn off notifications to limit EMFs. Studies have shown a link between exposure to radiation from cell phones in the three hours before bed and the difficulty to staying asleep or falling asleep. Try to use earthing sheets, which stimulate a similar reaction as if you were in direct contact with the ground, allowing you to receive energy that helps you sleep.

Avoid late night meals, as some studies have shown that food passes through the digestive system slower at night, and this leads to more fermentation of bacteria that live there as well as bloating, gas, constipation and even small intestinal bacterial overgrowth. Late night eating can increase the risk of insulin resistance, fat gain and accelerated aging and can even possibly cause certain types of cancer. The aim should be to stop eating about ninety minutes before going to bed; if you have to eat, the food should be high in fat and low in carbohydrates, to limit the insulin spike.

Also, if you can't fall asleep after forty-five minutes, its best to get up and try again an hour later – don't just lie there. Make sure to perform minor ritual ablution (*wuḍū*) before going to sleep, make supplications and sleep on the right side.

Whenever you go to bed, perform minor ritual ablution like you do for the prayer, and lie on your right side.' (Muslim) In description of the sleep of the Prophet peace and blessings be upon him, a *report* states, *'When the Prophet (peace and blessings be upon him) wanted to go to sleep, he puts his right hand under his cheek.'* (Muslim)

It is Allah Who receives the souls at the time of their death, and those that do not die during their sleep. He keeps those [souls] for which He has ordained death and sends the rest [back to their bodies] for a term appointed... (Qur'an 39: 42)

Upon assessing the autonomic effect of three sleep positions, some studies have shown that cardiac vagal activity was greatest when the subjects were sleeping on the right lateral position. Several studies have shown that recumbent positions affect the autonomic nervous system activity in patients with congestive heart failure.[17]

Create a Restful Room

In order to get restful, deep sleep, we need to prepare for it by creating an environment that is conducive to the best sleep. Keeping the room dark, quiet, clean and cool helps. This room should be kept for sleep only, or for sleep and conjugal relations for couples. The office should be kept out of the bedroom. Clear out the clutter, hang blackout curtains on the windows, set the night room temperature to between 60 - 67°F, limiting noise or using a white-noise fan to block background noise. Socks can help to keep your extremities warm. Adding a household plant to your room can improve the air quality and inhibit electromagnetic fields (EMFs). Try to eliminate electronics, as they do contain blue wavelengths that can suppress melatonin, the hormone needed for sleep and for stimulating the alert centers of the brain, so it is best to avoid blue light a few hours before bed. There are apps available that can change the colour temperature on your screen and use blue light blocking glasses to optimize sleep.

Live a *Ṭayyib* (Pure) Life for Optimal Sleep

What we do during the day can determine how we sleep – starting from the moment we wake up. Living a *tayyib* (pure) life helps to improve our sleep. Our target and mindset should be to wake up with prayer and gratitude. Thanking Allah for another day. Try to fast intermittently, focus on *tayyib* foods and limit daytime sleep disrupters such as caffeine, sugar, stress, lack of movement and too much artificial light or evening exposure to fluorescent light.

Foods that can help you sleep include walnuts, pasture raised eggs, avocados and green leafy vegetables (like kale and spinach). Melanopsin, the master time setter is a vitamin A based protein. You could get vitamin A from liver, trout, eggs, mackerel, salmon, sweet potatoes and carrots. Try to make sure to get EPA/DHA found in wild salmon and grassfed beef. Always stay well hydrated and replace caffeine with relaxing teas like chamomile and valerian (add in a teaspoon of gelatin). If you need caffeine, then limit its consumption to the morning hours only.

Increase your exposure to bright light for at least thirty minutes from 6:00 am to 8:30 am because this provides natural light cues for your circadian rhythms and keeps you alert. Try to walk to work or stand next to a window. Light boxes or visors and other gadgets can be used to stimulate sunlight even when you are stuck behind a desk. After sunset, avoid being on screen, replace all bright white lights with amber bulbs or wear amber glasses to reduce blue lights. This allows your body to shift into sleep mode. Try to make it a habit to also exercise regularly in the morning or afternoon. Periods of time with direct contact with the ground can help create an internal balance, thus optimizing sleep.

You need to go to the doctor if you have difficulty falling asleep, staying asleep, or you always feel sleepy during the day, act out your dreams during sleep, grind your teeth, snore frequently or wake up unrefreshed or with pain. When travelling, intermittent fasting optimizes the effects of jet lag and circadian rhythm, along with exercise and using melatonin 30 minutes before bedtime in the new time zone.

Pure Social Support

Islam teaches love. Allah loves each and every one of us even more than anyone ever possibly could, even our own mothers. Love really does heal. The feeling of being loved releases a flood of potent hormones into the bloodstream, which not only makes people feel better emotionally, but also significantly strengthens their immune systems. Giving and receiving love inspire healing – physically, emotionally, and spiritually. Humans are social creatures by nature and need each other to survive.

Prophet Muhammad, peace and blessings be upon him, said: "The most beloved of you to me is the one who has the best manners." (Bukhārī and Muslim)

He, peace and blessings be upon him, also said: "None of you (truly) believes until he loves for his brother what he loves for himself." (Bukhārī and Muslim)

Spread Love and Respect to All

Kindness increases oxytocin and serotonin, improves the immune system, and increases self esteem and heart rate variability. Oxytocin lowers stress hormones and oxidative stress. When we show kindness, everyone around us benefits from the same immune effects. Studies have shown that when a person sees someone showing an act of kindness, that person's immune antibodies IgA become elevated. Islam enjoins being kind to everything around us: animals, plants as well as all Allah's creations.

> The Prophet, peace and blessings be upon him, said: "All mankind is from Adam and Eve, an Arab has no superiority over a non-Arab nor a non-Arab has superiority over an Arab; also a white person has no superiority over a black person nor does a black person have any superiority over a white person unless it be for piety and good action." (Bukhārī and Muslim)

Allah, glorified and exalted is He, and His Prophet, peace and blessings be upon him, have taught people to treat others with love and kindness. They also taught to take care of our neighbours and families.

> *The believers are nothing else than brothers [in Islamic religion]. So make reconciliation between your brothers, and fear Allah, that you may receive mercy. O you who believe! Let not a group scoff at another group, it may be that the latter are better than the former; nor let [some] women scoff at other women, it may be that the latter are better than the former, nor defame one another, nor insult one another by nicknames. How bad it is, to insult one's brother after having Faith [i.e., to call your Muslim brother (a faithful believer) a sinner, or wicked, etc.]. And whosoever does not repent, then such are indeed wrong-doers. O you who believe! Avoid much suspicion, indeed some suspicions are sins. And do not spy, nor backbite one another. Would one of you like to eat the flesh of his dead brother? You would hate it [so hate backbiting]. And fear Allah. Verily, Allah is the One Who accepts repentance, Most Merciful.* (Qur'an 49: 10–12)

> The Prophet, peace and blessings be upon him, also said: "Do not hate each other, do not be jealous of each other, do not abandon each other and, O worshippers of Allah, be brotherly, for it is not permissible for any Muslim to abandon his brother for more than three days." (Bukhārī)

Prophet Muhammad, peace and blessings be upon him, also taught us: "It is not lawful for anyone to abandon his brother in Islam for more than three nights, that when they meet they ignore one another, and the best of them is the one who greets the other first." (Bukhārī, Muslim and Abū Dāwūd)

Islam has given clear instructions on how we should deal with other people. We must acknowledge them, respect them, avoid insulting, suspecting, backbiting or having jealousy towards them, etc.

Islam instructs Muslims to be kind to parents:

We have enjoined on man kindness to his parents; in pain did his mother bear him, and in pain did she give him birth. (Qur'an 46:15).

Thy Lord hath decreed that ye worship none but Him, and that ye be kind to parents. Whether one or both of them attain old age in thy life, say not to them a word of contempt, nor repel them, but address them in terms of honor. And out of kindness, lower to them the wing of humility, and say: 'My Lord! bestow on them Thy Mercy even as they cherished me in childhood.' (Qur'an 17:23–24).

We have enjoined on man and woman kindness to parents; but if they (either of them) strive (to force) thee to join with Me anything of which thou hast no knowledge, obey them not. (Qur'an 29:8).

We have enjoined on man and woman (to be good) to his/her parents; show gratitude to Me and to thy parents; to Me is (thy final) Goal. If they (parents) strive to make thee join in worship with Me things of which thou hast no knowledge, obey them not; yet bear them company in this life with justice (and consideration) and follow the way of those who turn to Me (in love). (Qur'an 31:14–15).

Prophet Muhammad, peace and blessings be upon him, has put a huge emphasis on treating our parents and family well.

He, peace and blessings be upon him, said: "Whoever desires an increase in their sustenance and age, should keep good relations with their kith and kin." (Bukhārī)

Prophet Muhammad, peace and blessings be upon him, said: "Heaven lies under the feet of mothers."

(Aḥmad, Nasā'ī)

A man came to the Prophet and said, "O Messenger of God! Who among the people is the most worthy of my good companionship?" The Prophet said: "Your mother." The man said, "Then who?" The Prophet said: "Then your mother." The man further asked, "Then who?" The Prophet said: "Then your mother." The man asked again, "Then who?" The Prophet said: "Then your father." (Bukhārī, Muslim)

'Abdullāh ibn 'Amr related that the Messenger of Allah said: "The major sins are to believe that Allah has partners, to disobey one's parents, to commit murder, and to bear false witness." (Bukhārī, Muslim)

It is reported by Asmā' bint Abū Bakr that during the treaty of Ḥudaybiyyah, her mother, who was then a pagan, came to see her from Makkah. Asmā' informed the Messenger of Allah of her arrival and also that she needed help. He said: "Be good to your mother." (Bukhārī, Muslim)

In Islam, the rights of neighbours are sacrosanct, we are commanded to honour and respect them.

Worship Allah and join none with Him in worship, and do good to parents, kinsfolk, orphans, the poor, the neighbor who is near of kin, the neighbor who is a stranger, the companion by your side, the wayfarer [you meet], and those [slaves] whom your right hands possess. Verily, Allah does not like those who are proud and boastful. (Qur'an 4: 36)

The Prophet, peace and blessings be upon him, said: "Whoever believes in Allah and the Last Day should honour his neighbour." (Bukhārī)

Abū Dharr related that the Prophet, peace and blessings be upon him, said: "O Abū Dharr, when you prepare broth put plenty of water in it and take care of your neighbours." (Muslim)

Prophet Muhammad, peace and blessings be upon him, said: "Gabriel continued to enjoin upon me to take care of my neighbours so much so that I thought that Allah would make neighbours the heirs of the deceased." (Bukhārī, Muslim, Abū Dāwūd and Tirmidhī)

Even when dealing with enemies, Allah, glorified and exalted, says,

... Either take them back in a good manner or part with them in a good manner... (Qur'an 65: 2)

Allah does not forbid you to deal justly and kindly with those who have not fought against you on account of religion and did not drive you out of your homes. Verily, Allah loves those who deal with equity. (Qur'an 60: 8)

.. Repel [evil] with that which is better [i.e., Allah orders the faithful believers to be patient at the time of anger, and to excuse those who treat them badly], then verily, the one who between you and him there was enmity, [will become] as though he were a close friend. (Qur'an 41: 34)

Ibn Mas'ūd related that the Messenger of Allah, peace and blessings be upon him, said: "After I am gone you will experience discrimination and will observe things that you will disapprove of." Someone asked: "O Messenger of Allah, what do you command us to do then?" He, peace and blessings be upon him, said: "Discharge your obligations and supplicate Allah for your rights." (Bukhārī and Muslim)

Islam has taught us to even respect those who work for us and treat others as we would like to be treated.

Anas ibn Mālik, the Prophet's peace and blessings be upon him servant, said: "The Prophet, peace and blessings be upon him, was not one who used to insult others or speak obscenities or curse, and when he wished to admonish anyone of us, he simply used to say: 'What is the matter with him, may his forehead be rubbed in dust.'" (Bukhārī)

Anas also said: "I served the Prophet for ten years and he never told me, 'Uff!' Nor did he ever scold me by saying, 'Why did you do such a thing or why did you not do such a thing?'" (Bukhārī)

The Prophet, peace and blessings be upon him, was love personified. We need to get back to living the Qur'an and Sunnah, spread love and respect, because our health and future depends on it. Love heals and empowers people.

Ṭayyib/Positive Support and Love Empower

Prophet Muhammad, peace and blessings be upon him, said: "The believers in their friendliness, compassion and affection are like the body, if one organ complains, all the other organs become dilapidated with insomnia and fever." (Bukhārī and Muslim)

Loving and respectful relationships heal from the inside out and create more positive relationships. Positive relationships with friends, family even or pets improve the immune system and can be healing. Friends prevent loneliness and offer us companionship. Positive company can increase our sense of belonging and purpose, boost our happiness, reduce our stress, improve our self-confidence and self-worth, and help us cope with any traumas. Based on the results of brain MRIs and blood and saliva tests, it is now known that feeling loved and supported releases hormones into the bloodstream. Such hormones include serotonin, relaxin, endorphins and oxytocin,[1] which keep us happy and healthy. These hormones lower cortisol,[1] improve blood circulation, lower blood pressure and heart rate, improve digestion, clear out toxins, increase natural killer cells, a number of white blood cells, red blood cells, IgA[2] and helper T cells. In brief they stimulate an activity that helps the immune system clear out infections and renew energy to repair cells and fight cancer. This helps lower overall inflammation, thus improving sleep, relieving feelings of restlessness and decreasing chronic pain as muscle tension and pain perception lower. Intimate contacts have been shown to increase the diversity and health of the microbiota. Hugs can stimulate the release of oxytocin, serotonin and dopamine which can elevate mood, lower cortisol and depression, improve sleep as well as immune function. Smiling has a direct effect on the immune system, as it stimulates a rise in the levels of immune antibodies and immune cells as well as the release of serotonin and dopamine, thus mitigating the effects of sleep. Mirror neurons found in the brain allow us to imitate the behaviour of those around us, so if we are around people who smile, we will also smile and reap the same biological effects.

Studies have shown that negative relationships and loneliness (one of the causes of stress) can lead to a premature death, increase cortisol levels and deplete the immune system. They are also associated with long term problems such as stress, anxiety and depression. A recent study looked at 10,000 individuals in Finland, Poland and Spain and found that loneliness was one variable that most strongly correlated with poor health. Studies have shown that the frequency of social contact was the only component of our social network that was correlated with improved health, while the quality of our social network or size didn't affect the level of loneliness. Some studies have shown that having pets releases the same hormones, and pet owners live longer than people who don't have pets. Other studies have also shown that friendly interactions in our neighbourhood, parks or local shopping areas are also important to protect against loneliness.

In one study which reviewed more than 40 studies on social support and inflammation, which covered more than 73,000 subjects, researchers found that the people with higher social support had lower levels of inflammation.[3] Another study looked at 2000 young black women (ages 24-34) in various social relationships (marriage, cohabitation, volunteerism, close friendships, religious houses attendance) and found that those with stronger integration had lower inflammation levels (measured by high sensitivity C-reactive protein.[4]

Creating a Ṭayyib/Pure Social Life

Try your utmost best to limit impure social relationships and increase the amount of *tayyib*/pure relationships. Stick with the people who fill your life with positivity and love.

Look for positive support in the following ways:

Volunteer

And they give food, in spite of their love for it [or for the love of Him], to the needy, the orphan, and the captive, [saying], "We feed you seeking Allah's Countenance only. We wish for no reward, nor thanks from you. Verily, We fear from Allah a Day, hard and distressful, that will make the faces look horrible [from their extreme dislike for it]." So Allah saved them from the evil of that Day, and gave them a light of beauty and joy, and their recompense shall be Paradise, and silken garments, because they were patient. (Qur'an 76: 8–12)

Prophet, peace and blessings be upon him said: "None of you truly believes until he loves for his brother (fellow human being) what he loves for himself." (Bukhārī and Muslim)

Volunteering makes an immeasurable difference in the lives of others and creates a sense of purpose. Science has also shown that volunteering can decrease depression, help us stay mentally and physically active, reduce stress and may even help us live longer. Volunteering helps to meet others, develop new relationships and even strengthen older relationships with those who have similar goals and mutual interests.[5] Finding volunteering opportunities in your community or volunteering at the hospital, mosque, community centre, museum or other charitable organizations are also great ways to connect.

Join Groups

Say, "Travel in the land and see how [Allah] originated creation, and then Allah will bring forth [resurrect] the creation of the Hereafter [resurrection after death]. Verily, Allah is Able to do all things." (Qur'an 29: 20)

Joining support groups, groups in the mosque, taking a class at a local gym or community venue, like a library, and finding travelling groups will help you locate people with similar interests. You can also invite acquaintances who have similar goals for a *tayyib* meal or green shake, if you'd like.

Joining a chat group or online community might help you make or maintain connections and relieve loneliness. As a rule of thumb always remember to exercise caution when sharing personal information or arranging an activity with someone you have just met online.

Reach Out

"The Muslim has six rights that other Muslims must fulfil: if you meet him, salute him (with the greeting of peace – saying, *al-Salām 'alaykum*); if he calls for you, answer his call; if he asks for advice, give him your advice; if he sneezes and thanks Allah, ask Allah to bless him; if he is sick, visit him; and when he dies, attend his funeral."

He, peace and blessings be upon him, also said: "Those who convey gossip from one person to another will not enter Paradise." (Bukhārī)

"Your smile for your brother is a charity." (Tirmidhī)

Random acts of kindness and generosity include smiling, holding the door open for someone and reaching out to loved ones. Chat with neighbours who are out when taking your child or pet for a walk, or pick up the phone to call those you love and tell them you were thinking of them. You can also call someone else the next day, and continue to repeat the process. Also, never be afraid to ask for help.

Give Zakāt

Take alms from their wealth in order to purify them and sanctify them with it... (Qur'an 9: 103)

Prophet Muhammad, peace and blessings be upon him, said: "The hand that gives is better than the hand that receives." (Bukhārī)

It is incumbent upon Muslims to give to those who are less fortunate. Zakāt is one of the five pillars of Islam. It is a fixed percentage that Muslims must give from their wealth annually to certain beneficiaries as stated in the Qur'an. Zakāt purifies the soul through the act of giving, kindness and charity. The word *zakāt* in Arabic means 'purification'; it purifies the donor's heart from greed, envy, hatred and selfishness. *Zakāt* is an act of kindness, comfort and love for the less fortunate.

Kind words and forgiving of faults are better than charity followed by injury. And Allah is Rich [Free of all needs] and He is Most Forbearing. O you who believe, Do not render in vain your charity by reminders of your generosity or by injury, like him who spends his wealth to be seen of people, and he does not believe in Allah, nor in the Last Day .. (Qur'an 2: 263–264)

If you disclose your charity, it is well, but if you conceal it, and give it to the poor, that is better for you. [Allah] will forgive you some of your sins. And Allah is Well-Acquainted with what you do. (Qur'an 2: 271)

Intimate Relationships

Advice to Couples

And among His Signs is this, that He created for you spouses from among yourselves, that you may find repose in them, and He has put between you affection and mercy. Verily, in that are indeed signs for a people who reflect. (Qur'an 30: 21)

O Humans revere your Guardian Lord, Who created you from a single person created of like nature its mate, and from this scattered (like seeds) countless men and women. Reverence Allah through Whom you claim your mutual rights. (*Qur'an 4:1*).

Marriage is hard and beautiful all at the same time. In marriage always remember Allah and pray that He puts love and mercy in your heart. First comes love, and then Allah knows that couples need mercy to help sustain their marriage.

They (your wives) are a clothing (covering) for you and you too are a clothing (covering) for them. (Qur'an 2:187)

The most complete of the believers in faith are those with the most excellent character, and the best of you are the best in behaviour to their women. (Tirmidhī)

Gratitude and positivity are key in marriage. Always focus on what the other spouse is doing right, not what he or she is wrong. Focus on what your spouse is doing for you. Be forgiving, don't stress about petty things, and pick your fights wisely. Always marry someone for his or her good heart. Communication and listening to each other are important; but also show love in sweet but simple ways. Laughter and play, for example, are magical ingredients in a happy and healthy marriage. Spend time with your spouse and continue saying "I love you", because these small words mean the world to them. The Prophet, peace and blessings be upon him, used to call his wives with the names they loved (a form of pampering and showing kindness to them), the Messenger of Allah, peace and blessings be upon him, used to feed his wives with his own hands.

Prophet Muhammad, peace and blessings be upon him, said: "*Whatever you spend is considered charity even the bite of food you put in your wife's mouth.*" (Bukhārī)

The Prophet, peace and blessings be upon him, was aware of his wives' feelings, understood their jealousy and love as well as their psychology and nature.

The Prophet, peace and blessings be upon him, said: "Treat women kindly; they were created from a rib, and the most crooked part of the rib is the highest part thereof; so, if you tried to rectify the rib it will be broken and if you leave the rib as it is, it will remain crooked, and women are just like that; therefore treat them kindly." (Bukhārī)

The Prophet, peace and blessings be upon him, used to consult his wives, demonstrate his love and loyalty to them, even lean and sleep on their laps at the time of their menstruation periods. (Bukhārī)

The Prophet, peace and blessings be upon him, told 'Ā'ishah in a long tradition reported by Umm Zar': "I am in my love and loyalty to you just like Abū Zar' and Umm Zar'." 'Ā'ishah replied: "You are dearer to me than my father and my mother; and you are even more loyal and loving than Abū Zar' is to Umm Zar'." (Bukhārī)

The Prophet, peace and blessings be upon him, treated his wives fairly when he was angry or happy and helped them out with household duties.

'Ā'ishah was asked about the manners of the Prophet at home and so she said: "He used to help in the family chores but when he heard the call to prayer, he stopped and went out without delay." (Bukhārī)

The Prophet, peace and blessings be upon him, expressed his love to his wives and had the best of manners towards them: he protected their privacy, refrained from beating or abusing them, and even used to wipe away their tears.

'Ā'ishah said: "I have never been jealous of any woman more than I was with Khadijah despite having not seeing her. Whenever the Prophet, peace and blessings be upon him, slaughtered a sheep he would say: 'Send it to the friends of Khadijah.' One day I made him angry; I told him: 'Why Khadijah!' The Prophet, peace and blessings be upon him, said: 'I was endowed with her love.'" (Muslim)

The faithful husband should not hate his faithful wife, because if he hates certain things in her character, then he should not forget the other good things in her character. (Muslim)

The worst rank for a man on the Day of Judgment is the rank of the man who sleeps with his wife and then discloses her privacy. (Muslim)

The Prophet, peace and blessings be upon him, had never beaten any woman, servant or anything else with his hand except when he was fighting in the way of Allah, the Almighty. He did not take revenge on anyone who harmed him except when the orders of Allah, the Almighty, were breached, for then he took revenge (Muslim).

The Prophet, peace and blessings be upon him, played with his wives, travelled with them and shared happiness and joy with them.

Aisha narrated: "I saw the Prophet, peace and blessings be upon him, at the door of my room while the Ethiopians were playing in the mosque and so he, peace and blessings be upon him, covered me with his gown to allow me to see them playing." (Bukhārī)

The love shown by the Prophet, peace and blessings be upon him, to his wives was beautiful and if husbands and wives were to emulate his example, stability and balance would be found in every home and marriage.

Advice to the Youth

In the world we are living in, children are fast becoming adults in some areas while in other areas they remain children when they should be more mature. Sex is one of those areas that has overwhelmed the youth. The temptation of the *Shayṭān* is drawing the youth to do everything that is against the Qur'an and Sunnah. So apart from reminding the youth of what Allah, glorified and exalted is He, has said, we should also tell them about the reasoning behind some of Allah's rulings.

And let those who cannot find someone to marry maintain chastity until Allah, glorified and exalted, makes them rich through His favours ... (Qur'an 24: 33)

And do not come near to unlawful sexual intercourse. Verily, it is a great sin, and an evil way [that leads one to Hell unless Allah forgives him. (Qur'an 17: 32)

Tell the believing men to lower their gaze [from looking at forbidden things], and protect their private parts [from illegal sexual acts]. That is purer for them. Verily, Allah is All-Aware of what they do. And tell the believing women to lower their gaze [from looking at forbidden things], and protect their private parts [from illegal sexual acts] and not to show off their adornment except only that which is apparent... (Qur'an 24: 30–31)

Prophet Muhammad, peace and blessings be upon him, said: "O young men, whoever can afford it, let him get married; and whosoever cannot afford, then let him fast, for fasting curbs his sexual desire." (Bukhārī)

Say [O Muhammad], '[But] the things that Allah has indeed forbidden are great sins [including every kind of unlawful sexual act] whether committed openly or secretly. (Qur'an 7: 33)

And she, in whose house he was, sought to seduce him [to do an evil act], she closed the doors and said, "Come on, you." He said, "I seek refuge in Allah [or Allah forbid]! Truly, he [your husband] is my master! He made my stay agreeable! [So I will never betray him]." Verily, the oppressors and evil-doers will never be successful. (Qur'an 12: 23)

A lot of people in this world are not looking for any real connections; they are only looking for joy which they can take from others. In order to know whether a person is worth sticking around for with, it is best to abstain from any intimate relationship in order to bless such a relationship. If the other person loves you and really wants to be with you, then they will respect your decision and wait. This will test the person to make sure she or he has the self-control and loyalty that you desire in a spouse. It is only through adapting the Qur'an and Sunnah that you can find the right spouse who, will support you, love you and treat you like you deserve.

A Word on Homosexuality and Gender Identity

Society's lines regarding what is acceptable and what isn't continue to change, but Allah's lines and limits do not change. Whether we agree and understand or not, Islam's position with regard to homosexuality is clear. It is mentioned in the Qur'an that it happened during the time of Prophet Lūṭ (Lot). Allah, glorified and exalted is He, clearly prohibits homosexuality.

Allah's fitrah [Allah's Islamic monotheism], with which He has created humankind. No change let there be in Allah's Creation [the Religion of Allah], that is the straight religion, but most people do not know. (Qur'an 30: 30)

Do you go in unto the males of the human species, and leave those whom Allah has created for you to be your wives? Indeed, you are a trespassing people! (Qur'an 26: 165–166)

And [remember] Lut [Lot], when he said to his people, "Do you commit evil [great sin, including every kind of unlawful sexual intercourse and sodomy] while you see [one

171

another doing evil without any screen]? Do you approach men in your lusts rather than women? Indeed, you are a people who behave senselessly." (Qur'an 27: 54–55)

People are all tested with different things. Some are tested with death in the family, some with lust and others with financial hardship. Adhering to Allah's directives is a test of *'ibādah* and commitment, whether we understand them or not. Society will continue to bend the lines of wrong vs. right, but that is where Allah's book comes to provide a timeless guidance.

The world is pigeonholing people and defining their existence, not through their brains or what they are able to accomplish in their lives, but rather through their sexual preferences. Why has society chosen to label people according to a specific action rather than according to their identity? People are much more than a mere label, and they are certainly much more than their sexual preferences.

Everyone has all kinds of desires; and the same applies with homosexuality. The problem does not lie in having a desire towards the same gender; the problem lies in acting upon those desires. If we have a desire that goes against the guidance of Islam, and we don't act on it, we are rewarded for that. And the more we struggle against and resists such a desire, the more reward we get from Allah.

If a person has a desire towards another person of the same sex, he or she should pray to Allah, glorified and exalted is He, to help him or her to get over such a desire and to give him or her the patience to persevere in their restraint and not act on their inclinations and whims. Being grateful for all the things we have is the best way to start focusing on something other than sex. Desire doesn't define an individual.

Parenting

Your wealth and your children are only a trial, whereas Allah! With Him is a great reward [Paradise]. (Qur'an 64: 15)

Allah, glorified and exalted is He, has given us an amazing gift – children – but it is our responsibility to protect them by all means because they are a trust placed in our hands. The intention and main aim in raising children is to give them the tools they need to succeed in this life and the next.

When a man dies, his deeds stop except for three things: an ongoing *ṣadaqah* (charity), knowledge by which others benefit, or a pious child who prays for him. (Abū Dāwūd)

Tarbiyah (Arabic for development/growth, the development and training of people in various aspects) and educating children from the very beginning are important for their overall health. This includes teaching them to take care of the gift Allah, glorified and exalted is He, has given them: their bodies and health. Children are pure, so to educate them is easy. If they misbehave, look at their food and environment for a possible cause. When a child lives a *tayyib* life, his or her prefrontal cortex and amygdala work better, and they make better decisions. A child is born with a lot of cells and limited connections, and our parenting can determine these brain connections. If a child lives a balanced life, he or she will have a balanced brain and connections. If a child lives an imbalanced life, it is more likely she or he will have an imbalanced brain and connections. Digestive health, detoxification, avoiding the four kinds of stress as well as sleep, social and spiritual health can all help to keep a child balanced, healthy and happy. I have dealt with this topic in detail in *The Holistic Rx for Kids: Parenting Healthy Brains and Bodies in a Changing World.*

> No child is born except on *al-fitrah* (the primordial human nature) and then his parents make him Jewish, Christian or Magian, as an animal produces a perfect young animal: do you see anything wrong with any part of its body? (Muslim)

Nourish The Bodies of Children with Rainbow Foods

> Each one of you is a guardian and is responsible for his charges. The ruler who has authority over people is a guardian and is responsible for them; a man is a guardian of his family and is responsible for them; a woman is a guardian of her husband's house and children and is responsible for them; a slave is a guardian of his master's property and is responsible for it; so all of you are guardians and are responsible for your charges. (Bukhārī)

Children are constantly growing and need high-nutrient foods to sustain their energy and growth. Nutrients regulate every single chemical reaction in the child's body. Children need to be mindful of the food they eat, how their bodies feel and how they should learn to live in the moment. They need to understand that eating chemicals, sugar and other toxins will kill the bacteria that are protecting them and keeping them healthy.

In the same way we teach children about gelatin and alcohol, we need to teach them to look for artificial and GMO foods because they are clearly not *tayyib*. We need to also teach them to "go down the list" every time they want to eat. We need to make them understand the importance of eating the rainbow of veggies, clean protein, healthy fats, fruit, as they should have optimal hydration, which are all critical for growing strong brains and bodies. Drinking juice is best to be limited as these displace nutrient rich foods and lower immunity. Most importantly, they have to limit screen time and instead play outside, as the microbes that live in the soil can increase their biodiversity for optimal health and happiness. When children are mindful, they are resilient. They are able to read labels, think for themselves, reflect on how the food affects their bodies and make food choices to nourish their bodies, not hurt them. Role modeling that behaviour is key to raising mindful children.

Cleaning Up Your Children's Surroundings

Children's bodies are continuously developing and because of this they are vulnerable to environmental toxins. To optimize a child's brain and body health, it is important to lower environmental toxins. First, locate the toxins, then make sure that your child is moving the body fluids and have him or her eat in order to detoxify, just like adults. Swap out toxic items used by your children for cleaner and pure items and products.

Managing Stress with Proper Parenting

Managing stress is essential for raising resilient mindful children as thoughts, feelings and emotions directly affect children's physical health. The quality of parenting can directly affect the child's brain chemicals.

Developing bonds of love, respect and honour with our children and being involved in their life can help to activate a sensory nerve in the their brain that releases oxytocin and natural opioids, which decrease their stress response and provide them with the feeling of well-being and thus help the brain develop.

'Ā'ishah narrated that a bedouin came to the Prophet, peace and blessings be upon him, and said, "I see that you kiss your children! But we don't kiss ours." The Prophet, peace and blessings be upon him, therefore said: "What can I do if Allah, glorified and exalted is He, has taken mercy away from your heart?" (Bukhārī)

Help your children with their emotions, help them use their words and take time to understand their painful feelings. It's important to get down and cuddle, play, look them in the eyes when they talk, laugh, read to them, and provide them with imaginative, explorative activities. The Prophet, peace and blessings be upon him, was kind to children; he let his grandchildren, Hasan and Husayn, climb on him while he was in prostration in the prayer.

'Abdullāh ibn Shaddād related that his father said: "The Messenger of Allah, peace and blessings be upon him, came out to us for one of the nighttime prayers carrying Ḥasan or Ḥusayn. The Messenger of Allah, came forward and put him down, then he said the *Takbīr* and started to pray. He prostrated during his prayer, and made the prostration lengthy. My father said: 'I raised my head and saw the child on the back of the Messenger of Allah, peace and blessings be upon him, while he was prostrating so I went back to my prostration.' When the Messenger of Allah, peace and blessings be upon him, finished praying, the people said: 'O Messenger of Allah peace and blessings be upon him, you prostrated during the prayer for so long that we thought that something had happened or that you were receiving revelation.' He said: 'No such thing happened. But my son was riding on my back and I did not like to disturb him until he had had enough.'" (Nasā'ī)

Place Order

Order needs to put in our children's lives by establishing family rules and clear boundaries. This will actually lower the level of stress for all members of the family and help children feel secure offer them an encouraging, safe, serene and well-structured environment, all while keeping the lines of communication with them open and being careful not to judge or negate their feelings as well as disciplining them in ways to preserve their dignity. This will deepen the emotional bond between you and your children. Children like logical reasoning, but it's important to make it simple when talking to them. Give your children a schedule for when to wake up, eat, play, exercise, go out, clean up, complete chores and sleep.

Give Children Responsibilities

Nay, and by the moon, And by the night when it withdraws, And by the dawn when it brightens, Verily, it is but one of the greatest calamities. A warning to mankind, To any of you that chooses to go forward (by doing righteous deeds), or to remain behind (by committing sins), Every person is beheld (accountable) on his own deeds. (Qur'an 4:32–38)

Giving children responsibilities at an early age and age-appropriate tasks helps them to realize that they can help the family, be leaders and accomplish anything they want. Some studies have shown that giving children responsibilities helps them to become successful adults.

Older children can learn to manage stress and reduce the effects of stress by practising abdominal breathing or mindfulness techniques such as meditation, praying, *du'a'* and *dhikr*. Establish a specific time for going to bed so that the adrenal glands don't go into overtime and cause undue stress. It is also important to focus on gratitude to build the children's sense of humour and optimism. Always be aware and honest about your causes of stress and emotions as children are like sponges and can sense and absorb even subtle changes in our mood or behaviour.

Sleep

Children aged 9-12 need an average of 9-12 hours of sleep while teens from 13-18 need around 8-10 hours of sleep per night. The brains of children and teens develop at a rate of 800 synapses per second, and when children sleep, their brains continue to form and strengthen these connections. A bedtime routine is the best way to help children develop healthy sleep habits. A good bedtime routine promotes the well-being of children.

Social Health

Love is the most important element in children's brain and body health. A secure attachment releases oxytocin, aka the "love hormone", which significantly strengthens the immune system, develops empathy and promotes emotional strength and self-regulation in children. Always give children unconditional love, honour and love them despite their mistakes and imperfections, make frequent eye to eye contact, spend family time with them, and be a teacher and role model for them and instil in them empathy and mindfulness.

Build Gratitude

Grateful children are the ones who are resilient, happy and healthy. Try to teach your children to wake up and think about all the things they are grateful for that day. Always aim to offer them words of encouragement and appreciation, teach them how to forgive and help them find their purpose.

Taking Care of Someone with Chronic Conditions

The one who stays with the one who is sick, and takes care of him and looks after him has done good by serving him and caring for him, and Allah, may He be glorified and exalted, says (interpretation of the meaning): *"and do good. Truly, Allah loves Al-Muḥsinūn (the good-doers)."* (Qur'an 2:195)

Ibn 'Umar narrated that the Messenger of Allah, blessings and peace of Allah be upon him, said: "The Muslim is the brother of his fellow Muslim; he does not wrong him or let him down. Whoever meets the needs of his brother, Allah will meet his needs. Whoever relieves a Muslim in distress, Allah will relieve him of distress on the Day of Resurrection." (Bukhārī and Muslim).

It can be taxing on your relationship and body when you are taking care of someone with chronic conditions. Taking care of someone sick is one of the greatest deeds in the eyes of Allah, but always make sure to take time to take care of yourself as well. Patience and love are important when taking care of people with a chronic disease. Tenderness and empathy will never fail you. In order to optimize that relationship, it is important to listen attentively, not be judgmental, answer questions as they come up, work to clear up misunderstandings, validate and respect their feelings, help them to relax, and always allow for setbacks and regressions. But to get the support you need, it is important to join a support group, so you can continue your good work.

Nurturing Your Relationships

If Allah loves a person, He calls out to Gabriel saying, "Allah loves so and-so, therefore do love him." So Gabriel loves him, and makes an announcement to the inhabitants of heaven, "Allah loves so-and-so, therefore do love him too." And the inhabitants of heaven would love him, and he is then granted the good pleasure and acceptance of the people on earth. (Muslim)

In order to nurture your relationships, try and feel love for Allah with all your strength. Take your time to look for quality friendships, focusing on the positive aspects of every relationship. Open yourself up by listening and sharing, but you should also respect boundaries and privacy as well as accept others for who they are.

The Prophet, peace and blessings be upon him, taught: "By the One Who holds my soul in His Hand, you will not believe until you love each other. Shall I tell you about something that if you do it you will love each other? Spread peace (i.e., saying, 'al-Salām 'alaykum') amongst you." (Muslim, Abū Dāwūd, Tirmidhī)

Allah, glorified and exalted is He, has put a huge emphasis on who we keep as friends and how we treat each other. So focus on building loving, *tayyib*/pure relationships because the latter, when in accordance with the Qur'an and Sunnah, heal from the inside out. It is never too late to build a new friendship or reconnect with old friends, as maintaining a healthy friendship or relationship is always a process of mutual giving and taking. Always let our friends know that they are appreciated.

Tayyib/Pure Spiritual Health to Optimize Physical Health

When I have fashioned him [in due proportion] and breathed into him of My spirit, then prostrate in obeisance unto him. (Qur'an 15: 29)

All human beings are creations of Allah whose hearts/souls need Him. When the hearts/bodies aren't filled with Allah, they look for other things to fill the void, such as material things, people, drugs, sex, etc. In order to stay balanced, we need to increase our spiritual connection with Allah to allow the healing of the soul. Some scientific studies have underscored the positive connection between spirituality and health. Spirituality affects the physical body by improving blood circulation, decreasing blood pressure, improving digestion and detoxification, turning off unhealthy genes and helping in the improvement of the overall immune system.

In order to be truly connected with Allah and with our spirit, we must be grateful. Muslims are supposed to be a people of gratitude, but society has brainwashed people to believe the opposite. Because happiness doesn't sell, people are told that they are not good enough until they get the next best product. Negativity is felt everywhere and this weakens the heart and soul of the believer. The only way out is going back to being truly grateful to Allah.

The strong believer is more beloved to Allah than the weak one, but there is good in both. (Muslim)

Ṣuhayb reported that the Prophet, peace and blessings be upon him, said: "The believer's affair is amazing: it is all for the good, and that is not the case for anyone except the believer. If something pleasing comes his way, he is thankful and thus it is good for him; and if something bad befalls him, he is patient, and thus it is also good for him." (Muslim)

And [remember] when your Lord proclaimed, 'If you are grateful, I will surely increase you [in favour]; but if you deny, indeed, My punishment is severe. (Qur'an 14:7)

The importance of positivity and thankfulness is underscored all over in the Qur'an. In *Sūrah* Ibrāhīm, verse 7, Allah, glorified and exalted is He, uses the strongest language as He promises and swears to it that He will increase us if we are grateful. The beauty of this is that Allah, glorified and exalted is He, doesn't specify what He will increase us in or towards whom we should be thankful to. Allah provides no specification, which makes it even more beautiful since our expressions of gratitude then become endless.

The Healing Power of Gratitude

O mankind! There has come to you a direction from your Lord, and a healing for (the disease in your) heart, and for those who believe in guidance, and mercy. (Qur'an 10:57)

Prophet Muhammad, peace and blessings be upon him, said: "There is an organ in the body which causes the health of the whole body when it is healthy; and when it is sick, it causes the sickness of the whole body; this organ is the heart." (Bukhārī and Muslim)

Gratitude is an expression of appreciation for what we have – a universal concept in nearly all the world's spiritual traditions. We experience a sense of deep spirituality when the feelings of gratitude are expressed. Giving thanks to Allah, our benefactors or others is one of the most effective ways to get in touch with our soul. Being thankful helps create a subconscious world of positivity that governs our thoughts and actions. In a 2019 World Happiness Report survey by the United Nations, the top 10 happiest nations in the world were also among the top 20 percent countries in which the life expectancy of their citizens was high.

Gratitude has been proven to have a physiological effect on the brain and body. It helps lower inflammatory markers, influences epigenetics, and even helps the heart, adding years to life. When we feel positive emotions, our brain instantly releases healing hormones like oxytocin, dopamin, serotonin, endorphins and relaxin into the blood stream, and this leads to improved blood circulation and slower digestion allowing the body to absorb more nutrients and lower stress levels, blood pressure and heart rate, thus deepening our breathing and strengthening our immune system by increasing the activity and the number of NK cells, white and red blood cells and destroying cancer cells and getting rid of infections. Positive energy boosts optimism, which in turn helps prevent disease and improve the immune system, well-being and sense of happiness.[1] A recent study found that an intervention designed to elicit gratitude by keeping a daily gratitude journal for two weeks increased the subjects' happiness, satisfaction with life and positive feelings, thus reducing their depression symptoms and negativity. Daily purposeful gratitude has been shown to improve sleep and overall physical health. Research has shown that those who were more grateful had better health and participated in healthy activities compared to people who were not grateful.

According to a study published by the *American Psychological Association* in 2015,[2] a grateful heart is also a happier and healthier heart. It was found that higher gratitude scores were proportional to a better mood, higher quality sleep, more self-efficacy, less inflammation and improved heart health. Gratitude makes us optimistic. Being optimistic improves our health and has been also proven to improve the immune system and lower inflammation. When we are stressed, gratitude helps us bounce back faster through focusing on what is going well in our life. It is predicted that cancer patients who were optimistic had less disruption of their normal lives as well as less distress and fatigue while those who were pessimistic were likely to experience the thickening of their arteries. Optimism has been found to be positively correlated with satisfaction with life and self-esteem. We need to take and appreciate every moment as

Attitude of Gratitude
Ways to cultivate gratitude and positivity

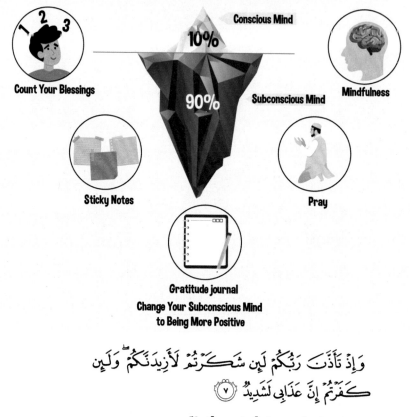

"And [remember] when your Lord proclaimed,
'If you are grateful, I will surely increase you [in favor];
but if you deny, indeed, My punishment is severe.'" (Quran 14:7)

Time to Get Back to Being a People of Alhumdulillah!

PICTURE 4.2   ATTITUDE OF GRATITUDE

it comes, and embrace thankfulness not only to affect our mind but also to influence our genetic composition and heart. "Heartfelt" emotions – like gratitude, love, and care – produce sine wave or coherent waves which radiate to every cell of the body. This is determined through technology that measures changes in heart-rhythm variation and coherence. Some research shows that "depleted" emotions – like frustration, anger, anxiety, and insecurity – make the heart-rhythm pattern erratic and the brain recognizes this as stress. This in turn creates a desynchronized state, raising the risk of developing heart disease and increased blood pressure, weakening the immune system, impairing cognitive function, and blocking the ability to think clearly.

Changing the Subconscious from *Khabīth* to *Ṭayyib*

Prophet Muhammad, peace and blessings be upon him, said: "If the son of Adam (that is, a human being) had two valleys full of gold, he would wish for a third one!" (Bukhārī and Muslim)

It is in the nature of human beings to want more. The first sin committed was the sin of wanting more. It is very easy to become preoccupied with chasing our dreams or working hard just to get by. It is also very easily to become oblivious of our quality of life, how we treat others, how we feel and the present moment. Stress, work and family responsibilities as well as routines can trap us in a pattern of negative thinking that feeds on itself and creates more stress and unhappiness. This negativity is what makes us unable to show gratitude or excel in this world and the next.

Truly humans were created very impatient; fretful when evil touches them; and grudging when good touches them. (Qur'an 70: 19–21)

The Prophet, peace and blessings be upon him, said: "I saw Hellfire and I never saw a scene like it, and I saw that most of its people are women." They (the Companions) asked, "O Messenger of Allah! Why?" He said: "Because of their disbelief." They asked: "Do they disbelieve in Allah?" He replied: "They are ungrateful to their spouses for what they provide for them; if one were to be kind to one of them for ages, and then she sees one make a mistake just once, she would say: 'I never saw any good from you.'" (Bukhārī)

Our subconscious mind is constituted of "neural pathways" that are established in the brain as a result of our conditioning and past beliefs, and it governs 90 percent of our thoughts, actions and drive us to survive and thrive, thus shaping our behaviour. The subconscious relies on our perception of the world. We are constantly bombarded with negativity, so training the subconscious to be more positive is important for our overall health. Because negativity is all around us, we have to make a conscious effort

181

to keep our mind and heart positive on a daily basis so that we can truly be people of gratitude.

When we consciously turn negativity into positivity, the neural pathway associated with negativity takes time to come down fully, so it is critical to continue showing gratitude on a regular basis. Our thoughts and subconscious are powerful, as unconscious negative thoughts can undermine our health, while positive thoughts can boost the immune system and heal disease.

And He gave you of all that you asked for, and if you count the Blessings of Allah, never will you be able to count them ... (Qur'an 14: 34)

The Prophet, peace and blessings be upon him, advised: "Look at those who are inferior to you and do not look at the ones above you, for this is more likely to make you not despise Allah's blessings." (Muslim)

- Training the subconscious.

As soon as you wake up in the morning, take a moment to think about ten things you are grateful for. You should start your morning on a positive note because this will influence the rest of your day. Be thankful for simple things, things that you take for granted, things that go well, people and events from the past that have helped you be who you are today. Focus on happy memories.

Prophet Muhammad, peace and blessings be upon him, taught us: "He who wakes up in the morning healthy in his body, safe in his residence and having his day's sustenance, is as if the entire world has been granted to him." (Tirmidhī, Ibn Mājah and Ibn Ḥibbān)

Keeping a journal and writing about the things that you are grateful for also increases your gratitude. You could decorate your journal with things that remind you of your purpose in life and help you feel positive, like pictures and inspirational quotes. After writing about what you are grateful about, you can write down all your negative thoughts and then change them by finding what is positive in those situation that prompted these negative thoughts.

- Expressing gratitude.

Showing appreciation to those who have helped you in your daily life will help you and motivate others, thus creating a peaceful environment. You can easily incorporate gratitude in any situation, and, especially when you combine it with relaxation techniques, like deep breathing and walking outside, the effects then can be powerful. That positive attitude should always be a part of us, even when visiting the sick.

The Messenger of Allah, peace and blessings be upon him, said: "When you visit a sick person, say good words to him for the sake of Allah, for although that does not prevent any harm, it still brings relief to the patient's heart." (Tirmidhī)

In a sound hadith, the Messenger of Allah, peace and blessings be upon him, used to supplicate for the sick or afflicted person by say to them: "It is all right, you will be purified (through this affliction), Allah willing." (Bukhārī)

Trusting in Allah – Surrender to Allah's Will

Say, "Nothing shall ever happen to us except what Allah has ordained for us. He is our Mawla [Master, Helper and Protector]. And in Allah let the believers put their trust." (Qur'an 9: 51)

And Mūsā [Moses] said, "O my people! If you have believed in Allah, then put your trust in Him if you are Muslims [those who submit to Allah's Will]." (Qur'an 10: 84)

As discussed above, trusting in God helps us feel light and spiritually connected, allowing us to increase resilience to the world around. Studies have shown that trust in God improved mental health indices.[3]

Forgiveness Frees the Soul

Whoever forgives and makes reconciliation, his reward is due from Allah. (Qur'an 42: 40)

.. And that which Allah has is better and more lasting for those who believe ... and when they are angry, they forgive. (Qur'an 42: 36–37)

The believers are truly brothers. So make reconciliation between your brothers, and fear Allah, that you may receive mercy. (Qur'an 49: 10)

Acts that have offended or hurt us can always remain part of our life, thus smouldering our health. But these can increase inflammation, preventing us from completely healing from chronic disease. Forgiveness involves a decision to let go of resentment and thoughts of revenge, and this lessens our hurt. Forgiveness helps us focus on other positive episodes of life, which can lead to feelings of understanding, empathy and compassion for the ones who hurt us.

Don't Get Angry

Those ... who repress anger, and who pardon people; verily, Allah loves the doers of good. (Qur'an 3: 134)

First, we need to control anger, forgive and then be good. Islam teaches us to respond to evil with good actions, which then purifies the heart and spirit, so we can get back in control of our life. Always aim to resist getting angry, just as we should consign our hurt and pain to Allah.

A man came to the Prophet, peace and blessings be upon him, and asked him for advice and so the Prophet, peace and blessings be upon him, said to him three times repeatedly: "Do not get angry." (Bukhārī)

Controlling our temper is not an easy task: it needs patience, wisdom and struggle against our ego.

This is why Prophet Muhammad, peace and blessings be upon him, said: "Who do you count as strong among you?" The Companions said: "The one who throws people down (during fights)." He, peace and blessings be upon him, said:

No! The strong one is the he who controls his temper when he gets angry. (Muslim)

The Prophet, peace and blessings be upon him, taught Muslims how to control anger and rage with this advice:

Anger is from the Devil, and the Devil is made of fire, and fire is extinguished by water; so if anyone of you gets angry, let him perform minor ritual ablution. (Aḥmad)

Those ... who repress anger, and who pardon people; verily, Allah loves the doers of good. (Qur'an 3: 134)

Learning to Forgive

Scientists have shown that suppressing emotions (fear, grief, worry, stress, trauma) can supress the immune system and contribute to disease. Learning to forgive is essential to our spiritual health and it gives us inner peace. Forgiveness is far from easy, especially when a great deal of trauma is involved.

Allah, glorified and exalted is He, rewards those who forgive with a tremendous reward.

And whosoever is patient and forgives, indeed that is of the steadfast heart of things. (Qur'an 42: 43)

Whatever is with you, will be exhausted, and whatever is with Allah [of good deeds] will remain. And those who are patient, We will certainly pay them a reward in proportion to the best of what they used to do. (Qur'an 16: 96)

... Let them pardon and forgive. Do you not love that Allah should forgive you? And Allah is Oft-Forgiving, Most Merciful. (Qur'an 24: 22)

... If you pardon [them] and overlook, and forgive [their faults], then verily, Allah is Oft-Forgiving, Most Merciful. (Qur'an 64: 14)

In order to forgive, try to understand the others' actions and bring compassion and understanding to the situation. Trauma is part of one's life, and most people have dealt with it in some form- add statistics- 70% of adults in the U.S. have experienced some type of traumatic event at least once in their lives. More than 2/3rds of children report at least one traumatic event by the age of 16, Trauma should not drag one down.

In order to learn to forgive, it is imperative to address the present, acknowledge that it existed, and change the situation. Always aim to change to a situation that is better. This helps to assign a new meaning to your hurt and pain and assign a new positive label to them. Be grateful for every moment of hurt or pain, because they complete your identity. Other ways to release suppressed emotions are daily prayers, crying to Allah, and even writing a letter to those who caused the hurt. When you write it down, it can help you release the pain from the body. You do not need to send the letter; in fact, you can throw it away or burn it after writing it. Pain and hurt may take a long time to subside and be forgiven, but once it is done, it will be the biggest burden ever lifted from your shoulders.

Daily Prayers and Asking Allah for Forgiveness

[The believers whose lives Allah has purchased are] those who repent to Allah [from polytheism and hypocrisy, etc.], who worship Him, who praise Him, who fast [or go out in Allah's Cause], who bow down [in prayer], who prostrate themselves [in prayer], who enjoin doing good [all that Islam ordains] and forbid [people] from evil [all that Islam has forbidden], and who observe the limits set by Allah [do all that Allah has ordained and abstain from evil deeds which Allah has forbidden]. And give glad tidings to the believers. (Qur'an 9: 112)

Praying five times per day is meant to heal our souls. In prayer, concentrate on connecting with the Divine. Surrender all your worries and hurt to Allah, Who has the power to heal you.

Not so those devoted to Prayer: those who remain constant in their prayers. (Qur'an 70: 22–23)

And those who [strictly] guard their worship. (Qur'an 70: 22)

Seeking Allah's forgiveness (*istighfār*) is a gift for all Muslims. Through asking for forgiveness, we return to our Lord whenever we step out of bounds.

And [commanding you]: Seek the forgiveness of Allah, and turn to Him in repentance, that He may grant you good enjoyment for a term appointed, and bestow His abounding Grace to every gracious one [i.e., those who help and serve the needy and deserving, physically and with their wealth, and even with good words]. (Qur'an 11: 3)

Prophet Muhammad, peace and blessings be upon him, said: "By Allah, I seek Allah's forgiveness and repent to Him (saying, *Astaghfir Allāh wa atūbu ilayhi*) more than seventy times a day." (Bukhārī)

And Allah would not punish them while you [Muhammad] are amongst them, nor will He punish them while they seek [Allah's] Forgiveness. (Qur'an 8: 33)

... And enter the gate in prostration [or bowing with humility] and say, 'Forgive us', and We shall forgive you your sins and shall increase [reward] for those who do good. (Qur'an 2: 58)

Then Adam received from Allah Words. And Allah pardoned him [accepted his repentance]. Verily, He is the One Who forgives [accepts repentance], the Most Merciful. (Qur'an 2: 37)

... And all of you repent to Allah, O believers, that you may be successful. (Qur'an 24: 31)

The Prophet, peace and blessings be upon him, once told his Companions: "A man went to a vast field with a camel loaded with food and fuel. He fell asleep, and when he awoke, he did not find his camel. He began to search for it, running to and fro, and after the sun and his hunger had exhausted him, he said: 'I will go back to the place from where I started my search to sleep such a sleep that it may cause my death.' Then, he placed his head upon his hands and slept there waiting for his death. When he awoke, he found his camel standing before him with the food and water. His joy then knew no bounds to the extent that he said in confusion: 'O Allah! You are my slave and I am your Lord!' Allah becomes more pleased with the repentance of the believer than this man's joy." (Muslim)

Prayer and *isthigfār* bring us closer to Allah and relieve our hearts from worry. Religious/spiritual beliefs and practices improve mental health and make us adapt more quickly to health problems compared to those who are less religious/spiritual.[4]

Reading and Contemplating the Qur'an

Had We sent down this Qur'an on a mountain, you would surely have seen it humbling itself and being torn asunder by the fear of Allah. Such are the parables which We put forward to humankind that they may reflect. (Qur'an 59: 21)

The miraculous Qur'an is a Book of guidance and instruction for Muslims. As our understanding increases, we start to understand the Qur'an, which is timeless for all generations and walks of life. The Qur'an is beautiful in its words, rhythm and meanings, all of which lead to peace.

Allah, glorified and exalted is He, says in His Holy Book:

Has not the time come for the hearts of those who believe [in the Oneness of Allah] to be affected by Allah's Reminder [this Qur'an], and that which has been revealed of the truth? (Qur'an 57: 16)

Allah asks His created beings over and over again to use their understanding and learn more. The more we learn, the more we understand the Book that Allah, glorified and exalted is He, has sent down to mankind. This Book is a complete guidance and healing, physically, spiritually and mentally.

Know that Allah gives life to the earth after its death! Indeed We have made clear the Āyāt [proofs, evidences, verses, lessons, signs and revelations] to you, so that you may understand. (Qur'an 57: 17)

[This is] a Book, the Verses of which are perfected [in every sphere of knowledge], and then explained in detail from One [Allah], Who is Most Wise and Well-Acquainted [with all things]. (Qur'an 11: 1)

....it is (the Qur'an) to those who believe a guidance and a healing... (Qur'an 41: 44)

And We send down from the Qur'an that which is a healing and a mercy to those who believe [in Islamic monotheism and act on it], and it increases the oppressors and wrong-doers in nothing but loss. (Qur'an 17: 82)

To begin this healing journey and optimize your spiritual health, you must open up the Qur'an. Studies have shown that listening to the Qur'an lowers stress, anxiety and optimizes healing for the mind, soul and body.[5] Some studies have shown the beneficial effect of listening to the Qur'an on patients who are on hemodialysis.[6] Another study proved that the sound of the Qur'an is an effective treatment for those who suffer from spiritual and psychological issues.[7]

187

Ḥajj - from Materialism to Gratitude and Inner Peace

Ḥajj, the pilgrimage to Makkah, to the House of Allah, glorified and exalted is He (Kaʿbah), is an obligated duty on all Muslims, and is the ultimate spiritual experience.

In it are clear signs [such as] the standing place of Abraham. And whoever enters it shall be safe. And [due] to Allah from the people is a pilgrimage to the House – for whoever is able to find thereto a way. But whoever disbelieves – then indeed, Allah is free from need of the worlds. (Qur'an 3:97)

When we begin the *Ḥajj* we leave all worldly things behind and embark on a journey to seek Allah's forgiveness and mercy. We leave behind our family, children, wealth and all our comforts to please Allah, glorified and exalted is He, and Allah alone. *Ḥajj* is attended annually by about 3 million Muslims from all corners of the earth. The rituals of *Ḥajj* commemorate the struggles of Abraham, his wife Hagar and their son Ishmael and their surrender to God. *Ḥajj* reminds us of the Day of Resurrection, when mankind will be gathered under the blazing sun.

Prophet Muhammad, peace and blessings be upon him, said: "Whoever performs the pilgrimage and does not commit an obscenity or wickedness will return as (pure and free of sin as) on the day that his mother gave birth to him." (Bukhārī, Muslim, Aḥmad and Tirmidhī)

"Whoever performs the pilgrimage and does not commit any obscenity or wickedness will return (from it) as (pure and free of sin as) on the day when his mother gave birth to him." (Bukhārī and Muslim)

Reflections on *Ḥajj*

Then, when they had both submitted themselves [to the Will of Allah], and he had laid him prostrate on his forehead [or on the side of his forehead for slaughtering]; and We called out to him, 'O Ibrāhīm! You have indeed fulfilled the vision!' Thus do We reward the doers of good. Verily, that was a manifest trial, and We ransomed him with a great sacrifice. (Qur'an 37: 103–107)

.. And whosoever honors the Symbols of Allah, then it is truly from the piety of the heart. (Qur'an 22: 32)

With constant prayer and submission, Muslims forget their worldly luxuries and become in direct contact with people from all over the world. The *Ḥajj* is a reminder that all human beings are equal in the sight of Allah. The pilgrims learn about unity, love and respect for all of humanity. *Ḥajj* teaches us that Allah, glorified and exalted is He, loves simplicity.

By leaving their material belongings behind, Muslims come out of *Hajj* more grateful, realizing that materialism doesn't bring happiness while gratitude does.

Gratitude in → Love, Happiness and Inner Peace in!

O you who believe! Bow down, and prostrate yourselves, and worship Allah and do good that you may be successful. (Qur'an 22: 77)

We fill our mind every single day with worries, thoughts and dreams, but when we fill our mind, soul and body with gratitude and prayer, our body starts to feel inner balance, allowing us to lower inflammation.

Verily, in the heavens and the earth are signs for the believers. And in your creation, and what He scattered [through the earth] of moving [living] creatures are signs for people who have Faith with certainty. And in the alternation of night and day, and the provision [rain] that Allah sends down from the sky, and revives therewith the earth after its death, and in the turning about of the winds [sometimes towards the east or north, and sometimes towards the south or west, sometimes bringing glad tidings of rain, and sometimes bringing the torment], are signs for a people who understand. (Qur'an 45: 3–5)

Finding Your Purpose

Then did you think that We created you uselessly and that to Us you would not be returned? (Qur'an 23:115-116)

Each person has been placed on this earth for a special purpose which is different from one person to another. Once you clear out the clutter in your brain, focus on gratitude and start living mindfully according to the Qur'an and Sunnah and think beyond yourself, you can find your purpose. Research has shown that when we have a strong "purpose in life", we are less likely to develop mild cognitive impairment, heart attacks, strokes and Alzheimer's disease. In fact, such a strong purpose in life helps to keep our brain plastic and preserve our cognitive reserves and lower depression. A lack of purpose has been found to be linked to higher cortisol, more abdominal fat and other negative health markers.

Optimism and gratitude are among the most important elements of mental and physical well-being, along with self-acceptance and positive relationships. Studies have demonstrated the existence of a positive association between religion, good immune health, lower infection rates, lower use of drugs, cigarettes, healthy diet, more exercise, coping with stress, socializing more, experiencing a greater sense of peace and a greater satisfaction with life as well as being calmer.

The Four S's Prescription

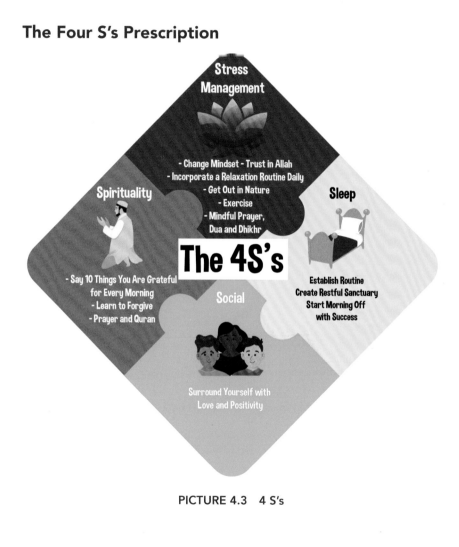

PICTURE 4.3   4 S's

PART 3

Using The Qur'anic Prescription For Healing

Getting Back to Qur'an for Ultimate Healing

And when I am sick, then He, Ever He, cures me" (Qur'an 26:80)

There is no disease that Allah has created except that He has also created its treatment. (Bukhārī)

...Say, O Prophet, "It is a guide and a healing to the believers. As for those who disbelieve, there is deafness in their ears and blindness to it ˹in their hearts˺. It is as if they are being called from a faraway place." (Qur'an 41: 44)

Do people think that they will be left alone because they say, We believe, and will not be tested? (Qur'an 29: 2)

Prophet Muhammad, peace and blessings be upon him, said: "No fatigue, disease, sorrow, sadness, hurt or distress befalls the Muslim, even if it be the prick of a thorn, except that Allah expiates some of his sins for it." (Bukhārī and Muslim)

There is no disease except that Allah, glorified and exalted is He, has made a cure for it; we have just to keep looking for it. We can do no worse than to start living the life that Allah, glorified and exalted is He, has intended for mankind, according to the Qur'an. Whether we are dealing with fatigue, digestive issues, skin problems, mental illness, instability, allergies, autoimmune diseases, chronic pain or even cancer, Allah, glorified and exalted is He, has provided a teacher for everyone.

And We send down from the Qur'an that which is a healing and a mercy to those who believe [in Islamic monotheism and act on it], and it increases the oppressors and wrong-doers in nothing but loss. (Qur'an 17: 82)

Your Body is Your Teacher

We are not here to fight against disease. I think that is where people have been wrong for so long. Disease and illness have been looked at as an enemy with which we are at war and, in a war, someone has to lose. So we need to look at disease and illness as a teacher, instead.

A teacher guides the student, even though such guidance may look too difficult. This teacher (aka the illness) simply tells us that our life is out of balance, and in order to heal and feel better, we need to restore that balance. Teachers don't give us all the answers, but guide us to make the correct ones. Our body does the same. Symptoms are signals from Allah, glorified and exalted, informing us that there is something "off" which needs fixing. These symptoms are due to the body's imbalance. Inflammation is a reaction that takes place when the body is off balance.

193

The Qur'an Brings Balance – Optimize the Elements of a Ṭayyib Lifestyle

This is the Book! There is no doubt about it—a guide for those mindful ˹of Allah˺. (Qur'an 2:2)

O humanity! Worship your Lord, Who created you and those before you, so that you may become mindful ˹of Him˺. (Qur'an 2:21)

A *ṭayyib* lifestyle will heal us and build *taqwā*. When we are mindful, we can put our body back in balance. This balance is restored by getting to the root cause (our individual imbalances) and fixing the deficiencies caused by an impure lifestyle. This lowers inflammation and heals not just one symptom but all of them.

What are the elements of a *ṭayyib* lifestyle? Let us recap here (for more detailed information, please see *The Holistic Rx: Your Guide to Healing Chronic Inflammation and Disease*):

Pure Food, Pure Environment, Pure Thoughts, Pure Words, Pure Friends, Pure Sleep, Positive Thoughts, a Pure Lifestyle = HEALING

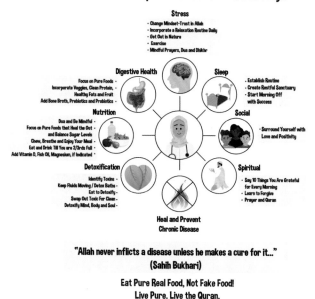

194

1. Optimizing Digestive Health and Detoxification - Purifying Our Food and Environment.
2. Optimizing Stress Management, Sleep, Social and Spiritual Health - Purifying Our Mind and Heart.

Keeping in Mind:

- Starting with *Bismillāh*, a *Du'ā'* and Setting the right Intention!
  In The Name of Allah, The Beneficent, The Merciful. (All) praise is (only) Allah's, the Lord of the Worlds. The Beneficent, The Merciful. Master of the Day of Judgement. Thee (alone) do we worship and of Thee (only) do we seek help. Guide us (O Lord) on the Straight Path. The path of those upon whom Thou hast bestowed Thy bounties, not (the path) of those inflicted with Thy wrath, nor (of those) gone astray. (Qur'an 1: 1–7)

    The end result is in Allah's hands, you just need to wake up every morning to make the most out of your day, and ask Allah for the best of paths. Then set your intention and remember that you are doing this for Allah and Allah alone.

- The "Root Cause" of Disease Differs from Person to Person.

    The root cause which puts an individual out of balance differs from one person to the next. You may be eating the best food, but the root cause lies in the trauma that you have experienced or it is due to an environmental toxin or you may have excellent stress management skills but you're negative-minded (that will definitely throw anyone off balance). Everyone is different.

    So ask yourself: What is making me out of balance? What changes can I do today to start moving a little closer to a *tayyib* lifestyle that will heal me?

- Planning Ahead and Setting a Date.

    You will need to find a period of time to dedicate for your healing. Find a four-week period in which you are able to prepare for and adapt to a different way of eating and living. The first week is usually the hardest and you may possibly experience withdrawal symptoms.

- Your Symptoms May Worsen *First* Before They Get Better.

    When you introduce healthy food and abstain from unhealthy food, the destruction of pathogenic bacteria and viruses begins, causing the release of toxins. You may notice a worsening in your symptoms. This is called a die-off reaction. Fatigue, digestive reactions, low-grade nausea, mild headaches and emotional irritability are common symptoms. Such a reaction depends on the individual. It usually lasts from a few days to a few weeks. Epsom salt baths, sea salt, seaweed, and/or sodium bicarbonate (baking soda) can help with the die-off reaction and speed up recovery. Half a cup in the bath water for thirty minutes is best. Again, do what you can do easily; if a daily use is too difficult, then start with whatever you feel comfortable with.

If you are starting a probiotic, go slowly with it and watch for a die off reaction. If no symptoms occur, then increase the dose of the probiotic gradually. If one notices a die-off reaction, then remain on that dosage until the symptoms disappear. If the symptoms are hard to deal with, you can space out the doses (that is, take the supplements less often) to help relieve some of the symptoms. Once the symptoms subside, gradually increase the dosage. Continue this process until you reach twenty billion organisms daily or whatever dosage keeps you feeling well. You have just to be patient and take it one day at a time.

- Healing Takes Time

If you have been dealing with chronic inflammation for a long time, then any improvement is better than no improvement – patience is key. Focus on all the symptoms that are improving, because if you focus only on symptoms which are not improving, then you will never get better. Take any and every improvement as a positive step in the right direction, but the process of healing takes time. It doesn't happen overnight, and everyone is different.

Part A: Optimizing Your Digestive Health and Nutrition for Healing

Whenever you put food in your mouth, you need to make sure it will heal you, not hurt. You need to make sure that it will lower inflammation, not increase it. So whenever you put food in your mouth, focus on the following:

1. *Tayyib*/pure foods that will heal the gut.
2. Eating *tayyib* foods in small quantities to keep glucose, insulin and hormones balanced.
3. Eating nutrient dense foods to give your body the nutrients it needs to heal.

Putting Out the Fire in the Gut

As 70–80 percent of the immune system is made of trillions of bacteria in the gut, putting out the fire in the gut will give the body a fighting chance to heal. Everyone is different, but start with the basics and then adjust as required. First, you will need to stop putting gasoline on the fire by avoiding all the foods that are likely to be causing problems. You will then need to take steps to restore a healthy balance of bacteria, replenish nutrients, repair the lining of the gut, and generally rebalance your system.

The idea of making a major change in your diet can be scary, but the sacrifice is worth it. Three to four weeks of a diet consisting of pure foods, and giving the body exactly what it needs for you to heal, is not going to hurt you; especially if you are doing this for the sake of Allah. Your goal is to regain proper balance of good bacteria, stamp out the bad microbes, heal the holes in the gut and lower its inflammation.

Once a minimum of three or four weeks have passed, and once your symptoms have improved/resolved (some might need a lot longer, everyone is different), you will need to be ready to take the next step – reintroducing other *tayyib* foods one at a time while carefully making note if any of them cause problems so that you can exclude them from the diet. A short-term gut healing diet is better than a lifetime of pain and suffering.

After a minimum of three to four weeks, you should feel better. You will know if your gut is healed once you start becoming less dependent on medications (only under doctor's supervision) and your symptoms have improved or disappeared.

Step 1: Remove the *Khabīth* and Some *Ṭayyib* Foods that May Be Bothering You

In order to put out the fire in the gut, you need first to remove ALL the possible offending triggers.

Food

Some of the foods below may be *tayyib*, but because you don't know which foods are causing problems, it is better to exclude all of them. This will take some of the igniter fluid off the fire in your gut, allowing it to calm down and then you can consider your options.

- Gluten/Grains.
  Avoid all gluten and if you can, grains, as they can damage the intestinal cells, feed the bad bacteria, leading to leaky gut.

The Gut Prescription:
5 Steps to Put Out the Fire

1. Remove Gasoline
Impure Foods / Processed Foods
- Gluten / Grains
- Dairy
- Processed Foods
- Sugar
- Food Sensitivities
- Infections

2. Replace
Pure Foods
- Nutrients
- Acid
- Enzymes

3. Repopulate
- Probiotics
- Prebiotics

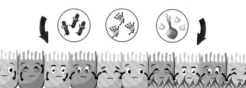

4. Repair Gut Lining
- Bone Broth
- Vitamin D
- Omega 3
- Supplements

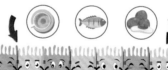

5. Rebalance
- Detoxification
- Stress Management
- Sleep
- Social Support
- Spiritual Health

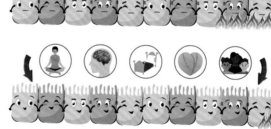

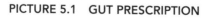

PICTURE 5.1   GUT PRESCRIPTION

- Dairy
- Sugar
- Soy
- All *khabīth* foods such as nutrient-depleted foods, processed foods (full of poor-quality fats and oils [commercial liquid vegetable oils, hydrogenated oils, and trans fats] and GMOs)
- Specific food sensitivities
- Other *khabīth* foods

You may be tempted to remove just one food at a time, but I recommend taking out all the foods that may bother you. Taking out one food at a time may not help you feel better and can be more discouraging and frustrating. Removing the foods all at once will help you feel better quickly. Once you feel better, you will then be ready to reintroduce each food one at a time to see how you are affected.

However, if removing all the food at once is too overwhelming, then avoid doing that. Stress causes more problems and inflammation, and it should be avoided. Hence, you can start with eliminating gluten, dairy and all the *khabīth* foods.

Most people start to see an improvement in their symptoms when they remove these foods from their diets. If after a couple of weeks you are still not seeing any improvement, then examine all the elements of a pure lifestyle to see which of them is off balance. Otherwise, you may also want to consider eliminating other problematic foods like beans/legumes (some people do well with lentils and navy beans), soy, eggs, nightshades, and nuts, as these can cause inflammation in some people.

Other Common Food Sensitivities

Eggs (organic and pasture-raised) are a great source of proteins but they contain lysozyme (protective enzyme that breaks down the cell membrane of the gram negative bacteria), which can increase intestinal permeability, and may even lead to allergies for some people.

Nightshade vegetables, like tomatoes, white potatoes, bell peppers, eggplant and spices, like cayenne pepper, paprika, and red pepper flakes, are to be avoided if you continue to have problems. They contain a variety of compounds like solanine, chaconine, and lectins which can worsen leaky guts.

Beans can be a great source of minerals, proteins and fibre, especially for vegetarians, but for some they may be inflammatory. First, they are pretty starchy, so for those with pre-diabetes or diabetes, it is best to limit them as much as possible. Moreover, beans and other legumes contain lectins,[1] phytates,[2] and saponins, which act like natural pesticides and are difficult to digest. They can also worsen the digestive function by causing an overgrowth of the bad bacteria, irritating the lining of the small intestine, leaky gut,[3] impairing the absorption of nutrients and minerals, and spiking blood sugar, which in turn creates inflammation[4] and autoimmunity.[5] Peanuts (a legume) can also lead to problems due to fungal aflatoxin.

For those with sensitivity to legumes and beans, pre-soaking, sprouting, fermenting and pressure cooking these foods can decrease the lectins and their harmful effects and improve digestion and absorption. Legumes to restrict include black beans, garbanzo beans, lentils, lima beans, soybeans and white beans.

Caffeine can be beneficial for some when taken in the right amounts, for others it may lead to more problems, especially if it leads to sleep problems. It should be avoided by those who have a mood disorder or insomnia, as it can lead to more anxiety and irritability. If you still need caffeine, then aim to drink it before 1 p.m. But if you are looking to wean off, try to make sure to take it very slowly, drink plenty of water and rest. Vitamin C may also help you decrease the withdrawal effects.

Nuts and seeds can also be problematic for some because of their lectins[6] leading to leaky gut[7] and nutrient deficiencies.[8] Soak and cook them to reduce their negative effects.

Other Sensitivities to Consider

You can also be sensitive to certain foods that may contain histamine (which can lead to headaches, allergy like symptoms, specifically after ingesting histamine foods like avocados, nightshades, fermented foods, bone broth, tea, and spinach), sulfates, salicylate, oxalate (compounds promoting kidney stones and inflammation) like spinach, rhubarb, beets, chocolate, pecans, almonds and beet greens. Cooking, sprouting and fermenting can reduce oxalates and lectins. Lectins are proteins that bind to sugars and may cause the inflammation of the digestive system and consequently, leaky guts, as well as symptoms like autoimmune conditions, aches and pains. Foods high in lectins are grains, pseudograins, legumes, eggplants, goji berries, peppers, nuts and seeds.

**If you have multiple food sensitives, or you are very frustrated with your condition, I highly encourage you to follow the GAPS introduction diet without dairy (see appendix).

Remove Infections

You will also need to remove infections that increase intestinal inflammation and stop bacterial overgrowth – like viruses, parasites, yeast, and small intestinal bacterial overgrowth (SIBO: good bacteria in the wrong place). Find an integrative, holistic and functional medical practitioner who is able to help you figure out what other chronic infections you may be dealing with. Then you can use a pharmaceutical or natural combination like for example berberine (active against candida albicans and staphylococcus aureas), wormwood, caprillic acid, grapefruit seed extract (antimicrobial and antifungal), garlic (active against bacteria, fungi, viruses, and parasites), oregano oil, and peppermint oil.

Step 2: Replenishing with Ṭayyib Food and the Ability to Digest

After that, you need to proceed to restoring and replenishing the vitamins, minerals, nutrients and essential ingredients for proper digestion and absorption which have been depleted by a *khabīth* diet, medication, disease, and/or aging. To do this, incorporate healing *ṭayyib* foods that Allah, glorified and exalted is He, has provided and replace any deficiencies necessary for digestion.

Replenishing with Healing Ṭayyib Food

A. First replenish with nourishing food which are packed with fibre, polyphenols, prebiotics and probiotics that can strengthen your GI tract and help your brain function properly. Instead of focusing on what you can't eat, focus on what you can. The following need to be part of every meal:

- Vegetables
- Clean protein
- Healthy Fat
- Water
- Low glycaemic fruit

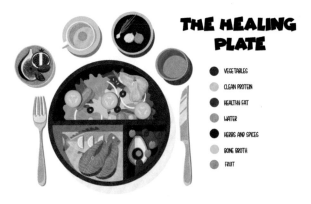

PICTURE 5.2   THE HEALING PLATE

Other foods for gut healing include:

> Abū Dharr related that the Prophet, peace and blessings be upon him, said: "O Abū Dharr, when you prepare broth put plenty of water in it and take care of your neighbours." (Muslim)

- Bone broth and collagen are rich in bioavailable, easily absorbed minerals like calcium, magnesium, phosphorus, silicon, and sulphur,[9] and these nutrients are necessary to support the immune system. Bone broth also contains amino acids like L-glutamine (energy source for your intestinal cells), glucosamine, chondroitin, collagen gelatin, proline, and glycine, all of which help repair, seal, soothe, and restore gut mucosal lining and lower inflammation. Try to have at least one cup a day of bone broth.
- Fermented foods should be added if tolerated. Fermented foods can actually feed the good and bad bacteria, so it is best to add fermented foods as you continue to heal your gut.
- Herbs that reduce inflammation include: black seeds, turmeric, rosemary, and ginger.

Optimizing the Ability to Digest

If you are eating healing foods, try to make sure that you are also digesting the foods you are eating. Keeping your stomach at an appropriate pH is key in optimal digestion.

Start the day with a glass of water mixed with lemon. With each meal, try to drink half a cup of water with half a teaspoon of raw apple cider vinegar. Digestive bitters (arugula, dandelion greens, wild berries, ginger, citrus peel, cocoa, tea, coffee and extra virgin olive oil) can also help to boost stomach acid, reduce inflammation and even manage blood sugar. If your symptoms don't improve within four weeks, you might need digestive enzymes to help break up macronutrients and absorb the nutrients you need from food. Try to have a plant-based enzyme formula along with an enzyme blend, especially the ones with protease, amylase, and lipase.

Too much stomach acid can cause reflux and other symptoms, but too little can cause bloating, an inability to break down food or activate digestive enzymes, as well as an overgrowth of yeast and bacteria. The means of decreasing stomach acid include alcohol, antibiotics, stomach medications, caffeine, hypothyroidism, imbalanced microbiome, nicotine, and chronic stress. You can easily check your acid level with a baking soda test. First thing in the morning, before eating or drinking anything, mix ¼ teaspoon of baking soda in 4–6 oz. of cold water and then drink the baking soda solution. Make a note of how long it takes you to belch, which should be up to five minutes. Any belching after three minutes indicates a low acid level. Betaine hydrochloric acid supplements can be helpful while your gut is healing if you carefully follow these guidelines: You should start with one capsule or tablet at the beginning of each meal, then increase the dose by one capsule per meal until you have a warm feeling in the stomach. You should then drop back down to the dose just before the warm feeling occurred. You should stay on it for one to two months, then stop and see how you feel.

Step 3: Repopulate

Restoring the balance of good bacteria in your gut is absolutely crucial to overall health. You can accomplish this by using probiotics (helpful bacteria) and prebiotic, fibre-rich foods.

Probiotics

Probiotics are found in fermented foods such as unpasteurized natural sauerkraut, kvass (fermented beet juice), fermented vegetables, kimchi, brined olives without vinegar, natto, miso and tempeh. They're also found in yoghurt and kefir, but these are dairy products, so you should not be eating them during this phase. Before refrigeration was invented, all cultures developed methods of making foods last longer, and one of these methods is fermenting foods. Vinegar, heat and pasturization kill bacteria in fermented foods, so avoid any probiotic food that has added sugar or vinegar. Most probiotic foods provide Lactobacillus and Bifidobacteria strains (natto offers Bacillus subtilis). Probiotics support and strengthen the gut lining, crowd out the bad bacteria and stop them from colonizing. They also improve the absorption of nutrients, reduce inflammation, nourish the cells in the colon and liver, create new compounds like B vitamins, vitamin K2, antioxidants, and enzymes, and lower the amount of harmful pathogens like candida, fungi, and parasites.[10]

Food is the best way to get probiotics and, in some cases, it is the only way to get certain bugs like Akkermansia. However, you can also take them through supplements (powder or capsule). These are generally safe but you should consult your physician if you are immunocompromised. It is best to take the probiotics with or after food.[11] You should look for a mixture with at least ten strains, like lactobacilli (especially plantarum and brevis), bifidobacteria (longem and lactis), and soil-based organisms, such as endospore probiotics like bacillus subtilis and bacillus coagulans. Soil bacteria have a number of added benefits. You should choose a product that is condition appropriate when it's available.

You should start slowly at one billion organisms daily and gradually go up to twenty billion organisms daily, or until you are rebalanced and feeling well. People are different in this respect, as they can need anything between fifteen billion to one hundred billion CFU, so you should find a dosage and supplement that is right for you. It is recommended that we keep taking the supplements for about six months in order to re-establish normal gut flora. You can even change them every three to six months, but you should remember that probiotic foods are key in optimizing gut health.

Mushroom mycelia and Saccaromyces boulardii are good yeasts that fight the bad yeast and restore normal flora in the intestinal tract. They help lower inflammation by having an antitoxin and antimicrobial effect and destroying pathogenic yeast like Candida albicans.[12] Yeast-based probiotics may improve SIBO, while spore-based probiotics can increase lactobacillius, thus improving gut diversity.

Prebiotics

Prebiotics are "food" for probiotics. They nourish and stimulate the growth of "good" bacteria while reducing disease-causing bacteria such as clostridia, klebsiella and enterobacter. They work with the probiotics to optimize gut healing. Prebiotics play an important role in healing the gut to decrease inflammation.[13] It is recommended to prebiotics found in green leafy vegetables and other high-fibre foods, which are especially good at promoting the growth of good bacteria, along with asparagus, carrots, garlic, leeks, raw onions, radishes, tomatoes, apples, flax seeds, garlic, Jerusalem artichoke, konjiac root, seaweed, pear, chicory root, cocoa, dandelion greens, and burdock root.

It is important to increase the biodiversity of the microbiome by exposing yourself to the external world and also by being cautious about the soil in which your foods grows.

Step 4: Repair

Repairing the gut lining is important to ensure the proper absorption of nutrients and gut function. You should eat lots of food that helps to repair the gut lining, such as foods with zinc (lean beef and poultry, nuts such as cashews and almonds) and vitamins A (carrots, dark leafy greens, winter squash, lettuce, dried apricots, cantaloupe, bell peppers, fish, liver, tropical fruits), C (bell peppers, dark leafy greens, kiwi, broccoli, berries, citrus fruits), and D (tuna canned in water, sardines canned in oil, beef or calf liver, egg yolks or cod liver oil), Omega-3, vitamin E and selenium, which improve inflammation and heal the gut lining. It is recommended that to continue drinking bone broth, a minimum of one cup per day. Bone broth is powerful in regenerating the gut wall lining. The following supplements can also help soothe inflammation and continue healing the gut:

- Probiotics are the most important part of resealing, through food or supplement.
- Omega-3 (2–4g per day with meals) improves inflammation and heals the gut lining.
- Digestive enzymes are nutrients that completely break down what we eat, which can reduce intestinal inflammation. You should look for the ones with protease (it breaks down proteins including gluten), amylase (breaks down starches), lipase (it breaks down fats), lactase (it breaks down lactose in dairy) and DDP IV.
- L-glutamine, 5g twice daily with meals, helps to preserve the gut lining, lowers inflammation 100. L-glutamine can be found in bone broth and also in animal proteins and raw spinach, red cabbage and parsley.
- Others include zinc carnosine (30 mg per day), colostrum powder, turmeric, slippery elm (200 mg per day), aloe vera (100 mg per day), licorice root, DGL (500 mg per day specifically for leaky gut exacerbated by emotional stress), frankincense (an essential oil that helps heal leaky gut and lower inflammation), quercetin (500 mg three times per day with meals), chamomile, organic sulphur compounds, methylsulfonylmethane (MSM), boswellia powder, marshmallow root (100 mg per day), butyric acid or butyrate, and plantain.

Ultimately, you should find what works best for you.

Step 5: Rebalance Through Living a *Ṭayyib* Life

Rebalancing by living a *ṭayyib* lifestyle can lower inflammation. Focus on activities that add diverse microbes from the soil which will help to balance the microbiome and lower stress. You should add activities like gardening, spending time walking barefoot outside (which will help improve sleep, raise energy, and lower inflammation by stabilizing the internal bioelectrical environment), shopping at local farmers markets for fresh produce, swimming in the ocean and fresh water lakes (decreases skin inflammation, RA, and psoriasis).[14] Getting a pet will also diversify the microbes in your home.[15]

Reintroducing Foods

When your symptoms have subsided or disappeared, you can begin reintroducing foods. You will need to listen to your body, as it will inform you whether you are ready for that food or not. If you are not, it is recommended that you stay on the healing diet and consult with a holistic or functional health care practitioner, as it may take time to heal, depending on your condition and how long you have been dealing with it. It's very important to re-introduce one food at a time and to pay careful attention to whether or not your symptoms return.

Start with the food that you miss the most. Eat that food in the most pure form for a couple of days and pay attention to how you feel. On day three, stop eating that food while continuing to observe how you feel. Because sensitivities can take up to seventy-two hours to manifest, it is important to wait and see if symptoms develop. When the re-introduction phase is complete, you will know exactly which foods you can eat and which ones cause problems. If you relapse, meaning you're your symptoms return, it could be because you have eaten a food which you are sensitive to, or it may happen because of deficit despite being on a good diet, as deficits in any of the other processes talked about in the first chapter may induce a relapse. Antibiotic therapy is another common reason for relapse. If you are prescribed an antibiotic and want to avoid a relapse, you should take a probiotic with 50–100 billion CFUs in between the antibiotic doses and stay on the probiotic for three times the length of the antibiotic course.

Here's what to do if you have a relapse:

- Make sure to implement all the elements of a *tayyib* lifestyle, to keep your body balanced.
- Cut out the food that leads to problem.
- Add digestive enzymes if needed, as you may not be digesting food properly which leads to further irritation.
- Continue with the probiotic.
- Monitor symptoms and stay as strict as you can for a couple of weeks, so you can get to where you would like to be and then start to re-introduce other foods again, when ready.

If your symptoms are not improving, then you may need to go back to the beginning of the gut healing diet (5 R program above) or start a stricter and more structured gut healing approach (like the GAPS introduction diet without dairy).

Other Tips for Health and Improving Insulin Resistance

- Begin the morning with water and lemon.
- Eat and drink until you are two-thirds full.
- Eat food mindfully. Remember to breathe, really enjoy meals, and chew every bite well.
- Fasting three to four hours in between meals (and up to two snacks per day).
- Stop eating and drinking at least three hours before going to bed; intermittent fasting can help to break the cycle of elevated insulin levels.

- Cutting out foods of a higher glycaemic load.
- Always combine carbohydrates with clean protein and healthy fats.
- Intermittent Fasting.

Living in a Pure Environment to Heal

Identify what is *khabīth* in the environment, move the liquids in your body, eat to detoxify and change what is *khabīth* in your food and lifestyle to that which is pure, because all this can help you heal, as discussed in Part 2, Chapter 1. But some people may need extra help in order to help them figure out the causes of their problems. And one of the common and overlooked problems that bother so many people is mould.

Mould

If you still do not feel adequate after a couple months, despite doing all the above, or perhaps you develop an autoimmunity in the process, then mould could be the cause of inflammation.

Mould is most common in damp and humid areas like the bathroom and basement, especially in older homes and in homes with basements, where there are known leaks, crawl spaces, flat roofs, and those built on a hillside. Some moulds are easy to detect, like black mould, but others are not so easy to detect. Mould can also be found under floorboards, anywhere there's a crack in the wall or window frame, making it even harder to detect or even on the carpet. Mould can also be ingested, such is the case with pistachios, cashews, peanuts, aged cheese, vinegars, pickled foods, dried fruit, and mushrooms. The symptoms of exposure to mould may include depression and other mood disorders, ADHD, skin rashes, headaches, autoimmunity, sleep issues, fibromyalgia or fatigue. Testing for mould is tricky because the typical mould test only focuses on air quality and the level of mould spores. Hence, you should find a functional medicine physician to assess this for you in a more detailed fashion. Sometimes it is best to find a mould-free place to stay for a while and see if one feel better. If you feel better away from home, and worse when returning home, then you could be reacting to mycotoxins. If this is the case, the approaches provided in this book will be helpful.

Optimizing Stress, Sleep, Social and Spiritual Health

Tackling Stress

As discussed above, stress leads to 80 percent of the complaints that come to primary care physicians, so no matter what you are doing, it all comes down to how you manage stress. Therefore make sure you incorporate stress management techniques and an exercise routine, spend time in nature, prayer, *dhikr* and du'ā' to really optimize your healing.

Optimizing Sleep

Sleep is key to the healing process, so if you are having problems with sleep, you need to figure out the underlying root cause. Being off balance can affect your sleep and if you are not sleeping, you can be thrown more off balance.

Stress and disease can lead to inflammation, causing sleep issues that further worsen the problem. So targeting the root cause is the key to sleeping better. The first thing to ask in such a scenario is whether you have been dealing with this problem recently or for a long time.

For short-term insomnia, you should then ask whether you are stressed out due, for example to an upcoming exam or performance, jet lag, change in work schedule or emotional stress. The problem could also be related to the way you sleep (sleep hygiene) as a sleep hygiene problem can lead to insomnia. Long term sleep issues can be due to chronic conditions, medication or sleep hygiene issues. For example, antidepressants, cold and flu medications that contain alcohol, pain relievers that contain caffeine (Midol, Excedrin), diuretics, corticosteroids, thyroid hormone, high blood pressure medications (beta blockers, calcium channel blockers), anticonvulsants, bronchodilators, decongestants, and stimulants all affect sleep. If you are having any of these medicaments then supplements may help to optimize your sleep until you are able to restore balance to your body.

If you are having sleep problems due to shift work or because of travel/jet lag issues, then you should try to adjust your sleep-wake cycle by exposing yourself to bright light while you are awake and wear dark glasses on the journey home. You should also try to keep your schedule as regular as possible. Sometimes you can take extra supplements to help you get sleep.

Social Health

The people around us can either make or break us, so try to keep friends and family around who will lift you up rather than drag you down. Remind yourself to follow the commands of Allah regarding how to treat those around you.

Spiritual Health

This is probably the most important part of your healing journey. Immediately after you wake up in the morning, say ten things you are grateful for every day. You need to shift your negativity by showing gratitude.

Fixing The Deficiencies

Living healthy and boosting our immunity always starts with diet, there is no other way round this. In 2014, the *Nutrition Journal* published an extensive review which showed that people who take vitamins and minerals delay the onset and severity of serious diseases, including heart disease, brain issues and even cancer. Supplements can give you the extra push in the right direction toward healing, support the immune system and allow it to be healthy and balanced. Nutritional deficiencies can interfere with your recovery, so taking supplements can give you the extra boost you need to expedite healing. Because of present toxic/*khabīth* conventional and commercial farming practices (as discussed in part 1), the standard American diet is full of processed foods and low on microbial diversity. Stress and toxins can decrease the absorption of nutrients and increase inflammation. Also, the older we get, the harder it becomes for the body to absorb nutrients. Medications can also lead to deficiencies; examples include the following:

- Proton pump inhibitors and H2 receptor antagonists cause depletions of beneficial flora; calcium; digestive enzymes; folic acid; B12; vitamin C, D, E, K; biotin; chromium; and zinc.

- Antidepressant medications like SSRIs diminish melatonin, iodine, selenium, and folate. You should not take St. John's wort, 5-HTP, or SAMe without talking to your healthcare provider first. Others diminish B2 and CoQ10.

- Oral contraceptive pills diminish vitamin B2, B5, B6, folate, B12, magnesium, zinc, vitamin C. You should avoid drinking grapefruit juice as it can increase oestrogen levels up to 30 percent.

- Antibiotics deplete good bacteria; vitamins B1, B2, B6, B3, B12, vitamin K (if antibiotic is taken for more than ten days); calcium; magnesium; and potassium.

- Antidiabetic drugs diminish coenzyme Q10, vitamin B12; metformin can deplete B9, B12, and possibly CoQ 10; insulin can deplete magnesium. Aspirin diminishes vitamin B1, biotin, folate, C, iron, and zinc. Take aspirin before taking niacin.

- Stronger anti-inflammatory drugs like steroids diminish potassium, vitamin C, zinc, vitamin D, selenium, calcium, folic acid, and magnesium.

- Medication which lowers blood pressure diminishes calcium, vitamin B6, B1, vitamin C, zinc, sodium, potassium, and magnesium.

- Oral contraceptive pills diminish zinc, vitamin B2, vitamin B3, B6, B12, folic acid, magnesium, vitamin C, and tyrosine.

- Thyroid replacements like Synthroid diminish calcium.

How to Choose a Supplement?

If you decide to use a supplement, you must remember that the supplements industry is largely unregulated, so you must be sure that you are using products made with integrity, and always read the labels. Look for large reputable brands and FDA approval and make sure it is third-party tested and follows good manufacturing practices. You should also check for the initials USP, GMP, or NSF to make sure the product doesn't contain additives, synthetic ingredients or colourings. Purchasing from supplements companies that use organic ingredients is an added bonus. Check the expiration date and make sure the product is fresh. Your best insurance is to purchase supplements from natural health stores or through a healthcare provider properly educated in quality professional supplements. Always check with a licensed primary care practitioner before starting a supplement. Moreover, you should not exceed the recommended dosage.

Vitamin D is a vitamin or prehormone which is an essential precursor to hundreds of disease-preventing proteins and enzymes, as it binds to many receptors and causes changes to cell function. D3 is made when the sunlight hits the skin. The liver and kidneys then transform vitamin D into a more active form, allowing the cells to read DNA instructions more effectively, which is important for your genetic code. Vitamin D regulates vital components of hormones and neurotransmitters, such as serotonin and helps control cell growth. It is also a cancer fighter and essential in mineral metabolism, as well as being a major player in bone strength, as it regulates the absorption and transport of calcium, magnesium and phosphorus for the mineralization and growth of bones. Vitamin D is a disease preventer and vital in decreasing inflammation and lowering insulin resistance.

Deficiency in vitamin D is strongly linked to autoimmune disease.[16] Most patients are deficient in vitamin D because of their lack of exposure to the sun and sunblock that blocks the ultraviolet B rays needed to convert vitamin D to its active form. There are two different types of vitamin D, vitamin D2 and vitamin D3. Vitamin D2 occurs in plants and vitamin D3 increases blood levels better than vitamin D2.

Look for a range of about 50–80 mg/ml to optimize health. It is best to have your physician check your vitamin D 25OH lab value. If you work closely with a professional, he or she can prescribe the appropriate dose to quickly increase your vitamin D level. Always make sure that you take vitamin D3, as vitamin D2 isn't metabolized by the body. Once it is optimized, you should continue a dosage which is about twenty times your weight in pounds daily or 2,000–4,000 IU per day is appropriate. A vitamin D overdose is rare but it is possible as a high vitamin D level (greater than 150 ng/ml) leads to excess calcium in the bloodstream, which can damage the kidneys and can even lead to psychosis. Remember to take vitamin D and other fat-soluble vitamins with meals containing fats. You should be cautious with vitamin D if you have hyperparathyroidism, Hodgkin's or non-Hodgkin's lymphoma, granulomatous disease, such as sarcoidosis and tuberculosis, kidney stones, kidney disease or liver disease. If you are looking for a natural way to optimize vitamin D, you will need to expose at least 40 percent of your skin to the sun, just until it turns pink or one shade darker. Try to sunbathe from around noon to 1 pm, using mineral-based sunscreens to help optimize vitamin D conversion. Foods that are also rich in vitamin D include sea vegetables, fish (especially sardines, salmons, and mackerel), beef liver, some cheeses, mushrooms like portabellos, eggs, raw milk, and cod liver oil yolks.

Cod liver oil provides DHA, vitamin A, and D3 and to a lesser extent vitamins K and E, which help in the absorption and utilization of minerals and nutrients, and fight inflammation, as it is fermented preserving the essential oils in the fish. Some don't tolerate vitamin D supplementation and do better with cod liver oil. Since fermented cod liver oil has twice the vitamin A and D3 of regular cod liver oil, only half the amount is needed. If you don't use fermented cod liver oil, it is recommend to have butter oil in conjunction with a high-vitamin cod liver oil. About 1 tsp high-quality cod liver oil is usually recommended.

Vitamin K, another nutrient that people don't get enough of, is necessary to prevent calcification and clotting and is essential in bone, brain and immune health. There are two forms: K1 and K2. Vitamin K1, important for blood clotting, is easier to get as it is found in most green vegetables like lettuce, broccoli and spinach. K2, important for cardiovascular protection, cancer and strong bone, is found in dietary sources like fermented foods and is produced by bacteria in the gut. Its function is to show calcium where to go, and in doing so it helps to reduce calcification in the arteries and improve the calcium intake into bones and helps restore the ability of cancer cells to die. Upon increasing your vitamin D intake through supplements, you can create a relative insufficiency of vitamins K, A, and E. Vitamin K2 or MK-7 is needed for vitamin D to work effectively. A dose of 100–250 µg K2 daily or 50 µg for every 5,000 IU of D3 is beneficial. So when you take vitamin D or calcium supplement, try to make sure that you meet your vitamin K needs, by eating enough greens, fermented foods, nuts, cod liver oil, liver, and organ meats. Please make sure that you don't mix vitamin K1 with warfarin.

Magnesium is an essential mineral especially for nerve cells, mood, cognition, muscles and bones and has a major role in immunity.[17] About 75–80 percent of people are deficient in magnesium because of their acidic diet and constant fluoride exposure.[18] Cells need magnesium to work, for it binds to 3,700 different sites in the body, including more than three hundred enzymes and hundreds of body processes that use or synthesize ATP, DNA and RNA, cofactors in methylation and detoxification. Magnesium is also vital in muscular contractions and in the production of testosterone and progesterone, the production and utilization of fat, protein and carbohydrates, in the metabolism of calcium, sodium, and potassium; and is a constituent of bone and teeth. You need magnesium to avoid premature aging in your fibroblasts, which are cells in the connective tissues like bones, cartilage and tendons. Magnesium can help to reduce spasticity in muscles; improve chronic pain; improve digestion, mood and sleep. : It will also help you relax and it widens blood vessels, lowers blood pressure, increases HDL, lowers TG and hsCRP, and improves cardiovascular health, arrhythmias and blood sugar.[19] Deficiency in magnesium is linked to heart disease.[20] Deficiency in magnesium can also accelerate aging in several cell types and interfere with the division and renewal of cells. When you are deficient in magnesium, you can feel fatigued, anxious, experience chronic pain or cramps, have difficulty sleeping, feel numbness and tingling in extremities, heart racing or abnormal heart rhythms, and also experience carbohydrate cravings, loss of appetite as well as problems in blood sugar regulation, leading to chronic illness.[21] Ideally, taking about 350–400 mg of elemental magnesium by mouth every day will help fix the deficiency. Even though magnesium glycinate, chelate and maleate are absorbed best, magnesium citrate is great for constipation and sleep issues. Try to avoid magnesium supplements if you have poor kidney function; and if you are constipated, then avoid magnesium oxide. Try to make it a habit to take magnesium and calcium at least two hours apart from your multivitamin/mineral supplement. Sources of magnesium are green leaves, like frozen spinach, Swiss chard, avocados, dark chocolate, artichoke hearts, almonds, cashews, pumpkin and squash seeds, salmon, halibut, sea vegetables, tea, legumes, quinoa and meat. One of the richest sources of dietary magnesium is coffee.

Fish Oil

Fish oils are rich in essential fatty acids, like Omega-3 and Omega-6 fatty acids, which are needed for the work of cell membranes, and can't be produced by the body so they need to be consumed. Their use has been beneficial for a wide array of medical conditions. Essential fatty acid, specifically Omega-3, helps to improve the immune system, improve blood chemistry, promote brain and heart health, lower triglycerides and increase HDL.[22] It also improves insulin sensitivity, protects against depression, digestive disorders, arthritis, asthma, and Alzheimer's, just as it improves skin, nail, and hair strength, increases nutrient absorption, improves fertility and prevents and heals chronic disease by lowering inflammation.[23] Some studies suggest that patients with breast, prostate and non-small cell lung cancer may derive benefit from a supplementation of fish oil.[24]

Sixty percent of the brain weight is made up of fat, and 25percent of that fat is DHA. Omega-3s are predominantly anti-inflammatory because they reduce the expression of inflammatory genes and molecules in the body, while Omega-6 promotes the expression and release of pro-inflammatory prostaglandins and interleukins. Omega-3 foods include coldwater fatty fish like sardines, herring, wild caught salmon, lake trout, mackerel, shellfish, clams, oysters, mussels, pasture-raised chickens, grass-fed meat (grass-fed beef has fewer Omega-6s compared with soybean- or corn-fed cattle), antelope, shrimp, squid, organic, eggs, walnuts, and flax and chia seeds. DHA is found in algae. If you are a vegetarian, eating a seaweed salad several days a week or taking a seaweed supplement with DHA is an effective way to benefit from Omega-3s. The body needs docosahexaenoic acid (DHA) to make myelin, and eicosapentaenoic acid (EPA), is very helpful in lowering inflammation. Omega-3 acid supplementation has been found to be helpful in a variety of autoimmune conditions.

Doses of 1–4 grams are recommended when taking fish oil supplements. For rheumatoid or other arthritis, 3,000 mg per day of EPA plus DHA is suggested. For general support of the immune system, try 1,000–2,000 mg per day. If you are a vegetarian, you can take 1,000–3,000 mg of flaxseed oil, but it isn't as potent as taking fish oil. Krill oil can also be good, because it is low in toxins and heavy metals and has the same level of EPA and DHA as fish oil.[25]

Always be sure to get fish oil that's clear of heavy metals, PCBs, pesticides and other toxins, because if the fish is contaminated, then the fish oil is contaminated too. Omega-3 causes platelet inhibition, so common side effects can be belching, halitosis, heartburn, nausea, loose stools, rash, increased bleeding and bruising (mostly seen with 3g or more a day). The risk of bleeding in patients on blood thinners shouldn't be a concern because of the low dosage. Do make sure to check with your physician first, as INRs should be carefully monitored in patients who start taking Omega-3.

Our Balanced Children

One of parents' worst nightmares is seeing their children consumed by a chronic health condition. The bodies of our children are very similar to our own bodies, but just a little smaller. Look for any subtle signs that indicate that the health of your child may be becoming imbalanced.

Normal children are full of fun and excitement; they are engaged and have the energy to keep up with those around them. They have eyes that are clear and bright with no dark circles, swelling or redness. They can fall asleep in less than thirty minutes, eat a variety of foods including vegetables and fruit. They have little or no gas, bellyaches, or snake-like poops.

If your child has any symptoms of colic, gas, spitting up, indigestion, congestion, rash or hives, cough, difficulty breathing, abdomen digestion, constipation or other digestive issues, chronic ear infections, cradle cap, projectile vomiting, fits/tics, sinus issues, or adenoids, these may be risk factors which can develop into bigger health problems such as autism, autoimmune disease, or mood disorders. So look out for these symptoms because they are signs that their little bodies are off balance.

If you notice such symptoms, remove one or two of the problematic foods at a time, starting from the food that your child eats the most, following the programme above. Though there is no standard protocol, for those with serious issues – like colitis, autoimmunity, seizures, or autism – a gut healing diet like GAPS (Gut and Psychology Syndrome Diet) along with avoiding food which causes sensitivities like dairy and following the foundations of good health (section one) is a great starting point. Breast-feeding mothers can follow the same protocol, eliminating and watching symptoms in their baby.

They may need extra supplements for digestive health:

- Probiotics can be given to babies born with C-section and/or had history of yeast, antibiotics or steroids during pregnancy, labour or while nursing. Probiotics can also be considered if there is a family history of increased intestinal permeability issues, like autoimmunity or metabolic syndrome. Keep a look out for lactobacillus acidophilus and bifidobacterium infantis. Dosage depends on age.
  - Infants up to twelve months: 1–2 billion of bacterial cells per day; one to two years of age: 2–4 billion per day; two to four years: 4–8 billion per day; four to ten years: 8–12 billion per day; and twelve to sixteen years: 12–15 billion per day.
- Digestive enzymes: younger than five years old: pinch of digestive enzyme powder with each meal; older than five: ½ teaspoon with each meal.
- Glutamine powder: 1.5g of glutamine powder twice daily if your child is over four years old. Supplements should be added slowly and gradually, as some children with autism may regress with certain supplements like B12 or GABA/glutamate. Children with folate deficiency should not have ANY kind of dairy, including camel's milk.

It is very important that you clean up your child's surroundings. The child's developing brain is very sensitive, so pesticides and other environmental toxins can disrupt the endocrine system and lead to neurodevelopemental disorders. Heavy metal detoxification is very important for improving autism and helping the body maximize glutathione. Optimizing gut health, limiting the daily toxin exposure and even integrative modalities (like homeopathy) will help protect against any adverse effects of vaccines.

Managing stress is very important for any child to learn early. Their thoughts, feelings and emotions directly affect their physical health. Your way of parenting can directly affect your child's brain chemicals. The bonds of love and respect that you can develop by being involved in his or her life can release oxytocin and natural opioids, which decrease stress response systems, providing the child with feelings of well-being, and help the brain to develop. It's important to get down and cuddle, play, look at your children in the eyes when they talk, laugh, read to them, and provide them with imaginative and explorative activities. Offer them an encouraging, safe, serene, well-structured environment, keeping the lines of communication with them open, all while being careful not to judge or negate their feelings, and also disciplining them in ways to preserve their dignity. Children need order in their lives with clear boundaries. Always be aware and honest about your own stressors and emotions as children are like sponges and can sense and absorb even subtle changes in your mood or behaviour. This will help lower everyone's stress.

While children are developing and learning, we should instill in them lifelong coping mechanisms, to increase their resilience in life. Try to help them to understand their feelings and use their words. When they are at an appropriate age, Teach them prayer, *du'ā'*, *dhikr*, and abdominal breathing, all with mindfulness meditation.

Sleep is just as important for children (maybe even more than it is for adults), and a bedtime routine is very important. They should end the day with prayer, meditation, words of encouragement and hope.

By starting and ending the day with gratitude, children are taught that everything they eat or wear is for Allah only and that they should take care of the gift that Allah has given them. Thus, you start changing your children's perspective on their bodies and relationship with the world around them.

When the gut microbiomes of children are balanced, their hormones, minds and bodies are balanced too.

Taking the Healing Further

As discussed above, the elements of a *tayyib* lifestyle are important and should be the starting-point.

Finding an Integrative, Holistic, Functional Medicine Physician

Try to find a practitioner through a referral from a friend, family member or your conventional doctor. It is important to always check education and credentials, then set up a pre-appointment phone call or appointment with the practitioner of interest to get a good idea of the practitioner and the practice. During this interaction, be prepared with a list of questions and concerns, and because most healthcare plans don't cover alternative integrative modalities, it is important to enquire about any upfront costs. Always be cautious of any practitioner makes excessive claims and insists on signing one up immediately for a specified number of treatments. It is important to be open with your primary care provider about what other modalities you are pursuing and any list of herbs and medications you are taking. This will keep an open and honest relationship with your providers.

Lab Tests

Once you have found a suitable health care practitioner who is willing to listen and spend the time needed with you, work with him or her to get an initial set of lab tests. This will help you address individual deficiencies and issues.

The following tests are those your primary care doctor should feel comfortable ordering, and if coded appropriately, most insurances cover them. To get these tests, just request them from your doctor. These tests can be repeated every one to three months depending on your personal situation.

However, there is a difference between optimal and normal. Optimal is what your body functions best at, as normal is anywhere within that large range that doesn't classify as low or high. I have provided the target/optimal ranges that I use and the interventions I typically recommend for my patients. Your personal physician may work with slightly different targets/ optimal ranges and interventions.

Base line labs I get on my patients are CBC, CMP, fasting insulin, fasting lipids, ferritin, homocysteine, hsCRP, vitamin D, HbA1c, TSH and thyroid antibodies, ANA, B12 and magnesium.

Labs	Target Fasting Levels	Interpretation/Suggested Intervention
Complete Blood Count (CBC)	Normal values for the target range.	If the levels become, anaemia and other abnormalities will need to be ruled out. Gut healing needs to be stressed.
Comprehensive Metabolic Profile (CMP)	Normal values for the target range. Fasting glucose: less than 90 mg/dL Calcium: less than 10 mg/dL	If fasting glucose is elevated, IR management is stressed. If calcium is higher than 10, carefully dose vitamin D, to prevent parathyroid issues. If liver tests are elevated, look for other causes and improve insulin resistance.
Thyroid Stimulating Hormone (TSH)	Ideally 0.5- 2.5 microIUu/mL	If abnormal, work with a physician to find the underlying root cause and proper treatment options. Work with your doctor to begin a combination of T3 and T4 medication such as compounded T3/T4 or natural desiccated thyroid.

Labs	Target Fasting Levels	Interpretation/Suggested Intervention
Free T4, Free T3, Reverse T3 TPO antibody Antithyroglobulin Antibody	Free T4 1.3-1.8ng/dL Free T3 3.0-4.5 pg/mL, Reverse T3 less than 20 ng/dL TPO antibody <9 IU/mL or negative ATA <4 IU/mL or negative	If elevated, address root cause. If the antibodies are elevated, address autoimmunity. Most hormones will decrease with age. If reverse T3 is elevated, it can be due to excessive exercise, starvation diets, stress, or heavy metals.
Magnesium	Serum Mg > 2 mg/dL RBC Mg 5-6.5 dL	There isn't a great test to check the exact levels in your blood. But practitioners can get a sense that you are deficient and if it is less, need to supplement 1000 mg of Mg for 3 weeks then maintain at 500 mg per day.
25-hydroxy Vitamin D (vitamin D25-OH);	50–80 ng/mL	Adjust vitamin D dose up or down according to level. There are multiple ways to dose vitamin D; work with your doctor to determine how much supplemental vitamin D you will need. Blood level more than 45 ng/ml or for maintenance: 2000–4000 IU daily depending on sun exposure, activity level, age, etc. Levels 35–45 ng/ml, correct with 5000 IU of D3 for 3 months. Levels <35 ng/ml correct with 10,000 IU of vitamin D3, depending on level. Best taken with food, calcium, and with vitamin K.

(continued)

Labs	Target Fasting Levels	Interpretation/Suggested Intervention
Folate and Vitamin B12	In the top quartile of the reference (range for that lab) B12 >500 pg/mL Folate 10-25 ng/mL	Interpret with homocysteine, if lower than 500 add 1000 mcg of B12 × 3 weeks and then maintain 500 mcg every day, but may need more; if you have SNPs, please check with your doctor.
Homocysteine	4–8 micromole/L	Homocysteine level reflects methylation, inflammation and detox. If elevated, that means you are not breaking down toxins well (i.e. not methylating well). Add B12 500 mcg q day, folate 50 mcg q day and B6 50mg q day and recheck in 3 months; if still high once folate and B12 are optimized, see a functional medicine practitioner for guidance. If low, add more protein to diet. If high, switch to the methyl forms of folate (methylfolate) and methyl forms of B12 (methyl B12). Also a vitamin B complex like B-100.
Highly Sensitive C-Reactive Protein (hs-CRP)	Less than 1.0 mg/L (milligram/liter) = low risk (ideal) 1–3 mg/L = intermediate risk Greater than 3 mg/L = high risk	These levels you want low. If high, follow the foundations of good health and see your practitioner for further guidance. Following a gut healing protocol and/or low glycaemic diet will help improve the inflammation. Stress can also lead to elevated hsCRP, so it is important to incorporate a relaxation technique into your daily routine.

Labs	Target Fasting Levels	Interpretation/Suggested Intervention
Fasting Lipids	Triglyceride/HDL cholesterol ratio less than 3	A ratio greater than three indicates probable insulin resistance. Decrease carbohydrate intake and increase intermittent fasting. This may indicate need for more fish oil. Advanced lipid evaluation measures cholesterol particle size and inflammatory markers. This test will also provide information about heart risk factors like Lipoprotein (a), Apolipoprotein A-1 and B, and if you are absorbing too much cholesterol or making too much cholesterol.
HDL Cholesterol (good cholesterol)	HDL cholesterol greater than , 60 mg/dL (milligram/deciliter)	If HDL is less than 60, decrease carbohydrates, increase vegetables and berries and other low glycaemic foods, increase fish oil, and increase exercise.
Fasting Insulin	Less than 10 microIU/mL, ideally below 5 microIU/mL	If higher, concentrate lowering insulin resistance by following a low glycaemic diet and intermittent fasting
HbA1c	Less than 5.4 percent	If higher, concentrate on lowering insulin resistance. If it remains elevated despite perfect diet and lifestyle.
Antinuclear Antibodies	Negative	For all autoimmunity, gut healing is very important. If positive, discuss with your doctor.

(continued)

Labs	Target Fasting Levels	Interpretation/Suggested Intervention
Other Hormones	DHEA Sulfate: 300-450 mcg/dL Pregnenolone: 50-150 ng/dL Total testosterone:500-1000 ng/dL Free Testosterone 6.5-15 ng/dL Progesterone- vary with age and cycle Estradiol- vary with age and cycle	
Other Vitamin	RBC Zinc 12-14mg/L Serum selenium: 110-150 ng/mL	If low, supplement zinc with 30-60 mg of zinc daily. If low in selenium, start consuming selenium rich foods.
Other Inflammatory Markers	Interleukin-6: < 3 pg/mL TNF-alpha: <6pg/mL	
Ratio of Omega 3s to Omega 6s	At least 3:1	If not ideal, cook with healthier oils, don't eat fake food and take a fish oil supplement
Insulin Like Growth Factor 1	Less than 200	As we grow older, we don't want this number to increase, as it could point to cancer if it is increasing.

Any Change is a Good Change!

Any change is a good change! But if after three months you have still not seen enough changes, then go through the following checklists on Digestive Health and Detoxification and The Four S's. Instead of getting frustrated, keep looking for what your teacher is trying to teach. What is still out of balance in your life? What can you do today to get healthier than you were yesterday?

Digestive Health and Detoxification

- I am complying with all the recommendations of the foundations of good health.
- I have followed the Gut Prescription or other gut healing diets.
- I am successfully avoiding all trace exposure to gluten and other grains.
- Could legumes/lentils, nightshades, nuts, seeds, and eggs be causing problems? Or could there be other food sensitivities (e.g., histamine or salicylate intolerance)?
- I have double-checked ingredients on supplements, medications, spices, and prepackaged and prepared foods.
- I eat a large variety of vegetables, with other green foods, proteins, and healthy fats at each meal.
- I am drinking broth regularly.
- I am moderating my intake of high-glycaemic-load foods.
- I am fasting three hours between meals and intermittent fast when I can.
- I am not eating three hours before bed.
- I eat appropriately sized meals with an appropriate amount of time between them.
- I am drinking enough water but avoid excessive liquids with meals.
- I eat probiotic foods or take a probiotic supplement.
- I use sea salt or Himalayan salt.
- My environment is toxin free.
- I have asked my doctor to check genetics and methylation issues.
- I am taking gut healing supplements as needed.
- I am taking the appropriate supplements for optimal general health and organ function support.
- I have identified my possible toxic exposure.
- I am eating to detoxify.
- I am taking Epsom salt baths as often as I can.
- I am dry brushing, finding ways to sweat and keeping my fluids moving.
- I have swapped toxic for clean.

The Four Big S's: Stress, Sleep, Social Health, and Spirituality

- I am learning to relax and use my breath.
- I am respecting my boundaries, and I say no when I need to and ask for help and accept it.
- I make sure I am having fun every day.
- I offer mindful prayers, *du'ā'* and *dhikr* every day on time.

- I spend time in nature.
- I am engaging in some sort of mild to moderate intense activity every day.
- I make sure I get eight to twelve hours of quality sleep every night and nap when I need to.
- I practice good sleep hygiene (sleeping in a cool, quiet, dark room and making positive sleep associations).
- I sleep and wake up the same time each day.
- I make time to nurture positive social connections.
- I am practising gratitude daily.

Let's Take it a Step Further

Sometimes even the best intentions aren't enough, and it is important to find the right person to guide you and help you get organized because this will help you get and stay on the path toward healing. Hence, go to a functional medicine or holistic practitioner, nutritionist or health coach to help you figure out the right food/lifestyle plan. It is important to work with your doctor to assess food allergies/sensitivities, supplements/medications to support organ function, any persistent infections, GI tests to assess your individual gut imbalances, your toxic load/liver detoxification/ heavy metal poisoning, mould exposure, hormone regulation and sometimes checking your specific genetic profile, with the help of a practitioner who can tailor a specific plan that will work best for you.

1. Food Sensitivities and Gut Testing:
   To help guide treatment, there are a number of testing methods for gut issues – some of which have been around for decades, others are very new, and always changing to help guide treatment.
   - Listen to your body.
   - Food Sensitivity Testing: IgG and IgE tests can check for food sensitivities. Once you find out what you are sensitive to, you can then try to avoid it for a certain period, and add in a gut healing diet, so you can continue the healing process.
   - Comprehensive Stool Testing: A comprehensive stool test is a non-invasive test that gives a picture of some of the organisms present in a patient's GI tract, as well as some sense of bacterial balance as well as the presence of yeast.
   - SIBO Testing: A lactose breath test or hydrogen or methane breath test can check for SIBO (small intestinal bacterial overgrowth), the leaky gut and an organic acids test reveals vitamin and mineral deficiencies.

If there is SIBO or SIFO (small intestinal fungal overgrowth), it is best to start treatment right away. You can start by switching to a spore form- ing probiotic or even adding in saccharomyces boulardii, stop any fer- mented foods and stay on a lower carb gut healing diet. Then you will need to eradicate the bacteria that is growing in the wrong place, by anti-microbial herbs like oil of oregano or biocidin. It is important to find out what led to the SIBO. Are there problems with digestion? For instance, low stomach acid may lead to SIBO so you may need to add more stomach acid or digestive enzymes. Surgery? Drugs (like opiates)? Magnesium deficiency? Slow gut motility (diabetes or thyroid issues)? Or even pancreatic insufficiency? Therefore talk to your healthcare prac- titioner to address appropriately your individual situation.

2. Nutritional Evaluations
The body needs nutrients to work appropriately, and these tests will determine what nutrients you are deficient in. These tests will give you a report of what the nutrient levels look like in your body.

3. Environmental Toxins
If you are still not feeling better, environmental toxins may be the culprit, as you could be exposed to something that is putting you out of balance. There are so many tests to see what exact toxin you may be exposed to. For those with high toxic load, it may be beneficial to add supplements to optimize healing.

It is important not to detoxify too early, as you need a healthy gut and adre- nal system for detoxification not to backfire. As discussed previously, probiot- ics and digestive enzymes (specifically with lipase) optimize gut healing and improve the digestion of fats. Glutathione (600–1,200 mg acetyl-glutathione daily), or N-acetyl cysteine (600–1,800 mg daily), along with vitamin C (2000 mg daily), and a liver support blend with alpha lipoic acid (300–600 mg daily) and milk thistle (150 mg twice daily) – all can be taken on an empty stomach. If you are diabetic, be aware that ALA can lower blood sugar levels. R-alpha- lipoic acid is more active and better absorbed.

If it is felt that you have a high toxic load, it can be very difficult to do a detox programme on your own, therefore find a professional. A professional can test for genetic mutations or other errors in liver detoxification that can also slow the recovery, like single nucleotide polymorphisms (SNPs) (MTHFR, GSTMI, and COMT SNP gene mutations). If any level is positive, then tak- ing large doses of a premethylated B vitamin (B6, B12, and folinic acid) and glutathione will help optimize function and detox, along with everything else above. B12 also is needed for proper functioning of the brain and nervous system. Chelation, by your practitioner with dimercaptosuccinic acid (DMSA), may need to be done, especially if you have constant yeast infections, spent time in China, have amalgam fillings, eat tuna more than once a week, work with toxins regularly, or have SNPs. It is important to make sure that you have fully healed your gut before chelation.

4. Chronic Infections

Certain microbes can be causing your symptoms. Chronic infections, specifically viral ones, can be dormant and get activated or triggered with an inflammatory response and a weakened immune system. Viruses like herpes (e.g., 1, 2, 6), Epstein-Barr virus, hepatitis etc., and certain bacterial infections which can go along with autoimmune conditions include yersinia enterocolitica, H. pylori, SIBO/SIFO, Chlamydia pneumoniae, bartonella, mycobacterium avium subspecies paratuberculosis (MAP), mycoplasma, streptococcus, babesia and borrelia burgdorferi (Lyme), fungal infections like candida, and parasitic infections like toxoplasmosis and blastocystis hominis.

5. Genetic Testing

This test will help guide the practitioner to a specific nutritional plan and targeted nutrients you may need. Genetic testing will help you adjust your lifestyle to optimize your gene function, and upregulate different genes for health. A professional can test for genetic mutations/variations or other errors in liver detoxification that can also slow the recovery, like single nucleotide polymorphisms (SNPs) (MTHFR, GSTMI, and COMT SNP gene mutations). If you have genetic variations in B vitamin genes, you may need higher doses and special forms of these nutrients.

6. Stress Issues

This healing journey can be frustrating and you can feel very lonely. This is true especially in times of chronic stress when your body requires extra nutrients to support the adrenals, as stress in and of itself can deplete vital nutrients like magnesium, vitamin C, Omega-3 and the B vitamins.

Certain plant compounds and supplements known as adaptogens can help balance and modulate the stress response, helping to lower some of the negative effects of chronic stress. Ashwagandha (500mg once or twice daily) lowers cortisol and balances hormones. Other adaptogenic herbs are Asian ginseng root extract (200 mg twice daily), cordyceps (containing both cordycepic acid and adenosine, 400 mg twice daily), rhodiola root extract (50 mg twice daily), and holy basil. Homeopathy and acupuncture are also great options.

If you start to notice warning signs like an inability to sleep, depression, using drugs or alcohol to cope with stress, negative and self-destructive thoughts or fears that are beyond your control, or thoughts of suicide, it is time to seek immediate professional help.

Always Remember: You may need medications to put out the fire before you control the blaze. As an adjunct to the foundations of good health, aim to apply these additional integrative modalities in conjunction with the advice of your doctor.

Integrative Modalities

Along with the pillars of optimal health, integrative modalities are great tools to expedite healing, if alongside a practitioner. For an acute or chronic issue, work with your doctor to address the issues medical and holistically, using modalities that I will discuss here to adjunct your conventional care. There is so much more we can do to adjunct healing by investigating and addressing your underlying root causes and improve current symptoms, with conventional and integrative modalities like supplements, homeopathics, acupressure, aromatherapy, cupping, ruqyah, mind-body medicine and so much more. For a deeper dive into integrative modalities for 80 + conditions, please see *The Holistic Rx: Your Guide to Healing Chronic Inflammation and Disease.* There are so many other integrative modalities and practitioners that one can see and incorporate into their care, so the options are endless. Alhamdulillah!

Staying Motivated – With So Much Hope

When you don't feel well, the motivation to implement what we just learned is hard. Taking it one step at a time – preparing the mind, body, and soul – can help you succeed.

1. *Cultivate a grateful mindset and surrender to Allah's will.* You deserve a happier and healthier life, so much to already be thankful for. You are doing this for Allah, everything you do or spend is for Allah, may He be glorified and exalted.

   So keep your duty to Allah and fear Him as much as you can; listen and obey; and spend in charity; that is better for yourselves. And whosoever is saved from their own covetousness, then they are the successful ones. If you lend to Allah a goodly loan [i.e., spend in Allah's Cause] He will double it for you, and will forgive you. And Allah is Most Ready to appreciate and to reward, Most Forbearing. (Qur'an 64: 16–17)

2. *Discovering your reason.* Your body is a gift which has a right over you. So why do you want to do this now? To be pain-free, to achieve your dreams? What do you want to accomplish when you are healed? Do this only to be the best that you can be for the sake of Allah.

225

3. *Set goals and targets.* Setting achievable goals and targets, with set specifications and dates, will help to optimize your success.

4. *Identify your obstacles.* What is stopping you from doing this right now? After identifying those obstacles, come up with a plan of action that will help you overcome them, taking it one day at a time, one obstacle at a time.

5. *Out with the khabīth and in with the ṭayyib.* Now, bid farewell to all the inflammatory *khabīth* foods that keep sabotaging you.

6. *Set a routine.* Routines work! Find what works for you and stick to it. What is the best time for exercise? Meal planning? Grocery shopping? You should plan your meals ahead of time. On the weekend, plan your food for the upcoming week so that you can go shopping and have everything you need. Every minute in between can be used to your benefit, fit in more walking, do some deep breathing, *du'ā'*, *dhikr*, mindful meditation and gratitude – any of these can be done anywhere!

7. *Build your own positive support system and be prepared.* Inform those around you that you are trying to eat healthy, and let them know their help and support would be appreciated. Try to bring your own food to events and stick to "the list" when going to any event. Never go completely hungry, and say no to food pushers.

8. *Don't overwhelm yourself.* Take one meal at a time, one day at a time. Going down that list will make it less overwhelming.

9. *Setbacks are actually steps forward.* If you slacken in following all the instructions, it's fine, just get back on track. Your setback is the platform for a stronger comeback. Every setback is an opportunity to grow and realize that you are human!

10. *Be patient.*
.. *Only those who are steadfast shall receive their rewards in full, without reckoning.* (Qur'an 39: 10)

And We made from among them [Children of Israel], leaders, giving guidance under Our Command, when they were patient...(Qur'an 32: 24)

Whatever is with you, will be exhausted, and whatever with Allah [of good deeds] will remain. And those who are steadfast, We will certainly pay them a reward in proportion to the best of what they used to do. (Qur'an 16: 96)

And certainly, We shall test you with something of fear, hunger, loss of wealth, lives and crops, but give glad tidings to the steadfast ones. Who, when afflicted with calamity, say: Truly, to Allah we belong and truly, to Him we shall return. They are those on whom are the blessings [i.e., who are blessed and will be forgiven] from Allah, and [they are those who] receive His Mercy, and it is they who are the guided ones. (Qur'an 2: 155–157)

Prophet Muhammad, peace and blessings be upon him, said: "Wondrous is the case of the believer; there is good for him in everything, and it is so for (the believer) only. If he experiences something agreeable, he is grateful to Allah and that is good for him; and if he experiences adversity, he is steadfast (patient) and that is good for him." (Muslim)

Growing and Learning – Trusting in Allah

And they ask you, [O Muhammad], about the soul. Say, "The soul is of the affair of my Lord. And mankind have not been given of knowledge except a little." (Qur'an 17:85)

You should never give up. Keep praying for Allah's guidance. You can try your best, the rest is up to Allah.

Prophet Muhammad, peace and blessings be upon him, said: "The likeness of the believer is as a stalk of com which the wind does not cease to blow down; even so trials do not cease to fall upon the believer. The likeness of a hypocrite is as a cypress tree which does not bend (or shake) unless it is felled." (Bukhārī and Muslim)

In a similar hadith, he, peace and blessings be upon him, said: "The parable of the believer is that of a herb, the wind pushes it over and straightens it in turn, until it strengthens." (Bukhārī)

.. It may be that you dislike a thing and Allah brings through it a great deal of good. (Qur'an 4: 19)

It may be that you dislike a thing which is good for you and that you like a thing which is bad for you. Allah knows but you do not know. (Qur'an 2: 216)

After applying the elements of a *ṭayyib* lifestyle, any little improvement in the right direction is a HUGE improvement. Small improvements are better than no improvement, and one step in the right direction is better than no steps. Even a step backward can make you stronger!

Verily! In the creation of the heavens and the earth, and in the alternation of night and day, there are indeed signs for people of understanding. Those who remember Allah [always, and in prayers] standing, sitting, and lying down on their sides, and think deeply about the creation of the heavens and the earth, [saying], 'O Allah! You have not created [all] this without purpose, glory to You! [Exalted be You above all that they associate with You as partners.] Give us salvation from the torment of the Fire. (Qur'an 3: 190–191)

Healing Prescription Recap

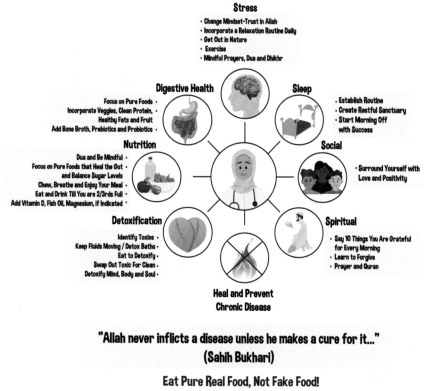

PICTURE 5.3 QUR'ANIC PRESCRIPTION

228

Conclusion

"...And whosoever fears Allah...He will make a way for him to get out (from every difficulty). And He will provide him from (sources) he never could imagine." (Qur'an 65:2–3)

"Verily, His Command, when He intends a thing, is only that He says to it: Be! And it is" (Qur'an 36: 82)

Time to Start Living Qur'an and Sunnah and Take Back Control!

"And I [Allah] created the jinns and humans only so they should worship Me [Alone]." (Qur'an 51: 56)

"Satan threatens you with poverty and orders you to commit sins; whereas Allah promises you Forgiveness from Himself and Bounty, and Allah is All-Sufficient for His creatures' needs, All-Knower" (Qur'an 2: 268)

We live in a world where we are no longer truly the slaves of Allah, we are slaves to the food industry, we are slaves to the economy, we are slaves to the material goods we possess or run after, and we are slaves to the pharmaceutical industry. We are all stuck on this hamster wheel just trying to get by. But as we try to get buy, we are destroying our bodies, increasing climate change, killing plants and animal species to extinction, disrupting the soil and threating our future.

"... Verily Allah will never change the condition of a people until they change what is in themselves ... " (Qur'an 13: 11)

To truly get back to Allah, so to change ourselves, we must step off the hamster wheel and get back to truly living the Qur'an and Sunnah. Allah (SWT) has sent down

229

this book and His example as a timeless guidance for all of mankind. Society will continue to change its rules, confusing us all of what is right and what is wrong, what is best for the human souls and the planet and what is wrong for the human souls and the planet. Allah (SWT) has given us the clear instructions to ensure we are no longer slaves to society but slaves to Allah (SWT) alone, to help us succeed in this life and the next, to save our planet and our future.

"Say [O Muhammad to people], 'If you [really] love Allah, then follow me [accept Islamic monotheism, follow the Qur'an and the Sunnah], Allah will love you and forgive you your sins. And Allah is Oft-Forgiving, Most Merciful." (Qur'an 3: 31)

The world around us is telling us we have no control over our health, as we simply need to trust the pharmaceutical industry. Don't let the hamster wheel own you! But we do have control. We have control to take care of our bodies and environment the best we can and the rest we leave up to Allah (SWT).

Allah Chose YOU!

Allah chose you, out of a billion and plus people in the world, Allah chose YOU to be guided. Most will look past this or skim it without understanding.

"The example of those who disbelieve is like that of one who shouts at what hears nothing but calls and cries cattle or sheep - deaf, dumb and blind, so they do not understand." (Qur'an 2:171)

But Allah chose YOU to understand. Take that as a medal of honor. Allah has a purpose for each and every one of us- we just need to find it. You can change the circumstances of our present and future, we can work on becoming the very best version of ourselves, to heal humanity and the planet one step at a time.

So ask yourself, who are you? What shaped you? Who do you want to be? What you have already been through can shape you, can change you, but they are not what you have decided to be. They can shape you, not break you. You can't control the past, you can give it to Allah, but you alone can decide what it meant. You are always bigger than the parts that you play, and Allah (SWT) knows that. All your struggles are only the beginning of an amazing transformation—a transformation to find the better you, a healthier you, and a stronger you! Because you are not broken, you are unbreakable.

"...Allah puts no burden on any person beyond what He has given him ..." (Qur'an 65: 7)

"No disaster strikes except by permission of Allah . And whoever believes in Allah – He will guide his heart. And Allah is Knowing of all things." (Qur'an 64:11)

Give yourself permission to heal your wounds, a chance to change for the better, a chance to turn your life around, and the boost you need to get yourself off the ground running! That fall was a blessing in disguise as it gave you the power and motivation to escape the wheel for good! I'm sooo proud of you, as you already took the first, most difficult step— to acquire knowledge and understanding—the most important key that will help you to unlock unimaginable doors, as Allah (SWT) has all the power to change anything and any circumstances.

"Say: Whether you hide what is in your hearts or you reveal it, Allah knows it all. He knows what is in the Heavens and what is on Earth. And Allah has power over all things" (Qur'an 2:29)

Your name is not Muhammad Migraines, Amina Asthma, Idrees IBS, or Haala Hashimotos. These conditions don't have to define you. You can finally take charge of your own health! The fire that rages within your body has kept you stuck—despite that, look at all you have accomplished! It takes someone very special to have done all that you have done, competing with those who are not fighting a battle within! You are a gem—I can't say that enough. Now imagine a life when we actually are not slaves to society, we are slaves to only Allah, when we actually live the Qur'an and Sunnah, with no fire that burns within, a life full of peace, a life full of energy, a life full of unlimited possibilities—what can you accomplish, what will you do? OOO it's already giving me goose bumps because the sky's the limit, I can't wait to watch you fly!

" ... Allah intends for you ease, and He does not want to make things difficult for you ... " (Qur'an 2:29)

With no other distractions and nothing to drag you down, with Allah's help anything you put your mind to could be yours. Your once-distant dreams can now be your reality! You are a blessing to this world and those around you—that is why Allah chose YOU! We need you to change the future of our planet, but it time to first start with you. Let's begin that transformation, it is finally time to start living ṭayyib/pure, and finally escape the hamster wheel for good!

Put Your Trust in Allah (SWT) for True Success

"O you who believe! Be patient and excel in patience and remain steadfast, and be careful of (your duty to) Allah, that you may be successful." (Qur'an 3:200)

When you remember that every bite you are taking, every dollar you are spending, every action is for Allah and only Allah, to take care of the gift that Allah has given us, our bodies, children and our planet, the reward is 1000s fold. The first couple weeks are going to be hard, but if you take one step towards Allah, Allah (SWT) promises he will run towards you (Bukhari). Once you get the hang of it, as the energy and pain improve, it will not be so bad—it's actually quite rewarding. I am here for you! We can do this together! Take it one day at a time, one meal at a time! Slowly you will transform into who you were meant to be, the real and authentic you! Transform to a more energetic you! Transform to a pain-free you! Transform into a happier you! The ups and downs in your journey will only make you stronger!

"To those who do right is a goodly [reward], Yes, even more [than in measure]!.." (Qur'an 10: 26)

"Allah will establish in strength those who believe, with the word that stands firm, in this world and in the Hereafter.."(Qur'an 14: 27)

You are so worth it, do this for Allah, do this for yourself, do this for your families, do this for the planet. Haven't you waited long enough? Put all your trust in Allah, as He has provided us with the information you need to set yourself free—imagine the places you could go! Look out world, here you come!!! Alhumdulliah!

Gratefully, Madiha Saeed, MD " And when I am sick, then He, Ever He, cures me" (Qur'an 26:80)

Pure Food, Pure Environment, Pure Thoughts, Pure Words, Pure Friends, Pure Sleep, Positive Thoughts, a Pure Lifestyle = HEALS

Allah (SWT) Knows Best

Appendix

Sample Gut Healing Diet

So for those who are truly suffering, have multiple ailments, hives, foods and chemical sensitivities, autistic, etc, I recommend the GAPS diet without dairy initially. The GAPS diet includes dairy, but I find my patients heal and do better faster off dairy initially; later it can be added in as tolerated. This diet helps to heal with *tayyib* food and lifestyle. There are two parts of the GAPS diet, the full GAPS diet and the introduction GAPS diet. For those with serious issues, I have them start off with the introduction GAPS, as it takes away most food and layers then slowly allows the gut to heal faster, and you can easily find out what foods you may be sensitive to. Below, I have laid out what the GAPS diet entails.

Gut And Psychology Syndrome (GAPS) Diet

The GAPS diet, by Dr. Natasha Campbell, helps to heal the digestive tract from disease. It is split up into two parts: introduction and full. Foods not allowed on GAPS are grains, sugar, processed foods, beans and legumes (except for lentils and navy beans), starchy veggies (corn, potatoes, okra, and parsnips), and soy. Dairy and other items should be avoided if there's intolerance. The diet focuses on homemade broths, healthy fats, and veggies. See a full list of foods to include/avoid in Dr. Campbell's book, pages 159–67.

GAPS Introduction Diet The introduction GAPS diet is designed to heal and seal the gut lining quickly to allow the body to recover. The foods are introduced gradually, structured in stages, and it's like a "boot camp" for the gut to heal. It provides foods that are gentle and healing for the gut lining, providing the beneficial microbes needed, removing food intolerances quickly, but it does require patience. The introduction diet is structured in six stages, adding new foods gradually over weeks to months, depending on your body's response. You are expected to stay on each stage for about three to five days, progressing when your body is ready (with no die off like digestive issue or rashes). If your symptoms worsen in the next stage, return back to the previous stage for a few more days. Most importantly, you should listen to your body. This diet does include some dairy, but this should be avoided if you have intolerances; like most foods, dairy can eventually be reintroduced back into the diet as tolerated (there is a step-wise approach for that introduction, starting from organic ghee, then unsalted butter, homemade yoghurt, fermented kefir and cream, homemade cheese, traditional cheese, cream, and then raw milk). Foods included in each stage:

- Start every day with a glass of filtered water with fresh lemon juice.
- **Stage 1:** homemade stocks and soups with well-boiled veggies and meats, chopped liver, well-cooked vegetables (with fibrous stems removed and peeled), animal fats, coconut oil, sea salt, peppercorns, probiotic foods, filtered water, teas (turmeric, loose herbal like chamomile and fresh ginger root), lemon juice, and raw, organic cold pressed honey.
- **Stage 2:** continue with foods from previous stage and include fermented cod liver oil, fermented fish and gravlax, raw egg yolks, stews and casseroles (with boiled meats and veggies), fresh herbs, dairy if tolerated (like homemade whey, yoghurt, sour cream and kefir), increased fermented juices, homemade ghee (if tolerated, start with one teaspoon per day and gradually increase).
- **Stage 3:** continue with previous stages and then gradually add ripened avocado, pancakes (made with squash, nut butter [optional], eggs, and a small amount of honey), almond butter, eggs, fully cooked vegetables (celeriac, asparagus, and cabbage), probiotics, fermented vegetables, and sautéed onion in animal fat.
- **Stage 4:** continue with previous foods, and start to simmer stocks longer, gradually add roasted and baked meats, cold pressed olive oil (start with one teaspoon per day), fresh pressed juices (on an empty stomach, start with one teaspoon a day of fresh carrot juice and then add celery, lettuce, and mint), walnut and almond flour, and nut/ seed flour breads.
- **Stage 5:** continue with previous foods and gradually add raw vegetables and cooked apples in coconut oil and ghee, spices, fruit as a juice ingredient (avoid citrus), and pecan flour.
- **Stage 6:** continue with previous foods and gradually add raw fruits, honey, Brazil nuts, sweet treats, and baked goods with GAPS-approved ingredients.

Full GAPS Diet

Aim to keep a diary through the introduction phase, where you record the whole process of food introduction and the individual symptoms and reactions.

- Start the day with a glass of still mineral or filtered water with a slice of lemon or teaspoon of apple cider vinegar (warm or cold) or glass of freshly pressed fruit/vegetable juice.

- The body is detoxifying from 4:00 am to 10:00 am; eating fresh fruit, drinking water and freshly pressed juices, and having probiotic foods will assist in this process, so have breakfast at around 10:00 am.

Digestive Health and Detoxification

Continue juicing and bathing (in Epsom salt alternating with bicarbonate of soda, sea salt, seaweed powder, and cider vinegar) as it is an excellent way to detox and reduce toxic load as discussed in chapter 2, along with having natural chelators (like juice, seaweed, coriander and other herbs, fermented foods, etc.).

Supplements

GAPS children and adults should have a group of essential supplements: essential therapeutic-strength probiotic, essential fatty acid, cod liver oil, digestive enzymes, and vitamin and mineral supplements.

Essential Fatty Acid

a. A seed/nut blend of Omega-3 and 6 (ratio 2:1). Start with a small amount (depending on the age of child) – start with a few drops building up to 1–3 tablespoons a day.
   - For children under the age of eighteen months: 1–2 teaspoons.
   - Adults: build up to 4–5 tablespoons a day.

b. Fish oil (high EPA/DHA). Adults: start with a small dosage and build up to 3–4 teaspoons a day. Children under two: gradually increase to 1 teaspoon per day. Children over two: start small and gradually increase to 1–3 teaspoons daily.

Cod Liver Oil

- (ratio of A:D is 10:1)
- Adults: Start with 2–2.5 mL (about ½ tsp/day) and gradually increase to 1 tsp daily.
- Lactating or pregnant women: gradually increase to 1.5–2 tsp per day.
- Children: Start half that dose and gradually increase to ½ tsp.
- For babies and very small children: Rub cod liver oil onto their skin (diaper area), gradually increase to 1/3 tsp.

Digestive Enzymes

- Betaine HCl with added pepsin (200–300 mg of betaine, 100 mg pepsin)
- Child: eighteen months to twenty-four months: 1 pinch
- 1–2 years: 2–3 pinches
- 4–6 years: half a capsule
- 6–10 years: half to a full capsule
- 11 years and older: at least one capsule at the beginning of each meal

Other ways to increase acidity and optimize digestion: cabbage juice and stock with your meals.

GAPS Feeding Schedule

For children and families who are prone to disease, when they are ready to introduce foods, they should do so according to the GAPS introduction schedule (minding sensitivities).

Week 1: Start with homemade meat stock with the fat, and freshly pressed vegetable juice mixed with warm water between meals (start with carrot juice then add cabbage, celery, and lettuce).

Week 2: Continue with previous foods, add probiotics gradually, homemade sauerkraut juice, soups with pureed non-starchy vegetables. If yoghurt is well tolerated, gradually increase its daily amount, introduce sour cream, fermented with yoghurt culture.

Week 3: Continue with previous foods; add boiled meats (starting with chicken); introduce ripe avocado, starting with a teaspoon added to the vegetable puree, gradually increasing the amount. Increase amount of yoghurt and sour cream to 1–2 tsp with meals.

Weeks 4 and 5: Continue with previous foods; add raw egg yolks to vegetable puree (do a sensitivity test first); add cooked apples; increase amount of butter, coconut oil, or ghee.

Weeks 6 and 7: Carry on with previous foods, increase the amount of homemade yoghurt or sour cream to 3 tsp with every meal. Gradually increase raw egg yolks to two a day, adding to your baby's soup or cups of meat stock. Increase the meat intake, particularly gelatinous meats around the joints and bones (well cooked in water).

Weeks 8 and 9: Continue with previous foods. Add pancakes made with nut butter and eggs. Increase the amount of freshly pressed juices, add some yoghurt to the juice. Try to add some fresh apple to the juice mixture. Add raw vegetables starting with lettuce and peeled cucumbers (blended in a food processor and added to soup or vegetable puree). After these two vegetables are well tolerated, gradually add other raw vegetables, finely blended.

Week 10 and onward: Carry on with previous foods, add scrambled egg with raw butter or animal fat, with avocados and raw or cooked vegetables. Try some ripe raw apples (without the skin), ripe banana with all fruit given between meals. Introduce gradually your homemade cottage cheese (made from homemade yoghurt) starting with a tiny amount and gradually increasing. When on full GAPS diet, you can start adding small amounts of natural salt to the food.

Resources

Madiha Saeed, MD HolisticMom, MD @HolisticMomMD www.holisticmommd.com

My Shopping List and What I Feed My Family

After years of researching food and its nutritional value, to keep the body and mind as healthy as possible, combining limited time with kids, work and busy lifestyle – this is what my meals look like with four young boys.

I focus on the most nutrient dense *tayyib* foods that will optimize digestive health, and maintain glucose and hormone balance. I ask my family and patients to always go down the list every time they want to put something in their mouth. Have them ask themselves: What is my veggie, clean protein and healthy fat at this meal/snack?

Breakfast

- Fruit with nuts (my kids love dates with nut butter)
- Pancakes (eggs, pb and banana or eggs, pumpkin and banana)
- Waffles (almond flour, coconut flour or cassava flour)
- Muffins, banana bread/zucchini bread (almond, coconut flour, cassava flour)
- Eggs/Quiche
- Kabobs
- No grain cereal in almond milk with fresh or frozen berries
- Chia seed pudding with berries and seeds
- Smoothies, green, fruit and/or nut butter
- Fresh fruit
- Sautéed greens
- Veggie/protein hash

The options are endless.

School Lunch

Here are some ideas that work well with my children, and can be assembled by them with limited stress in an already busy school day morning. We pack in little glass storage containers and stainless steel food jars that stack in their lunch boxes.

1. Veggies 2. Clean Protein 3. Healthy Fat

- Egg or chicken or salmon/sardine salad
- Meat roll ups with veggies
- Soup/chili (made with tons of different kinds of veggies and beans/lentils in bone broth),
- Zucchini pasta with meat sauce,
- Unwich (lettuce wraps)
- Stir fry with meat and veggies (I try to make extra dinner to save for fast lunches),
- Kebab's, burger patties, meatballs,
- Unwrapped egg roll in a bowl
- Fajitas
- Tacos served with lettuce to make wraps or in cassava flour taco shells
- Barbequed leftovers, soups, etc.
- Falefels
- Fish
- Lentils or bean salad
- Veggies (carrots, broccoli, sweet peppers, cucumbers, cauliflower, etc) with avocado oil dressing or guacamole
- Olives, nuts and seeds or baked good that I have made with it (usually left over from breakfast), no grain crackers and no grain chips
- Dark chocolate

Snacks

- Veggies, Clean Protein and Healthy Fat
- Fruit or veggies with nut butter
- Nuts with dairy free dark chocolate or raisins
- Sugar snap peas with hummus
- Jerky
- No grain bars
- No grain granola
- Olives and other veggies, options are endless!
- Veggies, Clean Protein and Healthy Fat Dill Salmon with cauliflower rice and sweet potato fries No grain fried fish with coleslaw Curries with Cauliflower

rice Curries with no grain wraps or chick pea naan Chili/Soup Dessert- Fruit or baked goods made from almond or coconut flour Options are endless!

Lunch & Dinner

Eating Out: We only eat out at organic restaurants or those certified as non-GMO restaurants.

- Focus again on a ton of veggies, clean protein, healthy fat and fruit.

Shopping List

- Vegetables
- like asparagus, bok choy, celery, kiefer, kimchi, sauerkraut and fermented vegetables, cruciferous vegetables (broccoli, brussels sprouts, beets, cauliflower, watercress, cabbage, kale, swiss chard, and collard greens, onions, mushrooms, etc.).
- Prebiotic and probiotic foods
- Clean Protein
  - Wild Caught Seafood
  - Eggs (preferably pasture-raised)
  - Chicken (preferably pasture-raised)
  - Turkey
  - Beef (preferably grass-fed)
  - Lamb
  - Goat
  - Jerkies without preservatives.
  - Bones for broths
  - Others
- Healthy Fat
  - Avocados/Guacamole
  - Olives (canned or jarred kalamata olives)
  - Coconut Products
  - Nuts (walnuts, pecans, macadamia and walnuts) and Nut/Seed Butters (raw if possible, cashew, walnut, macadamia, almond, sesame seed paste)
  - Seeds (like pumpkin, flax, chia, hemp and sesame)
  - Oils (Coconut Oil [extra-virgin], Olive Oil [extra-virgin], Grass-fed Butter, Ghee, Walnut, Flax, Sesame, MCT or Avocado Oil)
- Fruits
- Beans and Lentils (if tolerated)
- Flours

- Almond Flour
- Coconut Flour
- Tapioca Starch
- Chick Pea (Garbanzo Bean) Flour
- Arrowroot
- Cassava flour
- Tigernut flour
- Milk
  - Almond Milk (unsweetened without carageneen)
  - Canned Coconut Milk (BPA free, full fat, unsweetened, preferably without gaur gum)
  - Hemp Milk (unsweetened)
  - Baking Items
  - Unsweetened Cocoa Powder
  - Sugar free/Dairy free Dark Chocolate Chips
- Sweeteners (most cost-effective at Costco)
  - Raw Honey
  - Organic Stevia
  - Maple Syrup
- Protein Powder
  - Beef Gelatin
  - Collagen
  - Pea Protein Powder (if tolerated)
- Condiments
  - Mustard
  - Ketchup (No sugar)
  - Mayonnaise (Avocado Mayo – most cost-effective at Costco)
  - Sea Salt/Himalayan Sea Salt
  - Salad Dressings (Made with Avocado oil)
  - Apple Cider Vinegar
  - Balsamic Vinegar
  - Coconut Aminos
  - No Grain, No Dairy Dips
- Snacks
  - Almond Flour or Seed Crackers
  - No Grain Chips (usually made with cassava flour)
  - Seaweed (preferably with olive oil)
  - Chips fried in coconut oil
- Pastas
  - Chick pea or lentil pasta
  - Almond flour lasagna sheets

- Cheese
  - Nut cheese
  - Nut ricotta
- Taco shells
- Cassava flour taco shells and no grain tortillas
- Spices/Herbs
  - Sea Salt (Himalayan or Celtic)
  - Pepper
  - Turmeric
  - Garlic
  - Others like cayenne pepper, black seeds, rosemary, ginger, cilantro, oregano, sage, cumin, thyme, paprika, parsley, cinnamon, onion powder and so many more (Love the seasoning blends)
- Beverages
  - Herbal Teas (like green, dandelion, milk thistle, chamomile, turmeric, etc.)
  - Filtered/Purified Water
  - Seltzer
- Bars
  - Nut and Seed Bars
  - Paleo Bars
- Candy
  - Three ingredient chocolate treats and mints
  - No sugar chocolate
- Swap *Khabīth* for *Ṭayyib*
  - All natural soaps, lotions, shampoos, Make-up, cleaners, toilet paper, laundry detergent, dishwashing detergent, unbleached parchment paper, non-toxic shower curtain liners etc
  - Cast-iron, glass and ceramic cookware
- Epsom Salt, Baking Soda, Sea Salt for Baths
- Household plants

Tips For Picky Eaters

- Educate your child, IQRA
  - Stock up for success. Only stock your home with appropriate and healthy foods.
  - Set a good example. It is important to model healthy habits, as children imitate their guardians.
  - Family meal time is key. Set a standard of only having one meal as you are one family.

- Involve your children in picking out veggies, fruit, protein, and fat sources from the grocery store and in food preparation.
- Make it fun! Cut their veggies into shapes and arrange in colours of the rainbow.
- Stand your ground and be consistent – don't give in to allowing foods that aren't healthy. Be patient with new foods – one bite of good food is better than no bite of good food, but no bite of food is better than a bite of poison. Sometimes your children might need to go to bed hungry, but they won't let themselves starve, I promise!
- Educate your children about the relationship between food and the body. Knowledge is power! Explain to them what happens when they eat good food versus bad food. Tell them about all the good bugs/pets in their belly that they have to feed and that they need to starve the bad guys.
- Switch their favourite foods with healthier options. If your kids likes brownies, give them brownies (just make it with almond flour). It's a great treat after they finish their veggies, protein, and fat!

A Week of Healing and Thriving

I have given you an example of a week's worth of food below (this is what we do in my house). To keep your stress levels low, keep it simple. Find one or two meals that you enjoy and eat that more often. Remember if you quickly get hungry again after a meal, you are likely not eating enough fat, protein or need to hydrate. You will notice as you eat more nutrient dense food, you will need to eat less food. Incorporate Qur'anic/Prophetic Foods When you can.

Meal	Sunday	Monday	Tuesday	Wednesday	Thursday	Friday	Saturday		
Breakfast Time	Blueberry waffles, scrambled eggs and veggies	Boiled eggs with an apple and nut/seed butter, sauerkraut	Super chocolate smoothie with extra greens	Kabobs, avocado with veggies and fruit	Chia pudding topped with seeds and blueberries with a green smoothie	No grain cereal with non-dairy milk with a green smoothie	Banana pancake with kabobs and boiled veggies		
Lunch Time	Thai soup with healing bone broth	Chicken salad, seed/nut crackers and a side salad	Vegetable, grass-fed beef chili made in broth	Canned salmon with salad drizzled with olive oil	Egg salad, seed/nut crackers and side salad	Mushroom burger with a salad and topped with avocado	Kabobs with broccoli slaw		
Dinner Time	Mushroom burger with salad, sweet potato fries	Shrimp fajitas on avocado with grain free tortilla chips	Pan grilled salmon with pineapple salsa and veggies	Organic hot dogs and boiled broccoli with avocado	Thai soup with healing bone broth	Blackened mahi-mahi with broccoli slaw	Paleo popcorn shrimp with boiled veggies		
Dessert	Healing brownies/fruit	Coconut cookie/fruit	Chocolate chip cookie/fruit	Chia pudding/fruit	Fruit	Blueberry cake	Cake/fruit		
Snack Time	Apple with nut/seed butter	Nuts/seeds and freeze dried blueberries	Ants on a Log	Carrots with guacamole and salsa	No grain cereal	Chia pudding	Nut/seed crackers with nut/seed butter, hummus or guacamole		
Drinks (number of cups) Water Broth									
Intermittent fasting? Fasted between meals?									

Supplements- Probiotic Vitamin D Omega-3 Magnesium Other						
Relaxation Strategy (with duration)						
Exercise Time/Steps						
Sleep Duration/ Quality						
Positive Social Interactions						
Gratitude Done?						
Environmental Detox?						
Detox Bath/ Fluids Flowing?						
How Many Prayers on Time?						
Time for Dua?						
Acts of Kindness?						
Qur'an?						

Nutrient and Foods

Vitamin A	Fish, shellfish, carrots, winter squash, lettuce, dried apricots, bell peppers, tropical fruit, cantaloupe and liver
Vitamin B1	Trout, sunflower seeds, acorn squash, peas
B2	Mushrooms, spinach, almonds, lean meats
B3	Yellowfin tuna, lean meats, peanuts, mushrooms, sunflower seeds, peas, avocado
B6	Root vegetables, red meat and leafy greens
B9	Avocados, beets, green vegetables
B12	Red meat, shellfish and fish
Vitamin C	Berries, green leafy veggies, yellow bell peppers, kale, broccoli, kiwi, citrus fruits, guava
Vitamin D	Sea vegetables, fish (salmon, sardines, mackerel), beef liver, mushrooms, eggs, raw milk and cod liver oil
Calcium	Green leafy vegetables, okra, broccoli, bok choy, flax seeds, sesame seeds, almonds, spinach, walnuts, sardines, brazil nuts, salmon, kale
Iron	Liver, red meat, squash, pumpkin seeds, nuts, lentils, shellfish, dark leafy greens
Magnesium	Avocados, green vegetables, dark chocolate, artichoke hearts, almonds, cashews, pumpkin and squash, meat and fish
Selenium	Fish, poultry and red meat
Zinc	Oysters, poultry and red meat
vitamin E	Avocados, leafy greens and fish
vitamin K2	Fermented vegetables, liver, fish
Copper	Mushrooms, organ meats, shellfish
Iodine	Fish, shellfish and sea vegetables
DHA/EPA	Fish and shellfish and sea vegetables
Glutamine	Fish, poultry and red meat, insoluble fibre is abundant in celery, cruciferous vegetables, leafy greens.
Folic acid	black beans, lentils, spinach, asparagus, sunflower seeds, romaine lettuce, broccoli, turnip greens, mango, peanuts

Books

Body Health

The Pegan Diet, Food Fix, What the Heck Should I Eat by Dr. Mark Hyman
The Obesity Code by Jason Fung, MD
The Autoimmune Solution and *The Thyroid Connection* by Amy Myers, MD
Hashimoto's Thyroiditis: Lifestyle Interventions for Finding and Treating the Root Cause and *Hashimoto's Protocol* by Izabella Wentz, PharmD
The Wahls Protocol: A Radical New Way to Treat All Autoimmune Conditions Using Paleo Principles by Terry Wahls, MD
Eat to Beat Disease by Dr William Li

Brain Health

This is Your Brain on Food by Uma Naidoo, MD
Grain Brain and *Brain Wash* by David Perlmutter, MD
A Mind of Your Own by Kelly Brogan, MD

Pediatrics

Super Nutrition for Babies by Katherine Erlich, MD
The Dirt Cure by Maya Shetreat Klein, MD
The Rule of Five: A Parent's Guide to Raising Healthy Kids in an Unhealthy World by Dr Ana Maria Temple
The Science of Parenting by Margot Sunderland
The Dirt Cure by Dr Maya Shetreat
Family Health Revolution by Carla Atherton
A Compromised Generation: The Epidemic of Chronic Illness in America's Children by Beth Lambert
The Wellness Mama 5 Step Lifestyle Detox: The Essential DIY Guide to a Healthier, Cleaner, All Natural Life By Katie Wells

Recipes

Meals

Breakfast

No Grain Granola

Ingredients

- ½ cup raw sunflower seeds
- ½ cup flax seeds
- ½ cup pumpkin seeds
- ½ cup unsweetened coconut flakes
- ½ cup cashew pieces
- 2 tbsp. coconut oil
- Honey, cinnamon, and vanilla

Directions

1. Mix all the ingredients together in a bowl.
2. Add honey, cinnamon, and vanilla to taste.
3. Bake at 325 degrees F until golden.

Chia Pudding

Ingredients

- ¼ cup chia seeds
- 1 cup coconut milk (or milk of your choice)
- 2 tsp. maple syrup, honey, or agave nectar, or to taste
- 1 tsp. pure vanilla extract (optional)
- Pinch of salt
- Sliced fruit, granola, jam, or nuts for serving

Directions

1. In a medium bowl, whisk to combine chia seeds, milk, sweetener of your choice, vanilla if using, and salt.
2. Cover and refrigerate until thick, 2 hours up to overnight.
3. Serve with mix-ins and toppings of your choice.

Blueberry Waffles

Ingredients

- 1 ½ cups almond flour
- 4 large eggs
- ¼ tsp. baking soda
- ¼ tsp. salt
- 2 ripe bananas, mashed
- ½ cup of blueberries
- Coconut oil spray

Directions

1. Plug in/preheat your waffle iron.
2. While that heats up, mix everything together.
3. Once the waffle iron is warm, spray on coconut oil to the waffle iron plate.
4. Pour the waffle batter onto the plate.
5. Close the waffle iron and allow it to thoroughly cook.
6. Once done (usually when the light turns on), take off the plate and enjoy! My kids love it with a drizzle of honey and/or butter.

This is my FAVOURITE recipe, because it is SOOOO easy and delicious! Best yet, I can change it regularly to what my kids are in the mood for, as I have made jelly cakes and blueberry muffins with this same recipe!! I love to make this ahead of time, and make it an easy suhoor recipe

Banana Pancake

Ingredients

- 1½ bananas
- 3 eggs
- 2 heaping tbsp. of a nut butter
- Dark chocolate chips (optional)

Directions

1. Mix all the ingredients together with a hand mixer, add in blueberries or chocolate at the end and mix them by hand.
2. Add butter to your fry pan and add about two tablespoons of batter to the pan. Fry at low heat as they cook very quickly.
   If I add two full bananas instead of the 1.5, I make crepes with this recipe and fill with fruit. Yum!
   Serve with scrambled eggs or homemade sausage.

Super Chocolate Smoothie

Ingredients

- 2 tbsp. nut butter
- 2 dates
- 3 cups almond milk
- 1 tbsp. unsweetened cocoa powder
- Ice
- Stevia to taste
- Handful of frozen greens

Directions

1. Blend and enjoy.
2. I add collagen, turmeric, L-glutamine and spirulina.

Halva Poori

Ingredients

- 1 cup almond flour
- 1 cup walnuts (pulsed in food processer)
- Honey to taste
- Water
- Cardamom

Directions

1. Heat oil in skillet.
2. Add cardamom seeds.
3. Add almond flour and walnut flour and sauté till golden brown.
4. Add in water and honey to taste.
5. Cover on low heat, stirring regularly.

Chick Pea Curry

Ingredients

- 1 cup of Masala (recipe below)
- 2 cans of chick pea

Directions

1. Cook together until the chick peas are soft.
2. Add more salt or spices as needed for taste.

Poori

Ingredients

- 2 cups of Arrowroot flour
- ½ cup of almond flour
- 2 eggs
- 1 cup of non-dairy milk
- ½ tsp. garlic
- ¼ tsp. black pepper
- 1 tsp. salt
- Cumin

Directions

1. Mix all ingredients together.
2. Make like a pancake on a ceramic skillet.
3. Turn over to cook both sides evenly.

Appetizer

Stuffed Samosas

Ingredients

- 2 cups arrowroot
- ½ cup almond flour
- 1 cup canned coconut milk
- 2 eggs
- ¼ tsp. pepper
- ½ tsp. salt
- ½ tsp. cumin seeds
- Filling of choice

Directions

1. Mix all together.
2. Pour batter onto a small skillet with oil and thin out like crepe. Partially cook both sides.
3. Cut in half.
4. Fold over in half or make into a cone. Seal edges with leftover batter and using a fork to press edges tightly.
5. Stuff with either seasoned ground beef or apples and cinnamon.
6. Fry in coconut oil on med/low heat.

Popcorn Shrimp

Ingredients

- Raw shrimp
- 1 tsp. salt
- ½ tsp. paprika
- ½ tsp. garlic
- ¼ tsp. pepper
- 2 tbsp. chickpea flour and more for dry coating

Directions

1. Mix spices and chickpea flour together.
2. Leave for 30 minutes.
3. Apply a dry coat of chick pea flour to each shrimp and fry!

Sardine/Chicken/Salmon Salad

Ingredients

- 2 cups cooked chicken breast, shredded or canned salmon or sardines
- ¼ cup avocado oil mayo
- ¼ cup celery
- ¼ cup yellow onion, finely chopped
- 3 green onions
- 2 boiled eggs, diced
- ¼ tsp. paprika
- Lemon juice
- 1 tsp. kosher salt
- Freshly ground pepper
- 1 tbsp. fresh parsley

Directions

1. Mix ingredients together.
2. Can serve on a bed of green leaves, avocado or a paleo seed/nut cracker.
3. Can also add ½ cup of grapes, thinly sliced almonds, 1 tablespoon of dill, Dijon mustard to taste and even finely sliced beef bacon…so many delicious options!

Dinner

Masala (Curry Base)

Ingredients

- 3 lbs onion
- 2 tbsp. garlic powder
- ½ tsp. cayenne pepper
- ½ tsp. black pepper
- 1 can of tomato paste
- 1 tsp. cumin powder
- 1 and ½ tsp. turmeric
- 2 tsp. salt
- ½ cup of oil
- 1 cup of water

Directions

1. Add all ingredients into a pressure cooker.
2. Pressure cook for 5–10 minutes.
3. After it is done, use the hand blender to blend it all into a paste.
4. Store in glass jars and store to use as a curry base.

This is a curry base. You can use this base for all veggie/meat curries. Add cauliflower, zucchini, squash, lentils, ground beef, chicken, spinach, etc.

Meat Curry Base

Ingredients

- 2 lbs onion
- 2 tbsp. garlic powder
- ½ tsp. cayenne pepper
- ½ tsp. black pepper
- 1 can of tomato paste
- 1 tsp. cumin powder
- 1 and ½ tsp. turmeric
- 2 tsp. salt
- ½ cup of oil
- 1 cup of water
- ½ tsp. of coriander powder
- ½ tsp. ginger

Directions

1. Add all ingredients into a pressure cooker.
2. Pressure for 5–10 minutes.
3. After it is done, use the hand blender to blend it all into a paste.
4. Store in glass jars and store to use as a curry base.

You can use this base for all meat curries. Add cauliflower, zucchini, squash, lentils, ground beef, chicken, spinach, etc. (in the above picture I have added turnips… my favourite!!! And actually my very first food!!! ☺

Stir Fried Okra

Ingredients

- One package frozen cut okra
- ¼ cup of oil
- 1.5 tomatoes chopped
- 1 medium onion sliced
- ¼ tsp. of ginger
- 1 tsp. of garlic
- 1 tsp. salt
- ¼ tsp. of black pepper
- ¼ tsp. turmeric powder
- ½ tsp. paprika
- ¼ tsp. cumin powder

Directions

1. Preheat oven to 400 F.
2. Bake okra on an unbleached parchment paper until lightly brown (can spray with a little bit of oil).
3. Remove from the heat and set aside.
4. In a medium ceramic skillet, sauté sliced onions until they start to become transparent in the oil.
5. Add in tomatoes and spices.
6. When it all starts to incorporate, add in previously baked okra to the tomato onion mixture.
7. Cook for another 25 minutes on low heat until it is done.
8. Enjoy!

Shrimp tacos with cilantro lime sauce

Ingredients

- Tortilla
- 2 cups of Arrowroot flour
- ½ cup of almond flour
- 2 eggs
- 1 cup of non-dairy milk
- ½ tsp. garlic
- ¼ tsp. black pepper
- 1 tsp. salt
- Shrimp
- 3 cups of cooked baby shrimp

Directions

1. Mix all the ingredients together.
2. Pour the mixture like a pancake on a ceramic skillet.
3. Turn over to cook both sides evenly.

You can fill it with a ground beef or cauliflower stuffing. Fold and cook each side well. This will create a delicious stuffed tortilla. Frying it in a little bit of oil, it will create a fried delicious bread that can be eaten with anything. You can use this for anything that requires a naan or tortilla… love them for tacos!!!

Spinach Curry

Ingredients

- 2 cups of masala/curry base
- 2 bags of frozen organic spinach
- 1 tsp. of salt, increase and decrease as needed
- 1 tsp. of paprika

Directions

1. Mix all ingredients together under moderate heat in pan.
2. Continue to cook, until water has dried and colour has changed to a darker green.

Yellow Anti-inflammatory Chicken Ingredients

Ingredients

- 2 lbs chicken cut up into 1-inch pieces
- 1 tsp. turmeric
- ½ tsp. salt
- ¼ tsp. black pepper
- Juice of one lemon
- ¼ tsp. cumin
- 1 tsp. garlic
- 1 tsp. ginger
- 1 small diced tomato (optional)
- ¼ cup oil

Directions

1. Heat oil in a skillet.
2. Mix ginger and garlic for one minute and add the rest of the ingredients except the tomatoes on high heat.
3. Five to six minutes before the chicken looks done, add the tomatoes.
4. Then cover till the water evaporates.
5. Yum!

Fried Fish

Ingredients:

- ¼ cup of cassava flour
- 1 egg
- 1 tbsp. of water
- ¼ tsp. cumin
- ½ tsp. salt
- ¼ tsp. corriander
- ¼ tsp. garlic

Directions

1. Mix the batter together.
2. Dip fish in the batter.
3. Shallow fry in coconut oil or avocado oil.

Butternut Veggie Soup

Ingredients

- 4 cups bone broth
- 1 can organic butternut squash
- 1 can pumpkin
- 2 cups cauliflower rice
- 2 cup carrots, chopped
- 1 cup celery, chopped
- 1 white onion, roughly chopped
- 1 tsp. garlic
- ¼ tsp. black pepper, freshly ground
- 2 tbsp. of avocado or coconut oil
- ½ tbsp. of rosemary
- Salt, to taste

Directions

1. Saute onions in a little oil to brown.
2. Add in broth.
3. Add veggies and spices to the broth, and bring it to a boil.
4. Reduce the heat and simmer till all the vegetables are cooked.
5. Let it cook and pour the soup into a blender, you can do this in batches if you need. If your soup is thick you can add more broth.
6. Serve with drizzled coconut milk, parsley or seeds! Delicious!

Lentil Tortilla

Ingredients

- 1 cup tapioca flour
- 1 cup urad flour
- 1 cup chickpea flour
- Cumin, to taste
- Salt, to taste

Directions

1. Mix the flours together.
2. Make like a pancake on a ceramic skillet.
3. Turn over to cook both sides evenly.

Can fill with ground beef or cauliflower stuffing, fold and cook each side well. This will create a delicious stuffed tortilla. Frying it in a little bit of oil, will create a fried delicious bread that one can eat with anything.

Arrowroot tortilla/Naan

Ingredients

- 2 cups of Arrowroot flour
- ½ cup of almond flour
- 2 eggs
- hs cup of non-dairy milk

- ½ tsp. garlic
- ¼ tsp. black pepper
- 1 tsp. salt
- 1 tsp. cumin

Directions

1. Mix all the ingredients together.
2. Pour the mix like a pancake on a ceramic skillet.
3. Turn over to cook both sides evenly.

You can fill this tortilla with ground beef or cauliflower stuffing. Once the stuffing is in, fold and cook each side well. This will create a delicious stuffed tortilla. Frying it in a little bit of oil, will create a fried delicious bread that you can eat with anything. You can use it for anything that requires a naan or tortilla…. I love them for tacos!!

Blackened Wild Caught Salmon

Ingredients

- 1 tsp. dried parsley
- 1 tsp. dried oregano
- 1 tsp. dried thyme
- 1 tsp. paprika
- 1 tsp. salt

- ½ tsp. onion powder
- ½ tsp. garlic powder
- ½ tsp. pepper
- 3(6oz) wild caught salmon
- 1 tbsp. coconut oil

Directions

1. Mix all the spices together in a plate.
2. Heat coconut oil in a skillet.
3. While it is heating up, evenly coat the filet in the spice rub.
4. Cook the spice rubbed fish until cooked through. The thickness of the fish will determine the cooking time.
5. Serve warm on top of broccoli slaw and a side of sweet potatoes! Yum!!!

Lentil Pasta

Ingredients

- 1 pound of grass fed, grass-finished ground beef
- 1 medium onion, chopped
- 1 box of already boiled lentil pasta
- 1 jar of mushroom or veggie pasta sauce
- 1 tsp. of Italian seasoning
- 1 tsp. garlic

- 1 tsp. salt
- ¼ tsp. black pepper
- ½ tsp. paprika
- One cup of cauliflower rice
- One cup of broccoli sprouts
- ½ cup of bone broth
- Two tbsp. avocado oil

Directions

1. In a hot skillet, add chopped onions and oil, till brown and translucent.
2. Add in the cauliflower rice and broccoli sprouts, heat till they whither down.
3. Add in ground beef, bone broth and spices. Cook on medium until the ground beef looks almost done.
4. Add the pasta sauce, cook till it simmers and thickens.
5. Add the cooked pasta and toss.
6. Serve to hungry kids who won't even know this is gut healing pasta!

Mushroom Burger

Ingredients

- 2 pounds grass-fed ground beef
- Salt and pepper to taste
- 3 portobello mushrooms
- Half an onion
- Fresh cilantro

Directions

1. Mix the ingredients together.
2. Form into patties.
3. Brown on a skillet with butter.

My kids love lettuce wrapped burgers! Serve with sweet potato fries.

Thai Soup with Healing Bone Broth

Bone Broth Ingredients

- 2 pounds (or more) bones from a healthy source
- Kosher salt and freshly ground black pepper, to taste
- 2 cloves of garlic, minced
- 1 onion, diced
- Four cups of water to yield four cups of broth
- A large stock pot to cook the broth in
- Strainer to remove the pieces

Thai Soup Ingredients

- 2 tbsp. unsalted butter
- 1 pound medium shrimp, peeled and deveined
- 1 can of mushrooms
- 1 tbsp. freshly grated ginger
- 2 tbsp. red curry paste
- 2 (12-ounce) cans unsweetened coconut milk
- Juice of 1 lime
- 2 tbsp. chopped fresh cilantro leaves

Bone Broth Directions

1. Place the bones in a large stock pot.
2. Pour water over the bones.
3. Add onion and garlic.
4. Boil for 3-8 hours.
5. Remove bones with fine metal strainer.

Thai Soup Directions

1. Melt butter in a large stockpot over medium-high heat.
2. Add onions and bell pepper in butter until soft.
3. Add onion and bell pepper to the pot.
4. Stir in ginger until fragrant for about 1 minute.
5. Add in mushrooms.
6. Add in curry paste until well-combined for about 1 minute.
7. Gradually whisk in coconut milk and bone stock, and cook.
8. Bring to a boil; reduce heat and simmer until slightly thickened for about 8-10 minutes.

9. Separately, cook shrimp with salt, garlic and pepper, to taste.
10. Stir in shrimp, lime juice and cilantro into the pot.
11. Feel the healing!

Blackened Mahi-Mahi

Ingredients

- 1 tsp. dried parsley
- 1 tsp. dried oregano
- 1 tsp. dried thyme
- 1 tsp. paprika
- 1 tsp. salt
- ½ tsp. onion powder
- ½ tsp. garlic powder
- ½ tsp. pepper
- 3(6oz) wild caught Mahi-Mahi filets, thawed and patted dry
- 1 tbsp. coconut oil

Directions

1. Mix all the spices together in a plate.
2. Heat coconut oil in a skillet.
3. While it is heating up, evenly coat the filet in the spice rub.
4. Cook the spice rubbed fish until cooked through. The thickness of the fish will determine the cooking time.
5. Serve warm on top of broccoli slaw.
6. Top with sautéed mushrooms and onions.

Broccoli Slaw

Ingredients

- One package broccoli
- 1 cup of coleslaw mix
- ½ cup all natural avocado mayo
- ¼ tsp. pepper
- 1 tsp. honey
- Sunflower seeds, as desired
- Raisins or grapes, as desired

Directions

Mix all the ingredients together and you have a delicious salad! Simple!

Shrimp Scampi

Ingredients

- 1 cup butter
- 2 tbsp. prepared Dijon-style mustard
- 1 tbsp. fresh lemon juice
- 1 tbsp. chopped garlic
- 1 tbsp. chopped fresh parsley
- 2 pounds medium shrimp (cooked, shelled and deveined)

Directions

1. In a small saucepan over medium heat, combine the butter, mustard, lemon juice, garlic, and parsley.
2. When the butter melts completely, add in shrimp, cook until mixture thickens.

Stuffed Paratha (Flatbread)

Ingredients

- ½ cup almond flour
- ½ cup tapioca
- 1 cup canned coconut milk
- 2 tbsp. already prepared ground beef
- Butter or coconut oil for frying

Directions

1. Mix almond flour, tapioca and coconut milk together into a thin batter.
2. In the fry pan, add a teaspoon of butter/coconut oil.
3. Add mixture and thin out like a pancake.
4. When one side starts to firm up, add in the ground beef.
5. Add another layer of batter to cover all the ground beef.
6. Flip.
7. Allow both sides to cook on low heat.
8. Enjoy!

The stuffing in this recipe can vary according to your preferences.

"Rice" and Meatball Curry

Ingredients

Curry
- 1 pound onions
- 1 tbsp. garlic powder
- ¼ tsp. cayenne pepper
- ¼ tsp. black pepper
- ½ can organic tomato paste
- ½ tsp. cumin powder
- ¾ tsp. turmeric
- ½ cup oil
- 1 cup bone broth
- ¼ tsp. coriander powder
- ¼ tsp. ginger
- 1 tsp. salt

Meatballs
- 1 ⅔ pounds beef or lamb
- ½ tsp. cumin powder
- ¼ tsp. salt
- ¼ tsp. black pepper

Directions

1. Combine curry ingredients and place in a pressure cooker for 10 minutes under pressure.
2. Release from pressure and use a hand mixture to liquefy all ingredients.
3. Boil until thickens.
4. Mix together meatball ingredients.
5. Roll into tablespoon-sized balls and drop into boiling curry.
6. Allow to continue to cook until the meat is all cooked.
7. Add fresh coriander to taste.
8. Thickness of curry is per your preference.
9. Add on top of cauliflower white rice.

Shrimp Fajitas

Ingredients

- 1 yellow bell pepper, sliced
- 1 red bell pepper, sliced
- 1 orange bell pepper, sliced
- 1 small red onion, sliced thin
- Wild caught shrimp
- ½ teaspoon cayenne pepper
- ½ tsp. garlic
- ½ tsp. onion powder
- ½ tsp. cumin powder
- ½ tsp. smoked paprika
- 1 tsp. fresh cilantro
- ½ cup oil

Directions

1. Cook shrimp with spices and set aside.
2. Sauté peppers and onions until soft in oil.
3. Mix together and serve over avocado.

Kefta Kababs

Ingredients

- 2 pound ground beef or lamb
- 1 tbsp. mint
- 1 grated onion
- 1 tsp. parsley
- ¼ tsp. cayenne pepper (or less depending on taste)
- ½ tsp. cinnamon
- 2 tsp. paprika
- ¼ tsp. pepper
- 1 tsp. salt
- ½ tsp. pomegranate seeds
- 1 tsp. cumin
- ¼ cup fresh cilantro

Directions

1. Mix all ingredients together.
2. Form kabob around a handle of a wooden spoon.
3. Cook in an iron skillet until done.
4. Garnish with sautéed onions.

Pan Grilled Salmon with Pineapple Salsa

Ingredients

Salmon

- 4 salmon fillets
- 1 tsp. paprika
- 2 tbsp. honey
- 1 tbsp. mustard
- 1 tsp. salt
- ½ tsp. black pepper
- Oil for grilling

Salsa

- 1 cup pineapple, fresh
- 1 tbsp. cilantro
- 1 tbsp. fresh lime juice
- ¼ cup red onion, finely chopped
- 2 tsp. jalapeño, minced (optional)
- Salt to taste

Directions

1. To prepare salmon, mix all spices and condiments together.
2. Refrigerate for one hour.
3. Grill on cast iron with a tablespoon of oil, over medium-high heat.
4. To prepare salsa, mix together ingredients. Add salt to taste.
5. Spoon salsa over the top of the salmon. Can serve with dill cauliflower rice.

Dessert

Basic cake/cookie recipes

- 3 cups almond flour
- ½ cup honey
- ½ cup oil/nut butter
- 1 tsp. baking soda
- 1 tsp. salt
- Eggs – 3 eggs for cookies, 5–6 eggs for cake

Chocolate Marble Cake

Ingredients

- 3 cups almond flour
- ½ cup avocado oil/coconut oil
- ½ cup honey
- 6 eggs
- 1 tsp. baking soda
- 1 tsp. salt
- 1 tbsp. of cocoa powder

Directions

1. Preheat oven to 350 degrees F.
2. In a large mixing bowl combine all of the ingredients until smooth.
3. Pour the mixture into a glass oven-proof rectangular pan or an unbleached parchment-lined cookie sheet, save about ½ cup of batter.
4. With the remaining batter, mix in the cocoa powder.
5. Drop a tablespoon of batter in six different spots on the cake.
6. With a fork, in an "S" pattern go through the chocolate batter into the vanilla batter then back again, to create a design.
7. Bake for 15 minutes.
8. Remove and let cool before cutting to serve.

Date Cookies

Ingredients

- 3 cups almond flour
- ½ cup nut butter
- ½ cup honey
- 3 eggs
- 1 tsp. baking soda
- 1 tsp. salt
- 1 tsp. cinnamon
- Baking dates (can increase as desired)

Directions

1. Preheat oven to 350 degrees F.
2. In a large mixing bowl combine all of the ingredients until smooth.
3. Line a cookie sheet with unbleached parchment paper.
4. Scoop up about a tablespoon of batter, roll into a round ball (may need to wet hands to make sure it doesn't stick).
5. In the middle of the cookie dough ball, add a ½ tsp. amount of baking dates to the centre, surrounded by cookie dough.
6. Place on cookie sheet, flattening slightly.
7. Bake for 15 minutes.
8. Remove and let cool before cutting to serve.

Chewy Coconut Cookies

Ingredients

- 1 cup almond flour
- 1 cup finely shredded coconut, unsweetened
- ¼ cup coconut oil
- ¼ cup honey
- ½ tsp. pure vanilla extract
- A pinch of sea salt

Directions

1. Mix all ingredients in a bowl.
2. Place batter into a tablespoon to help form the balls.
3. Turn the tbsp. over onto the pan; the batter should fall right onto the cookie sheet.
4. Slightly flatten the batter to form a cookie.
5. Bake them at 325°F for 15-20 minutes. Make sure you watch them. They will turn golden; take them out of the oven immediately.
6. Don't touch until cool.

Healing Brownies

Ingredients

- 2/3 cup honey
- 1 cup almond flour
- 3 eggs
- ½ cup cocoa unsweetened, raw
- ½ cup butter
- ¼ tsp. baking soda
- ¼ tsp. salt (if butter is unsalted)
- ½ cup walnuts

Directions

1. Mix together and bake at 350°F until knife comes out clean.
2. Add puréed/whole raspberries or strawberries and shredded coconut flakes for garnish.

Creamy Coconut with Fruit

Ingredients

- One can of coconut milk
- ½ cup blueberries or strawberries
- Nuts or seeds to top
- Stevia to taste

Directions

1. Mix together and enjoy!

Chocolate Chip Cookies

Ingredients

- 3 cups almond flour
- ½ cup honey
- ½ cup nut butter
- 1 teaspoon salt
- 1 tsp. baking soda
- 3 eggs
- Dark chocolate chips or raisins

Directions

1. Mix together.
2. Oil hands to make quarter size balls and flatten on cookie sheet.
3. Bake at 350°F until light golden brown.
4. Enjoy!

Chocolate Chip Cookie Bar

Ingredients

- 3 cups almond flour
- ½ cup avocado oil
- ½ cup honey or maple syrup
- 1 tsp. salt
- 1 tsp. baking soda
- 6 eggs
- Dairy free dark chocolate chips

Directions

1. Mix ingredients together.
2. Spread onto greased cookie sheet.
3. Bake at 350°F for 10-15 minutes or until golden.

Cashew Cake

Ingredients

- 3 cups almond flour
- ½ cup cashew butter
- ½ cup honey or maple syrup
- 1 tsp. salt
- 1 tsp. baking soda
- 6 eggs
- Add cashew pieces

Directions

1. Mix ingredients together.
2. Spread onto greased cookie sheet.
3. Bake at 350°F for 10-15 minutes or until golden.

Zebra sugar cookies

Ingredients

- 2 cups fine ground blanched almond flour
- Scant less than ¼ tsp. sea salt
- ¼ tsp. baking soda
- 3 tbsp. coconut oil, softened
- ¼ cup honey
- 1 - 2 tbsp. thick applesauce
- 1 tbsp. vanilla extract
- 2 tbsp. cocoa powder

Directions

1. Mix into two batches. One batch with vanilla and cocoa powder to the second.
2. To marble the dough, take the vanilla and chocolate dough and smash together gently.
3. Cut in half and smash together again, repeat again.
4. Roll into a log and wrap tightly in parchment paper.
5. Refrigerate for at least 1 hour before using.
6. Cut into cookies and bake at 325°F for 10-15 minutes.
7. Yum!!!

Endnotes

Introduction

1. *Health and Economic Costs of Chronic Disease | CDC.* (2019, October 24). https://www.cdc.gov/chronicdisease/about/costs/index.htm
2. *The Lancet: Latest global disease estimates reveal perfect storm of rising chronic diseases and public health failures fueling COVID-19 pan demic.* Institute for Health Metrics and Evaluation. (2020, November 21). http://www.healthdata.org/news-release/lancet-latest-global-disease-estimates-reveal-perfect-storm-rising-chronic-diseases-and.
3. *Obesity and overweight.* (n.d.). Retrieved February 24, 2020, from https://www.who.int/news-room/fact-sheets/detail/obesity-and-overweight
4. K. Weintraub, (2011). The Prevalence Puzzle: Autism Counts. *Nature* Nov 2;479(7371):22–4. doi:10.1038/479022a.

Part 1: Chapter 1

1. Gallagher, J. (2018, April 10). More than half your body is not human. *BBC News.* https://www.bbc.com/news/health-43674270
2. *Revised Estimates for the Number of Human and Bacteria Cells in the Body.* (n.d.). Retrieved February 24, 2020, from https://www.ncbi.nlm.nih.gov/pmc/articles/PMC4991899/
3. Gallagher, J. (2018, April 10). More than half your body is not human. *BBC News.* https://www.bbc.com/news/health-43674270
4. Centres for Disease Control and Prevention, Division for Heart Disease and Stroke Prevention Heart Disease Fact Sheet, http://www.cdc.gov/dhdsp/data_statistics/fact_sheets/fs_heart_disease.htm
5. *Suicide: One person dies every 40 seconds.* (n.d.). Retrieved February 25, 2020, from https://www.who.int/news-room/detail/09-09-2019-suicide-one-person-dies-every-40-seconds
6. World Health Organization Cancer Fact Sheet, http://www.who.int/news-room/fact-sheets/detail/cancer.

7. Centres for Disease Control and Prevention. Accessed January 5, 2020. http://www.cdc .gov/nccdphp/overview.htm. State of Obesity. (2017). "Obesity Rates by Age Group." Robert Wood Johnson Foundation. http://www.stateofobesity.org/obesity-by-age/., https://www.who.int/news-room/fact-sheets/detail/the-top-10-causes-of-death

8. State of Obesity. (2019). "Childhood Obesity Trends." Robert Wood Johnson Foundation. http://www.stateofobesity.org/childhood-obesity-trends/.

9. Andy Menke et al., "Prevalence of and Trends in Diabetes Among Adults in the United States, 1988–2012," *JAMA* 314, no.10 (September 2015): 1021–29. https://jamanetwork .com/journals/jama/fullarticle/2434682.

10. Sperm Counts Plummet In Western Men, Study Finds. (n.d.). NPR.Org. Retrieved February 26, 2020, from https://www.npr.org/2017/07/31/539517210/sperm-counts -plummet-in-western-men-study-finds.

11. Razzak JA, Khan UR, Azam I, Nasrullah M, Pasha O, Mālik M, Ghaffar A. Health disparities between Muslim and non-Muslim countries. East Mediterr Health J. 2011 Sep;17(9):654-64. Erratum in: East Mediterr Health J. 2011 Dec;17(12):948. PMID: 22259915.

12. Bethel, Christina D. A National and State Profile of Leading Health Problems and Health Care Quality for U.S. Children. Academic Pediatrics, 2011. Estimate of future impact is conservative given historical growth rates.

13. Musaiger AO, Al-Mannai M, Al-Lalla O, Saghir S, Halahleh I, Benhamed MM, Kalam F, Ali EY. Obesity among adolescents in five Arab countries; relative to gender and age. Nutr Hosp. 2013 Nov 1;28(6):1922-5. PMID: 24506370

14. One in Three Kids Will Develop Diabetes. (n.d.). Retrieved February 26, 2020, from https://www.webmd.com/diabetes/news/20030616/one-in-three-kids-will-develop -diabetes#1.

15. Li Y, Lv MR, Wei YJ, et al. "Dietary Pattern and Depression Risk: A Meta-Analysis."

16. Steelesmith DL, Fontanella CA, Campo JV, Bridge JA, Warren KL, Root ED. Contextual Factors Associated With County-Level Suicide Rates in the United States, 1999 to 2016. *JAMA Netw Open.* 2019;2(9):e1910936. doi:10.1001/jamanetworkopen.2019.10936

17. S.C. Curtin et al., "Recent Increases in Injury Mortality Among Children and Adolescents Aged 10–19 Years in The United States:1999–2016," *Natl. Vital Stat.* Rep.67, no. 4 (June 2018): 1–16.

18. National Centre for Health Statistics, *Health, United States, 2010: With Special Feature on Death and Dying*, Table 95 (Hyattsville, MD: US Department of Health and Human Services, 2011):319–21.

19. K. Weintraub, (2011). The Prevalence Puzzle: Autism Counts. *Nature* Nov 2;479(7371):22–4. doi:10.1038/479022a.

20. Firth J, Marx W, Dash S, et al. "The Effects of Dietary Improvement on Symptoms of Depression and Anxiety: A Meta-Analysis of Randomized Controlled Trials." *Psychosom Med.* 2019 Apr;81 (3): 265–80.

21. CDC. (2020, February 13). Promoting Health During the Holidays 7 Tips to Stay Healthy. Centres for Disease Control and Prevention. https://www.cdc.gov/chronicdisease /index.htm.

22. Chen S, Kuhn M, Prettner K, Bloom DE. "The Macroeconomic Burden of Noncommunicable Diseases in the United States: Estimates and Projections." *PLoS One.* 2018 Nov 1;13(11):e0206702. , *The Cost of Chronic Diseases in the U.S.* | *Milken Institute.* (n.d.). Retrieved February 25, 2020, from https://milkeninstitute.org/reports /cost-chronic-diseases-us

23. Recent responses to climate change reveal the drivers of species extinction and survival Christian Román-Palacios, John J. Wiens. Proceedings of the National Academy of Sciences Feb 2020, 201913007; doi:10.1073/pnas.1913007117

24. Food and Agriculture Organization of the United Nations. "What is Happening to Agrobiodiversity? Retrieved February 25, 2020, from http://www.fao.org/3/y5609e02 .htm

25. Food and Agriculture Organization of the United Nations. (2015). "Fertilizer Use to Surpass 200 Million Tonnes in 2018." http://www.fao.org/new/story/en/item/277488 /icode/.

26. Lehner P. "The Hidden Costs of Food." HuffPost. August 16, 2017. https://www.hufpost .com/entry/the-hidden-costs-of-food_b_11492520.

27. N.D. Mehta et al., "Inflammation Negatively Correlates with Amygdala-Ventromedial Prefrontal Functional Connectivity in Association with Anxiety in Patients with Depression: Preliminary Results," *Brain Behav. Immun.* 73 (October 2018): 725–30.

28. T.K. Inagaki et al., "Inflammation Selectivity Enhances Amygdala Activity to Social Threating Images," *Neuroimage* 59, no.4 (February 2012): 3222–26.

29. Pauline Anderson, "inflammatory dietary pattern linked to brain aging" Medscape, July 17, 2017, https://www.medscape.com/viewarticle/883038

30. Kolmychkova, K. I., Zhelankin, A. V., Karagodin, V. P., & Orekhov, A. N. (2016). Mitochondria and inflammation. Patologicheskaia Fiziologiia I Eksperimental'naia Terapiia, 60(4), 114–121.

31. J. Graham Ruby et al., "Estimates of the Heritability of Human Longevity Are Substantially Inflated Due to Assortative Mating, " *Genetics* 210, no. 3 (November 1, 2018): 1109–1124).

32. Life Expectancy by Country and in the World (2020) – Worldometer. (n.d.). Retrieved February 25, 2020, from https://www.worldometers.info/demographics/life -expectancy/

33. GBD 2017 Diet Collaborators, "Health Effects of Dietary Risks in 195 Countries, 1990–2017: A Systemic Analysis for Global Burden of Disease Study 2017." *Lancet* 393, no.10184(May 2019): 1958–72.

34. Schnabel, L., Kesse-Guyot, E., Allès, B., Touvier, M., Srour, B., Hercberg, S., Buscail, C., & Julia, C. (2019). Association Between Ultraprocessed Food Consumption and Risk of Mortality Among Middle-aged Adults in France. *JAMA Internal Medicine*, 179(4), 490–498. https://doi.org/10.1001/jamainternmed.2018.7289

35. Baraldi LG, Martinez SE, Cannella DS, Monteiro CA. "Consumption of Ultra-Processed Foods and Associated Sociodemographic Factors in the USA between 2007 and 2012. Evidence from a Nationally Representative Cross-Sectional Study." *BMJ Open* 2018;8:e020574.

36. Plumer B. "How Much of the World's Cropland Is Actually Used to Grow Food? *Vox*. December 16, 2014. https://www.vox.com/2014/8/21/6053187/cropland-map-food-feul-animal-feed.

37. Bird JK, Murphy RA, Ciappio ED, McBurney MI. "Risk of Deficiency in Multiple Concurrent Micronutrients in Children and Adults in the United States." *Nutrients*. 2017 Jun 24;9 (7).

38. Siegel KR, Ali MK, Srinivasiah A, Nugent RA, Narayan KM. "Do We Produce Enough Fruits and Vegetables to Meet Global Health Need?" *PLoS One*. 2014 Aug 6;9(8):e104059.

39. GBD 2017 Diet Collaborators. (2019). Health effects of dietary risks in 195 countries, 1990–2017: A systematic analysis for the Global Burden of Disease Study 2017. *Lancet* (London, England), 393(10184), 1958–1972. https://doi.org/10.1016/S0140-6736 (19)30041-8

40. S.Gill and P. Satchidananda, "A Smartphone App Reveals Erratic Diurnal Eating Pattern in Humans that Can be Modulated for Health Benefits," *Cell Metabolism* 22, no. 5 (2015): 789–98. doi:10.1016/j.cmet. 20015.09.005.

41. Ng M, Fleming T, Robinson M, et al. "Global, Regional, and National Prevalence of Overweight and Obesity in Children and Adults during 1980–2013: A Systemic Analysis for Global Burden on Disease Study 2013," *Lancet*. 2014 Aug 30;384 (9945):766–81.

42. Caballero B (2007). "The global epidemic of obesity: An overview". *Epidemiol Rev*. 29: 1– 5. doi:10.1093/epirev/mxm012. PMID 17569676.).

43. Schulte EM, Avena NM, Gearhardt AN. Which foods may be addictive? The roles of processing, fat content, and glycaemic load. *PLoS One*. 2015;10(2):e0117959. Published 2015 Feb 18. doi:10.1371/journal.pone.0117959

44. Schulte EM, Smeal JK, Lewis J, Gearhardt AN. Development of the Highly Processed Food Withdrawal Scale. Appetite. 2018 Dec 1;131:148-154. doi:10.1016/j. appet.2018.09.013. Epub 2018 Sep 15. PMID: 30227182

45. Arab countries- Abuvassin B, Laher I. "Diabetes Epidemic Sweeping the Arab World." *World J Diabetes*. 2016 Apr 25;7 (8):165–74.

46. GBD 2017 Diet Collaborators. (2019). Health effects of dietary risks in 195 countries, 1990–2017: A systematic analysis for the Global Burden of Disease Study 2017. Lancet (London, England), 393(10184), 1958–1972. https://doi.org/10.1016/S0140

-6736(19)30041-8 Mohajeri, M. H., La Fata, G., Steinert, R. E., & Weber, P. (2018). Relationship between the gut microbiome and brain function. Nutrition Reviews, 76(7), 481–496. https://doi.org/10.1093/nutrit/nuy009

47. M.Pall, "Scientific Evidence Contradicts Findings and Assumptions of Canadian Safety Panel 6:Microwaves Act Through Voltage-Gated Calcium Channel Activation to Induce Biological Impacts at Non-Thermal Levels, Supporting a Paradigm Shift for Microwaves/Lower Frequency Electromagnetic Field Action," *Reviews on Environmental* Health 30, no.2 (2015): 99–116. doi:10.1515/reveh-2015-0001.

48. N.E.Klepeis et al., "The National Human Activity Pattern Survey (NHAPS): A Resource for Assessing Exposure to Environmental Pollutants,") *J.Expo. Sci. Environ. Epidemiol.* 11 (2001):231–52.

49. L.T. Stiemsma et al., "The Hygine Hypothesis: Current Perspectives and Future Therapies," *Immunotargets Ther.* 4 (July 2015):143–57.

50. Centres for Disease Control and Prevention, "Short Sleep Duration Among U.S. Adults," https://www.cdc.gov/sleep/data_statistics.html.

51. C.S. Moller-Levet et al., "Effects of Insufficient Sleep on Circadian Rhythmicity and Expression Amplitude of the Human Blood Transcriptome," *Roc. Natl. Acad. Sci.* USA 110, no.12 (March 2013):E1132–41.

52. D. F. Kripke, "Hypotic Drug Risks of Mortality, Infection, Depression, and Cancer: But Lack of Benefit," version 3, FI000Res. 5 (2016):918.

53. "Ericsson Mobility Report:70 Percent of World's Population Using Smartphones by 2020," press release, June 3, 2015, https://www.ericsson.com/en/press-releases/2015/6/ericsson-mobility-report-70-percent-of-worlds-population-using-smarphones-by-2020.

54. "Americans Spend Nearly Half of Their Waking Hours (42 percent) Looking at a Screen, It's Been Revealed by new Research, " press release, August 13, 2018, survey conducted by OnePoll on behave of

55. R.J. Dwyer, K.Kushlev, and E. W. Dun, "Smartphone Us Undermines Enjoyment of Face-to-Face Social Interactions," *J. Exp. Soc. Psychol.* 78 (September 2018):233–39.

56. Shalini Misra, Lulu Cheng, Jamie Genevie, and Miao Yuan, "The iPhone Effect: The Quality of In-Person Social Interactions in the Presence of Mobile Devices," *Environment and behaviour* 48, no. 2 (2016).

57. M. G. Hunt et al., "No More FOMO: Limiting Social Media Decreases Lonliness and Depression," J. Soc. Clin. Psychol. 37, no.10 (November 2018):751–68.)(B. A. Primack et al.,"Social Media Use and Perceived Social Isolation Among Young Adults in the U.S," *Am. J. Prev.* Med. 53, no. 1(July 2017):1–8.

58. J. Gramlich, "5 Facts about Crime in the U.S.," Pew Research Centre, January 3, 2019, http://www.pewresearch.org/fact-tank/2019/01/03/5-facts-about-crime-in-the-u-s/.

59. A.Szabo, "Negative Psychological Effects of Watching the News in the Television: Relaxation or Another Intervention May Be Needed to Buffer Them!" *Int J. Behav. Med.* 14, no. 2 (2007):57–62.

Part 2: Chapter 3

1. Lesser LI, Ebbeling CB, Goozner M, Wypij D, Ludwig DS. Relationship between funding source and conclusion among nutrition- related scientific articles. *PLOS Med.* 2007 Jan;4 (1):e5.

2. "Inflammation: Maintaining the Mucosal Barrier in Intestinal Inflammation." *Nature Reviews, Gastroenterology & Hepatology,* http://www.ncbi.nlm.nih.gov/pubmed /26701373. Hadhazy, Adam. "Think Twice: How the Gut's 'Second Brain' Influences Mood and Well-Being." Scientific American. February 11, 2010. https://www .scientificamerican.com/article/gut-second-brain/.

3. NIH Human Microbiome Project defines normal bacterial makeup of the body | National Institutes of Health (NIH). (n.d.). Retrieved February 27, 2020, from https://www .nih.gov/news-events/news-releases/nih-human-microbiome-project-defines-normal -bacterial-makeup-body.

4. Your Changing Microbiome. (n.d.). Retrieved February 27, 2020, from https://learn .genetics.utah.edu/content/microbiome/changing/.

5. Le Chatelier, E., et al. "Richness of human gut microbiome correlates with/ metabolic markers." *Nature.* August 29, 2013; 500 (7464): 541–46.

6. Papel de la flora intestinal en la salud y en la enfermedad.F. *Guamer Nutr Hosp.* 2007 May; 22 (Suppl 2): 14–19.

7. McGough, G. (2011). Leaky Gut. Nursing Standard, 25(51), pp.30–30.

8. Arrieta, M. C., Bistritz, L., & Meddings, J. B. (2006). Alterations in intestinal permeability. Gut, 55(10), 1512–1520. https://doi.org/10.1136/gut.2005.085373.

9. Bischoff, Stephan C., Giovanni Barbara, Wim Buurman, Theo Ockhuizen, Jörg-Dieter Schulzke, Matteo Serino, Herbert Tilg, Alastair Watson, and Jerry M. Wells. "Intestinal Permeability – A New Target for Disease Prevention and Therapy." *BMC Gastroenterology.* 2014. http://www.ncbi.nlm.nih.gov/pmc/articles/PMC4253991/.

10. bid.

11. Bischoff, Stephan C., Giovanni Barbara, Wim Buurman, Theo Ockhuizen, Jörg-Dieter Schulzke, Matteo Serino, Herbert Tilg, Alastair Watson, and Jerry M. Wells. "Intestinal Permeability – A New Target for Disease Prevention and Therapy." *BMC Gastroenterology.* 2014. https://www.ncbi.nlm.nih.gov/pmc/articles/PMC4253991/.

12. Bouchaud, Gregory, Paxcal Gourbeyre, Tiphaine Bihouée, Phillippe Aubert, David Lair, Marie-Aude Cheminant, Sandra Denery-Papini, Michel Neunlist, Antoine Magnan, and Marie Bodinier. "Consecutive Food and Respiratory Allergies Amplify Systemic and Gut but Not Lung Outcomes in Mice." *Journal of Agricultural and Food Chemistry* 63, no. 28 (July 2015): 6475–483. doi:10.1021/acs.jafe.5b02338.

13. Campbell, A. W. (2014). Autoimmunity and the Gut [Review Article]. Autoimmune Diseases. https://doi.org/10.1155/2014/152428, Arrieta, M. C., Bistritz, L., & Meddings, J. B. (2006). Alterations in intestinal permeability. *Gut,* 55(10), 1512–1520. https://doi.org/10.1136/gut.2005.085373.

14. Camilleri, M., K. Madsen, R. Spiller, B. G. Van Meerveld, and G. N. Verne. "Intestinal Barrier Function in Health and Gastrointestinal Disease." *Neurogastroenterology & Motility* 24, no. 6 (May 2012): 503–12. doi:10.1111/j.1365-2982.2012.01921.x.

15. Nouri, Mehrnaz, Anders Bredberg, Björn Weström, and Shahram Lavasani. "Intestinal Barrier Dysfunction Develops at the Onset of Experimental Autoimmune Encephalomyelitis, and Can Be Induced by Adoptive Transfer of Auto-Reactive T Cells." *PLoS ONE* 9, no. 9 (September 2014). doi:10.1371/journal.pone.0106335.

16. Fresko, I. "Intestinal Permeability in Behcet's Syndrome." Annals of the Rheumatic Diseases 60, no. 1 (January 2001): 65–66. doi:10.1136/ard.60.1.65.

17. Bardella, Maria Teresa, Luca Elli, Sara De Matteis, Irene Floriani, Valter Torri, and Luca Piodi. "Autoimmune Disorders in Patients Affected by Celiac Sprue and Inflammatory Bowel Disease." *Annals of Medicine* 41, no. 2 (January 2009): 139–43. doi:10.1080/07853890802378817.

18. Lerner, A., & Matthias, T. (2015). Rheumatoid arthritis–celiac disease relationship: Joints get that gut feeling. *Autoimmunity Reviews,* 14(11), 1038–1047. https://doi.org /10.1016/j.autrev.2015.07.007.

19. PA, Jose, D, Raj. "Gut Microbiota in Hypertension." *Curr Opin Nehrol Hyperten* 2015; September 24 (5): 403–9. doi:10.1097/MNH.0000000000000149. https://www.ncbi .nlm.nih.gov/pubmed/26125644.

20. Bischoff, S.C., Barbara, G., Buurman, W. et al. Intestinal permeability – a new target for disease prevention and therapy. *BMC Gastroenterol* 14, 189 (2014). https://doi.org/10 .1186/s12876-014-0189-7.

21. Pike, Michael G., Robert J. Heddle, Peter Boulton, Malcolm W. Turner, and David J. Atherton.
"Increased Intestinal Permeability in Atopic Eczema." *Journal of Investigative Dermatology* 86, no. 2 (February 1986): 101–4. doi:10.1111/1523-1747. ep12284035.

22. Gérard, P. Gut microbiota and obesity. Cell. Mol. Life Sci. 73, 147–162 (2016). https:// doi.org/10.1007/s00018-015-2061-5.

23. Li, Xia, and Mark A. Atkinson. "The Role for Gut Permeability in the Pathogenesis of Type-1 Diabetes – A Solid or Leaky Concept?" Pediatric Diabetes 16, no. 7 (August 2015): 485–92. doi:10.1111/pedi.12305. Vaarala, O., M. A. Atkinson, and J. Neu. "The 'Perfect Storm' for Type 1 Diabetes: The Complex Interplay between Intestinal Microbiota, Gut Permeability, and Mucosal Immunity." *Diabetes* 57, no. 10 (September 2008): 2555–562. doi:10.2337/ db08-0331.

24. Gomes, J. M. G., J. A. Costa, and R. C. Alfenas. "Could the Beneficial Effects of Dietary Calcium on Obesity and Diabetes Control Be Mediated by Changes in Intestinal Microbiota and Integrity?" *British Journal of Nutrition* 114, no. 11 (September 2015): 1756–765.doi:10.1017/s0007114515003608.

25. Bischoff, S.C., Barbara, G., Buurman, W. et al. Intestinal permeability – a new target for disease prevention and therapy. *BMC Gastroenterol* 14, 189 (2014). https://doi.org/10 .1186/s12876-014-0189-7.

26. Lacy, B. E., Chey, W. D., & Lembo, A. J. (2015). New and Emerging Treatment Options for Irritable Bowel Syndrome. *Gastroenterology & Hepatology*, 11(4 Suppl 2), 1–19.

27. Camilleri, M., K. Madsen, R. Spiller, B. G. Van Meerveld, and G. N. Verne. "Intestinal Barrier Function in Health and Gastrointestinal Disease." *Neurogastroenterology & Motility* 24, no. 6 (May 2012): 503–12. doi:10.1111/j.1365-2982.2012.01921.x.

28. Morga, Yvette, Darry J. Campbell, and Jonathan M. Rhodes. "Mucosal Barrier, Bacteria and Inflammatory Bowel Disease: Possibilities for Therapy." *Digestive Diseases* 32, no. 4 (2014): 475–83. doi:10.1159/000358156

29. Bardella, Maria Teresa, Luca Elli, Sara De Matteis, Irene Floriani, Valter Torri, and Luca Piodi. "Autoimmune Disorders in Patients Affected by Celiac Sprue and Inflammatory Bowel Disease." *Annals of Medicine* 41, no. 2 (January 2009): 139–43. doi:10.1080/07853890802378817.

30. Bischoff, S.C., Barbara, G., Buurman, W. et al. Intestinal permeability – a new target for disease prevention and therapy. *BMC Gastroenterol* 14, 189 (2014). https://doi.org/10.1186/s12876-014-0189-7.

31. Brenner, D., Paik, Y.-H., & Schnabl, B. (2015). Role of Gut Microbiota in Liver Disease. Journal of *Clinical Gastroenterology*, 49. https://doi.org/10.1097/MCG.0000000000000391.

32. Mosci, Paolo, Elena Gabrielli, Eugenio Luciano, Stefano Perito, Antonio Cassone, Eva Pericolini, and Anna Vecchiarelli. "Involvement of IL-17A in Preventing the Development of Deep-seated Candidiasis from Oropharyngeal Infection." *Microbes and Infection* 16, no. 8 (August 2014): 678–89. doi:10.1016/j.micinf.2014.06.007.

33. Zhang, D., L. Zhang, F. Yue, Y. Zheng, and R. Russell. "Serum Zonulin Is Elevated in Women with Polycystic Ovary Syndrome and Correlates with Insulin Resistance and Severity of Anovulation." European Journal of *Endocrinology* 172, no. 1 (October 2014): 29–36. doi:10.1530/eje-14-0589.

34. Bischoff, S.C., Barbara, G., Buurman, W. et al. Intestinal permeability – a new target for disease prevention and therapy. *BMC Gastroenterol* 14, 189 (2014). https://doi.org/10.1186/s12876-014-0189-7.

35. Bekkering, Pjotr, Ismael Jafri, Frans J. Van Overveld, and Ger T. Rijkers. "The Intricate Association between Gut Microbiota and Development of Type-1, Type-2 and Type-3 Diabetes." Expert Review of *Clinical Immunology* 9, no. 11 (November 2013): 1031–41. doi:10.1586/1744666x.2013.848793.

36. Wu, S., Yi, J., Zhang, Y., Zhou, J., & Sun, J. (2015). Leaky intestine and impaired microbiome in an amyotrophic lateral sclerosis mouse model. *Physiological Reports*, 3(4), e12356. https://doi.org/10.14814/phy2.12356.

37. Forsyth, Christopher B., Kathleen M. Shannon, Jeffrey H. Kordower, Robin M. Voigt, Maliha Shaikh, Jean A. Jaglin, Jacob D. Estes, Hemraj B. Dodiya, and Ali Keshavarzian. "Increased Intestinal Permeability Correlates with Sigmoid Mucosa Alpha-Synuclein

Staining and Endotoxin Exposure Markers in Early Parkinson's Disease." *PLoS ONE* 6, no. 12 (December 2011).doi:10.1371/journal.pone.0028032.

39. Bischoff, S.C., Barbara, G., Buurman, W. et al. Intestinal permeability – a new target for disease prevention and therapy. *BMC Gastroenterol* 14, 189 (2014). https://doi.org/10 .1186/s12876-014-0189-7.

40. Leclercq, Sophie, Sébastien Matamoros, Patrice D. Cani, Audrey M. Neyrinck, François Jamar, Peter Stärkel, Karen Windey, Valentina Tremaroli, Fredrik Bäckhed, Kristin Verbeke, Philippe De Timary, and Nathalie M. Delzenne. "Intestinal Permeability, Gut-Bacterial Dysbiosis, and behavioural Markers of Alcohol-Dependence Severity. Leclercq, S., Matamoros, S., Cani, P. D., Neyrinck, A. M., Jamar, F., Stärkel, P., Windey, K., Tremaroli, V., Bäckhed, F., Verbeke, K., Timary, P. de, & Delzenne, N. M. (2014). Intestinal permeability, gut-bacterial dysbiosis, and behavioural markers of alcohol-dependence severity. *Proceedings of the National Academy of Sciences*, 111(42), E4485–E4493. https://doi.org/10 .1073/pnas.1415174111.

41. Kelly, John R., Paul J. Kennedy, John F. Cryan, Timothy G. Dinan, Gerard Clarke, and Niall P. Hyland. "Breaking Down the Barriers: The Gut Microbiome, Intestinal Permeability and Stress-Related Psychiatric Disorders." *Frontiers in Cellular Neuroscience* 9 (October 2015). doi:10.3389/fncel.2015.00392.

42. Vojdani, Aristo. "Immune Reactivity against Food Proteomes." *Journal of Food Processing & Technology* 6, no. 7 (2015). doi:10.4172/2157-7110.s1.019.

43. Bischoff, Stephan C., Giovanni Barbara, Wim Buurman, Theo Ockhuizen, Jörg-Dieter Schulzke, Matteo Serino, Herbert Tilg, Alastair Watson, and Jerry M. Wells. 25. Bischoff, S.C., Barbara, G., Buurman, W. et al. Intestinal permeability – a new target for disease prevention and therapy. *BMC Gastroenterol* 14, 189 (2014). https://doi.org/10.1186 /s12876-014-0189-7.

44. Maes, Michael, Ivana Mihaylova, and Jean-Claude Leunis. "Increased Serum IgA and IgM against LPS of Enterobacteria in Chronic Fatigue Syndrome (CFS): Indication for the Involvement of Gram-Negative Enterobacteria in the Etiology of CFS and for the Presence of an Increased Gut–Intestinal Permeability." *Journal of Affective Disorders* 99, no. 1–3 (April 2007): 237–40. doi:10.1016/j.jad.2006.08.021.

45. Goebel, A., S. Buhner, R. Schedel, H. Lochs, and G. Sprotte. "Altered Intestinal Permeability in Patients with Primary Fibromyalgia and in Patients with Complex Regional Pain Syndrome." *Rheumatology* 47, no. 8 (April 2008): 1223–227. doi:10.1093/ rheumatology/ken140

46. Galland, L. (2014). The Gut Microbiome and the Brain. Journal of Medicinal Food, 17(12), 1261–1272. https://doi.org/10.1089/jmf.2014.7000.

47. Julio-Pieper, M., J. A. Bravo, E. Aliaga, and M. Gotteland. "Review Article: Intestinal Barrier Dysfunction and Central Nervous System Disorders – A Controversial Association." *Alimentary Pharmacology & Therapeutics* 40, no. 10 (September 2014): 1187–1201. doi:10.1111/apt.12950.

48. 48Aubert, J.-P., Bayard, B., & Loucheux-Lefebvre, M.-H. (1976). Circular dichroism studies of some oligosaccharides containing 2-acetamido-2-deoxy-D-glucopyranose and D-mannopyranose residues. *Carbohydrate Research*, 51(2), 263–268. https://doi.org/10.1016/S0008-6215(00)83334-0.

49. Picca A, Pesce V, Lezza AMS. Does eating less make you live longer and better? An update on calorie restriction. *Clin Interv Aging.* 2017;12:1887-1902. Published 2017 Nov 8. doi:10.2147/CIA.S126458

50. Alcock, Joe, Carlo C. Maley, and C. Athena Aktipis. "Is Eating behaviour Manipulated by the Gastrointestinal Microbiota? Evolutionary Pressures and Potential Mechanisms." *BioEssays* 36, no. 10 (August 2014): 940–49. doi:10.1002/ bies.201400071.

51. Masharani, U., Sherchan, P., Schloetter, M., Stratford, S., Xiao, A., Sebastian, A., Nolte Kennedy, M., & Frassetto, L. (2015). Metabolic and physiologic effects from consuming a hunter-gatherer (Paleolithic)-type diet in Type-2 diabetes. *European Journal of Clinical Nutrition*, 69(8), 944–948. https://doi.org/10.1038/ejcn.2015.39.

52. 52 Ali, S. A., Parveen, N., & Ali, A. S. (2018). Links between the Prophet Muhammad (PBUH) recommended foods and disease management: A review in the light of modern superfoods. *International Journal of Health Sciences*, 12(2), 61–69.

53. Pandey KB, Rizvi SI. Planty polyphenols as dietary antioxidants in human health and disease. *Oxid Med Cell Longev.* 2009 Nov-Dec; 2 (5):270–78.

54. Heiman ML, Greenway FL. A healthy gastrointestinal microbiome is dependent on dietary diversity. *Mol Metab.* 2016 Mar 5;5(5):317–20.

55. Adults Meeting Fruit and Vegetable Intake Recommendations – United States, 2013. (n.d.). Retrieved February 28, 2020, from https://www.cdc.gov/mmwr/preview/mmwrhtml/mm6426a1.htm.

56. Holt, E. M., Steffen, L. M., Moran, A., Basu, S., Steinberger, J., Ross, J. A., Hong, C.-P., & Sinaiko, A. R. (2009). Fruit and vegetable consumption and its relation to markers of inflammation and oxidative stress in adolescents. *Journal of the American Dietetic Association*, 109(3), 414–421. https://doi.org/10.1016/j.jada.2008.11.036.

57. Kaczmarczyk MM, Miller MJ, Freund GG. The health benefits of dietary fibre: beyond the usual suspects of Type-2 diabetes mellitus, cardiovascular disease and colon cancer. *Metabolism.* 2012 Aug;61 (8):1058–66.

58. Zhang L, Hou D, Chen X, et al. Exogenous plant MIR 168a specifically targets mammalian LDLRAP1: evidence of cross-kingdom regulation by microRNA. *Cell Research.* 2012;22:107–2.

59. Holt, E. M., Steffen, L. M., Moran, A., Basu, S., Steinberger, J., Ross, J. A., Hong, C.-P., & Sinaiko, A. R. (2009). Fruit and vegetable consumption and its relation to markers of inflammation and oxidative stress in adolescents. *Journal of the American Dietetic Association*, 109(3), 414–421. https://doi.org/10.1016/j.jada.2008.11.036.

60. Elfiky, S. A., Elelaimy, I. A., Hassan, A. M., Ibrahim, H. M., & Elsayad, R. I. (2012). Protective effect of pumpkin seed oil against genotoxicity induced by azathioprine. *The*

Journal of Basic & Applied Zoology, 65(5), 289–298. https://doi.org/10.1016/j.jobaz
.2012.10.010

61. Yan, X., Wang, Y., Sang, X., & Fan, L. (2017). Nutritional value, chemical composition and antioxidant activity of three Tuber species from China. *AMB Express*, 7. https://doi
.org/10.1186/s13568-017-0431-0

62. Lindequist, Ulrike, Timo H. J. Niedermeyer, and Wolf-Dieter Jülich. "The Pharmacological Potential of Mushrooms." *Evidence-Based Complementary and Alternative Medicine* 2, no. 3 (2005): 285–99. doi:10.1093/ecam/neh107.

63. Lechner JF, Stoner GD. Red Beetroot and Betalains as Cancer Chemopreventative Agents. *Molecules*. 2019;24(8):1602. Published 2019 Apr 23. doi:10.3390/molecules 24081602

64. Hobbs DA, Kaffa N, George TW, Methven L, Lovegrove JA. Blood pressure-lowering effects of beetroot juice and novel beetroot-enriched bread products in normotensive male subjects. Br J Nutr. 2012 Dec 14;108(11):2066-74. doi:10.1017/S0007114512000190. Epub 2012 Mar 14. PMID: 22414688.

65. Gennari, L., Felletti, M., Blasa, M., Angelino, D., Celeghini, C., Corallini, A., & Ninfali, P. (2011). Total extract of Beta vulgaris var. cicla seeds versus its purified phenolic components: Antioxidant activities and antiproliferative effects against colon cancer cells. *Phytochemical Analysis: PCA*, 22(3), 272–279. https://doi.org/10.1002/pca.1276

66. Johnson, E. J. (2002). The role of carotenoids in human health. Nutrition in Clinical Care: An Official Publication of Tufts University, 5(2), 56–65. https://doi.org/10.1046/j
.1523-5408.2002.00004.x

67. Bolkent, S., Yanardağ, R., Tabakoğlu-Oğuz, A., & Ozsoy-Saçan, O. (2000). Effects of chard (Beta vulgaris L. var. Cicla) extract on pancreatic B cells in streptozotocin-diabetic rats: A morphological and biochemical study. Journal of Ethnopharmacology, 73(1–2), 251–259. https://doi.org/10.1016/s0378-8741(00)00328-7

68. Flynn, A. (2003). The role of dietary calcium in bone health. *The Proceedings of the Nutrition Society*, 62(4), 851–858. https://doi.org/10.1079/PNS2003301

69. Weber, P. (2001). Vitamin K and bone health. *Nutrition* (Burbank, Los Angeles County, Calif.), 17(10), 880–887. https://doi.org/10.1016/s0899-9007(01)00709-2

70. Kanner, J., Harel, S., & Granit, R. (2001). Betalains – A new class of dietary cationized antioxidants. *Journal of Agricultural and Food Chemistry*, 49(11), 5178–5185. https://doi
.org/10.1021/jf010456f

71. Johnson, E. J. (2002). The role of carotenoids in human health. *Nutrition in Clinical Care: An Official Publication of Tufts University*, 5(2), 56–65. https://doi.org/10.1046/j
.1523-5408.2002.00004.x

72. Morris, M. C., Wang, Y., Barnes, L. L., Bennett, D. A., Dawson-Hughes, B., & Booth, S. L. (2018). Nutrients and bioactives in green leafy vegetables and cognitive decline: Prospective study. *Neurology*, 90(3), e214–e222. https://doi.org/10.1212/WNL
.0000000000004815

73. Ekşi, G., Gençler Özkan, A. M., & Koyuncu, M. (2020). Garlic and onions: An eastern tale. *Journal of Ethnopharmacology*, 112675. https://doi.org/10.1016/j.jep.2020.112675

74. Nicastro, H. L., Ross, S. A., & Milner, J. A. (2015). Garlic and onions: Their cancer prevention properties. *Cancer Prevention Research* (Philadelphia, Pa.), 8(3), 181–189. https://doi.org/10.1158/1940-6207.CAPR-14-0172

75. Ashraf, R., Aamir, K., Shaikh, A. R., & Ahmed, T. (2005). Effects of garlic on dyslipidemia in patients with Type-2 diabetes mellitus. *Journal of Ayub Medical College*, Abbottabad: JAMC, 17(3), 60–64.

76. Josling, P. (2001). Preventing the common cold with a garlic supplement: A double-blind, placebo-controlled survey. *Advances in Therapy*, 18(4), 189–193. https://doi.org/10.1007/bf02850113

77. Ried, K., & Fakler, P. (2014). Potential of garlic (Allium sativum) in lowering high blood pressure: Mechanisms of action and clinical relevance. Integrated Blood Pressure Control, 7, 71–82. https://doi.org/10.2147/IBPC.S51434

78. Banerjee, S. K., & Maulik, S. K. (2002). Effect of garlic on cardiovascular disorders: A review. *Nutrition Journal*, 1, 4. https://doi.org/10.1186/1475-2891-1-4, Aged Garlic Extract Reduces Low Attenuation Plaque in Coronary Arteries of Patients with Metabolic Syndrome in a Prospective Randomized Double-Blind Study | *The Journal of Nutrition* | Oxford Academic. (n.d.). Retrieved February 25, 2020, from https://academic.oup.com/jn/article/146/2/427S/4584725

79. Oxidative insults to neurons and synapse are prevented by aged garlic extract and S-allyl-L-cysteine treatment in the neuronal culture and APP-Tg m... – PubMed – NCBI. (n.d.). Retrieved February 25, 2020, from https://www.ncbi.nlm.nih.gov/pubmed/21166677

80. Slimestad, R., Fossen, T., & Vågen, I. M. (2007). Onions: A source of unique dietary flavonoids. Journal of Agricultural and Food Chemistry, 55(25), 10067–10080. https://doi.org/10.1021/jf0712503

81. González-Peña, D., Checa, A., de Ancos, B., Wheelock, C. E., & Sánchez-Moreno, C. (2016). New insights into the effects of onion consumption on lipid mediators using a diet-induced model of hypercholesterolemia. *Redox Biology*, 11, 205–212. https://doi.org/10.1016/j.redox.2016.12.002

82. Matheson, E. M., Mainous, A. G., & Carnemolla, M. A. (2009). The association between onion consumption and bone density in perimenopausal and postmenopausal non-Hispanic white women 50 years and older. *Menopause* (New York, N.Y.), 16(4), 756–759. https://doi.org/10.1097/gme.0b013e31819581a5

83. Kook, S., Kim, G.-H., & Choi, K. (2009). The antidiabetic effect of onion and garlic in experimental diabetic rats: Meta-analysis. *Journal of Medicinal Food*, 12(3), 552–560. https://doi.org/10.1089/jmf.2008.1071

84. Jaber, R. (2002). Respiratory and allergic diseases: From upper respiratory tract infections to asthma. *Primary Care*, 29(2), 231–261. https://doi.org/10.1016/s0095-4543(01)00008-2

85. Khaki, A., Fathiazad, F., Nouri, M., Khaki, A. A., Khamenehi, H. J., & Hamadeh, M. (2009). Evaluation of androgenic activity of allium cepa on spermatogenesis in the rat. *Folia Morphologica*, 68(1), 45–51.

86. Hodgson, J. M., Ward, N. C., Burke, V., Beilin, L. J., & Puddey, I. B. (2007). Increased Lean Red Meat Intake Does Not Elevate Markers of Oxidative Stress and Inflammation in Humans. *The Journal of Nutrition*, 137(2), 363–367. https://doi.org/10.1093/jn/137.2.363.

87. D. Mozaffarian et al., "Plasma Phospholipids Long-Chain w-3 Fatty Acids and Total and cause-Specific Mortality in Older Adults: A Cohort Study," *Annals of Internal Medicine* 158, no.7 (2013): 515–525.

88. Miles EA, Calder PC. Influence of marine n-3 polyunsaturated fatty acids on immune function and a systemic review of their effects on clinical outcomes in rheumatoid arthritis. *Br J Nutr.* 2012 Jun;107 Suppl 2:S171-S184.

89. Kolahdooz F, van der Pols JC, Bain JC, et al. Meat, fish, and ovarian cancer risk: results from 2 Australian case-control studies, a systemic review, and meta-analysis. *Am J Clin Nutri.* 2010 Jun;91 (6): 1752–63.

90. Hites RA, Foran JA, Schwager SJ, et al. Global assessment of polybrominated diphenyl ethers in farmed and wild salmon. *Environ Sci Technol.* 2004 Oct 1; 38 (19): 4945–49.

91. Ponte PI, Prates JA, Crespo JP, et al. Restricting the intake of a cereal-based feed in free-range-pastured poultry: effects on performance and meat quality. *Poult Sci.* 2008 Oct;87 (10):2032–42. Ponte PI, Alves SP, Bessa RJ, et al. Influence of pature intake on the fatty acid consumption, and cholesterol, tocopherols, and tocotrienols content in meat from free-range broilers. *Poult Sci.* 2008; 87(1): 80–88.

92. Mutungi, Gisella, David Waters, Joseph Ratliff, Michael Puglisi, Richard M. Clark, Jeff S. Volek, and Maria Luz Fernandez. "Eggs Distinctly Modulate Plasma Carotenoid and Lipoprotein Subclasses in Adult Men Following a Carbohydraterestricted Diet." *The Journal of Nutritional Biochemistry* 21, no. 4 (April 2010): 261–67. doi:10.1016/j.jnutbio.2008.12.011.

93. Zeraatkar D, Han MA, Guyatt GH, Vernooij RWM, El Dib R, Cheung K, Milio K, Zworth M, Bartoszko JJ, Valli C, Rabassa M, Lee Y, Zajac J, Prokop-Dorner A, Lo C, Bala MM, Alonso-Coello P, Hanna SE, Johnston BC. Red and Processed Meat Consumption and Risk for All-Cause Mortality and Cardiometabolic Outcomes: A Systematic Review and Meta-analysis of Cohort Studies. Ann Intern Med. 2019 Nov 19;171(10):703-710. doi:10.7326/M19-0655. Epub 2019 Oct 1. PMID: 31569213.

94. Chwdhury R, Warnakula S, Kuntsor S, et al. Association of dietary, circulating, and supplement fatty acids with coronary risk:a systemic review and meta-analysis. *Ann Intern Med.* 2014 Mar 18;160 (6):398–406.

95. McAfee, A. J., McSorley, E. M., Cuskelly, G. J., Fearon, A. M., Moss, B. W., Beattie, J. a. M., Wallace, J. M. W., Bonham, M. P., & Strain, J. J. (2011). Red meat from animals offered a grass diet increases plasma and platelet n-3 PUFA in healthy consumers. *British Journal of Nutrition*, 105(1), 80–89. https://doi.org/10.1017/S0007114510003090.

96. Field, C. J., Blewett, H. H., Proctor, S., & Vine, D. (2009). Human health benefits of vaccenic acid. Applied Physiology, Nutrition, and Metabolism = Physiologie Appliquee, *Nutrition Et Metabolisme*, 34(5), 979–991. https://doi.org/10.1139/H09-079.

97. US Department of Agriculture. National Nutrient Database for Standard Reference. Beef, liver, raw. http://ndb.nal.usda.gov/ndb/foods/show/3787. February 18, 2017.

98. National Research Council (US) Committee on Drug Use in Food Animals. *The Use of Drugs In Food Animals: Benefits and Risks.* Washington, DC: National Academies Press; 1999.)

99. Schultz R Feeding Candy to cows is sweet for their digestion. *Wisconsin State Journal.* January 29, 2017.

100. Smith JS, Ameri F, Gadgil P. Effect of marinades on the formation of hererocyclic amines in grilled beef steaks. *J Food Sci.* 2008 Aug; 73 (6): T100-T105.

101. Van Vliet S, Burd NA, van Loon LJ. The skeletal muscle anabolic response to plant-versus animal based protein consumption. J Nutr. 2015 Sep; 145 (9): 1981–91.

102. Miller V, Mente A, Dehghan M, et al. Fruit, vegetable, and legume intake and cardiovascular disease and death in 18 countries (PURE): a prospective cohort study. *Lancet.* 2017 Aug 29.

103. Birt DF, Boylston T, Hendrich S, et al. Resistant starch: promise for improving human health. *Adv Nutr.* 2013 Nov 6;4 (6):587–601.

104. Craig WJ. Health effects of vegan diets. *Am J Clin Nutr.* 2009 May; 89 (5):1627S-33S.

105. Gardner, Christopher D., Alexandre Kiazand, Sofiya Alhassan, Soowon Kim, Randall S. Stafford, Raymond R. Balise, Helena C. Kraemer, and Abby C. King. "Comparison of the Atkins, Zone, Ornish, and LEARN Diets for Change in Weight and Related Risk Factors Among Overweight Premenopausal Women. The A to Z Weight Loss Study: A Randomized Trial." *Obstetrical & Gynecological Survey* 62, no. 7 (July 2007): 454–56. doi:10.1097/01.ogx.0000269084.43998.38.

106. Margioris, Andrew N. "Fatty Acids and Postprandial Inflammation." Current Opinion in Clinical Nutrition and Metabolic Care 12, no. 2 (March 2009): 129–37. doi:10.1097/mco.0b013e3283232a11.Masterjohn C. Saturated fat does a body good. Weston A. Price Foundation. May 6, 2016.

107. Innis SM. Dietary Omega-3 fatty acids and the developing brain. *Brain Res.* 2008 Oct 27;1237: 35–43.

108. Schwingshackl, L., & Hoffmann, G. (2014). Monounsaturated fatty acids, olive oil and health status: a systematic review and meta-analysis of cohort studies. *Lipids in health and disease*, *13*, 154. https://doi.org/10.1186/1476-511X-13-154

109. Majchrzak, T., Lubinska, M., Różańska, A., Dymerski, T., Gębicki, J., & Namieśnik, J. (2017). Thermal degradation assessment of canola and olive oil using ultra-fast gas chromatography coupled with chemometrics. *Monatshefte fur chemie*, *148*(9), 1625–1630. https://doi.org/10.1007/s00706-017-1968-y

110. Simopoulos, Artemis P. "Omega-3 Fatty Acids in Inflammation and Autoimmune Diseases." Journal of the American College of Nutrition 21, no. 6 (December 2002): 495–505. doi:10.1080/07315724.2002.10719248.

111. Chowdhury, R., Warnakula, S., Kunutsor, S., Crowe, F., Ward, H. A., Johnson, L., Franco, O. H., Butterworth, A. S., Forouhi, N. G., Thompson, S. G., Khaw, K.-T., Mozaffarian, D., Danesh, J., & Di Angelantonio, E. (2014). Association of Dietary, Circulating, and Supplement Fatty Acids With Coronary Risk: A Systematic Review and Meta-analysis. Annals of Internal Medicine, 160(6), 398. https://doi.org/10.7326/M13-1788. Dehghan M, Mente A, Zhang X, et al. Associations of fats and carbohydrate intake with cardiovascular disease and mortality in 18 countries from five continents (PURE: a prospective cohort study. *Lancet* 2017 Aug 29.) (Salim Y. Nutrition and CVD: data from 17 countries on 150,000 people. Cardiology Update 2017. Davos, Switzerlandl February 12, 2017.

112. Mozaffarian D, Wu JH. Omega-3 fatty acids and cardiovascular disease: effects on risk factors, molecular pathways, and clinical events. J Am Coll Cardiol. 2011 Nov 8;58 (20):2047–67. Nkondjock A, Receveur O. Fish-seafood consumption, obesity, and Type-2 diabetes: an ecological study. *Diabetes Metab*. 2003 Dec;29 (6):635–42. Simopoulos AP. Omega-3 fatty acids in inflammation and autoimmune diseases. *J Am Coll Nutr*. 2002;21(6):495–505. Li F, Liu X, Zhang D. Fish consumption and risk of depression: meta-analysis. *J Epidemiol Community Health*. 2016;70:299–304.

113. Hession, M., C. Rolland, U. Kulkarni, A. Wise, and J. Broom. "Systematic Review of Randomized Controlled Trials of Low-carbohydrate vs. Low-fat/lowcalorie Diets in the Management of Obesity and Its Comorbidities." *Obesity Reviews* 10, no. 1 (January 2009): 36–50. doi:10.1111/j.1467-789x.2008.00518.x.

114. Chowdhury R, Warnakula S, Kunutsor S, et al. Association of dietary, circulating, *Ann Intern Med*. 2014 Mar 18;160 (6):398–406.

115. Dreon DM, Fernstrom HA, Campos H, et al. Change in dietary saturated fat intake is correlated with change in mass of large low-density-lipoprotein particles in men. *Am J Clin Nutr*. 1998 May;67 (5): 828–36. Siri PW, Krauss RM. Influence of Dietary carbohydrate and fat on LDL and HDL particle distributions. *Curr Atheroscler Rep*.2005 Nov;7 (6):455–59.

116. Nickols-Richardson, Sharon M., Mary Dean Coleman, Joanne J. Volpe, and Kathy W. Hosig. "Perceived Hunger Is Lower and Weight Loss Is Greater in Overweight Premenopausal Women Consuming a Low-Carbohydrate/High-Protein vs High-Carbohydrate/Low-Fat Diet." *Journal of the American Dietetic Association* 105, no. 9 (September 2005): 1433–37. doi:10.1016/j.jada.2005.06.025.

117. Lawrence, G. D. "Dietary Fats and Health: Dietary Recommendations in the Context of Scientific Evidence." *Advances in Nutrition: An International Review Journal* 4, no. 3 (May 2013): 294–302. doi:10.3945/an.113.003657

118. Volk, Brittanie M., Laura J. Kunces, Daniel J. Freidenreich, Brian R. Kupchak, Catherine Saenz, Juan C. Artistizabal, Maria Luz Fernandez, Richard S. Bruno, Carl M. Maresh, William J. Kraemer, Stephen D. Phinney, and Jeff S. Volek. "Effects of Step-Wise Increases in Dietary Carbohydrate on Circulating Saturated Fatty Acids and Palmitoleic Acid in Adults with Metabolic Syndrome." *PLoS ONE* 9, no. 11 (November 2014). doi:10.1371/journal.pone.0113605.

119. Ameer, Fatima, Lisa Scandiuzzi, Shahida Hasnain, Hubert Kalbacher, and Nousheen Zaidi. "De Novo Lipogenesis in Health and Disease." *Metabolism* 63, no. 7 (July 2014): 895–902.doi:10.1016/j.metabol.2014.04.003.

120. Gausch-Ferre M, Hu FB, Martinez-Gonzalez MA, et al. Olive oil intake and risk of cardiovascular disease and mortality in the PREDIMED Study. *BMC Med.* 2014; 12:78.

121. Perez-Jimenez F, Ruano J, Perez-Martinez P, et al. The influence of olive oil on human health: not a question of fat alone. *Mol Nutr Food Res.* 2007 Oct; 51(10): 1199–1208.)

122. Elnagar, Ahmed, Paul Sylvester, and Khalid El Sayed. "(–)-Oleocanthal as a CMet Inhibitor for the Control of Metastatic Breast and Prostate Cancers." *Planta Medica* 77, no. 10 (February 2011): 1013–19. doi:10.1055/s-0030-1270724.

123. Romero, Concepción, Eduardo Medina, Julio Vargas, Manuel Brenes, and Antonio De Castro. "In Vitro Activity of Olive Oil Polyphenols against Helicobacter Pylori." Journal of *Agricultural and Food Chemistry* 55, no. 3 (February 2007): 680–86. doi:10.1021/jf0630217

124. Teres, S., G. Barcelo-Coblijn, M. Benet, R. Alvarez, R. Bressani, J. E. Halver, and P. V. Escriba. "Oleic Acid Content Is Responsible for the Reduction in Blood Pressure Induced by Olive Oil." *Proceedings of the National Academy of Sciences* 105, no. 37 (September 2008): 13811–16. doi:10.1073/pnas.0807500105.

125. Roos, Baukje De, Xuguang Zhang, Guillermo Rodriguez Gutierrez, Sharon Wood, Garry J. Rucklidge, Martin D. Reid, Gary J. Duncan, Louise L. Cantlay, Garry G. Duthie, and Niamh O'Kennedy. "Anti-platelet Effects of Olive Oil Extract: In Vitro Functional and Proteomic Studies." *European Journal of Nutrition* 50, no. 7 (January 2011): 553–62. doi:10.1007/s00394-010-01623.

126. Torres, N., Guevara-Cruz, M., Velázquez-Villegas, L. A., & Tovar, A. R. (2015). Nutrition and *Atherosclerosis*. Archives of Medical Research, 46(5), 408–426. https://doi.org/10.1016/j.arcmed.2015.05.010.

127. D'Imperio, Marco, Marco Gobbino, Antonio Picanza, Simona Costanzo, Anna Della Corte, and Luisa Mannina. "Influence of Harvest Method and Period on Olive Oil Composition: An NMR and Statistical Study." *Journal of Agricultural and Food Chemistry* 58, no. 20 (October 2010): 11043–51. doi:10.1021/jf1026982.

128. Givens, D. I. "Milk in the Diet: Good or Bad for Vascular Disease?" *Proceedings of the Nutrition Society* 71, no. 01 (October 2011): 98–104. doi:10.1017/s0029665111003223

129. Pimpin L, Wu JH, Haskelberg H, et al. Is butter back? A systemic review and meta-analysis of butter consumption and risk of cardiovascular disease, diabetes and total mortality. *PLoS One.* 2016 Jun 29;11 (6).

130. Pasture Butter, Cultured, 1 lb, 4 quarters | Buy Organic Valley Near You. (n.d.). Retrieved February 28, 2020, from https://www.organicvalley.coop/products/butter /pasture-butter/pasture-butter-cultured-1-lb-4-quarters/.

131. Watson, Stephen John, Gerald Bishop, Jack Cecil Drummond, Albert Edward Gillam, and Isidor Morris Heilbron. "The Relation of the Colour and Vitamin A Content of Butter to the Nature of the Ration Fed." *Biochemical Journal* 28, no. 3 (1934): 1076–85. doi:10.1042/bj0281076

132. Grosso, G., J. Yang, S. Marventano, A. Micek, F. Galvano, and S. N. Kales. "Nut Consumption on All-Cause, Cardiovascular, and Cancer Mortality Risk: A Systematic Review and Meta-analysis of Epidemiologic Studies." *American Journal of Clinical Nutrition* 101, no. 4 (February 2015): 783–93. doi:10.3945/ajcn.114.099515.

133. Estruch R, Sierra C. Commentary: frequent nut consumption protects against cardiovascular and cancer mortality, but the effects may be even greator if nuts are including in a healthy diet. *Int J Epidemiol.* 2015 Jun; 44 (3):1049–50.),51)

134. Pribis, P., & Shukitt-Hale, B. (2014). Cognition: The new frontier for nuts and berries. *The American Journal of Clinical Nutrition*, 100 Suppl 1, 347S-52S. https://doi.org/10 .3945/ajcn.113.071506.

135. Storniolo CE, Casillas R, Bullo M, et al. A Mediterranean diet supplemented with extra virgin olive oil or nuts improves endothelial markers involved in blood pressure control in hypertensive women. *Eur J Nutr.* 2017 Feb; 56 (1):89–97.

136. Jenkins, David J. A., Julia M. W. Wong, Cyril W. C. Kendall, Āmīn Esfahani, Vivian W. Y. Ng, Tracy C. K. Leong, Dorothea A. Faulkner, Ed Vidgen, Gregory Paul, Ratna Mukherjea, Elaine S. Krul, and William Singer. "Effect of a 6-month Vegan Low-carbohydrate ('Eco-Atkins') Diet on Cardiovascular Risk Factors and Body Weight in Hyperlipidaemic Adults: A Randomised Controlled Trial." *BMJ Open* 4, no. 2 (February 2014). doi:10.1136/bmjopen-2013-003505.

137. Dhiman, T. R., S. H. Nam, A. L. Ure. "Factors Affecting Conjugated Linoleic Acid Content in Milk and Meat." *Crit Rev Food Sci Nutr.* 2005;45(6):463–82. https://www .ncbi.nlm.nih.gov/pubmed/16183568.

138. Asghari G, Ghorbani Z, Mirmiran P, Azizi F. Nut consumption is associated with lower incidence of Type-2 diabetes: the Tehran Lipid and Glucose Study. *Diabetes Metab.* 2017 Feb;43 (1):18–24.)

139. Gopinath B, Flood VM, Burlutsky G, et al. Consumption of nuts and risk of total and cause-specific mortality over 15 years. *Nutr Metab Cardiovasc Dis.* 2015 Dec;25 (12): 1125–31.

140. Calani L, Dall'Asta M, Derlindati E, et al. Colonic metabolism of polyphenols from coffee, green tea, and hazelnut skins. *J Clin Gastroenterol.* 2012 Oct;46 Supple:S95-S99.

141. Guasch-Ferre M, Babio N, Martinez-Gonzalez MA, et al. Dietary fat intake and risk of cardiovascular disease and all-cause mortality in a population at high risk of cardiovascular disease. *Am J Clin Nutr.* 2015 Dec;102(6):1563–73.

142. Prior IA, Davidson F, Salmond CE, Czochanska Z. Cholesterol, coconuts and diet on Polynesian atolls: a natural experiment:the Pukapuka and Tokelau island studies. *Am J Clin Nutr.* 1981 Aug;34 (8): 1552–61.

143. Lipoeto, N. I., Agus, Z., Ocnzil, F., Wahlqvist, M., & Wattanapenpaiboon, N. (2004). Dietary intake and the risk of coronary heart disease among the coconut-consuming Minangkabau in West Sumatra, Indonesia. *Asia Pacific Journal of Clinical Nutrition,* 13(4), 377–384.

144. Ogbolu, D. O., A. A. Oni, O. A. Daini, and A. P. Oloko. "In Vitro Antimicrobial Properties of Coconut Oil on Candida Species in Ibadan, Nigeria." Journal of Medicinal Food 10, no. 2 (June 2007): 384–87. doi:10.1089/jmf.2006.1209.

145. Bergsson, G., J. Arnfinnsson, O. Steingrimsson, and H. Thormar. "In Vitro Killing of Candida Albicans by Fatty Acids and Monoglycerides." *Antimicrobial Agents and Chemotherapy* 45, no. 11 (November 2001): 3209–12. doi:10.1128/aac.45.11.3209-3212.2001.

146. Dulloo AG, Fathi M, Mensi N, et al. Twenty-four-hour energy expenditure and urinary catecholamines of human consuming low-to-moderate amounds of medium-chain triglycerides: a dose- response study in a human respiratory chamber. *Eur J Clin Nutr.* 1996 Mar; 50 (3):152–58.

147. Lindeberg, Staffan, Mats Eliasson, Bernt Lindahl, and Bo Ahrén. "Low Serum Insulin in Traditional Pacific Islanders – The Kitava Study." *Metabolism* 48, no. 10 (October 1999): 1216–19. doi:10.1016/s0026-0495(99)90258-5.

148. St-Onge MP, Jones PJ. Greater rise in fat oxidation with medium-chain triglyceride consumption relative to long-chain triglyceride is associated with lower initial body weight and greater loss of subcutaneous adipose tissue. *Int J Obes Relat Metab Disord.* 2003 Dec;27(12):1565–71. Assuncao ML, Ferreira HS, dos Santos AF, et al. Effects of dietary coconut oil on biochemical and anthropometric profiles of women presenting abdominal obesity. *Lipids.* 2009 Jul;44 (7):593–601.

149. Singh GM, Micha R, Khatibzadeh S, et al. Estimated global, regional and national disease burdens related to sugar-sweetened beverage consumption in 2010. *Circulation.* 2015 Aug 25;132(8):639–66.

150. Cheungpasitporn W, Thongprayoon C, O'Corragain OA, Edmonds PJ, Kittanamongkolchai W, Erickson SB. Associations of sugar-sweetened and artificially sweetened soda with chronic kidney disease: a systemic and meta-analysis. *Nephrology* (Carlton). 2014 Dec; 19 (12) 791–97.

151. Cheungpasitporn W, Thongprayoon C, Edmonds PJ, et al. Sugar and artificially sweetened soda consumption linked to hypertension: a systemic review and meta-analysis. *Clin Exp Hypertens.* 2015;37 (7):587–93.

152. Greenwood DC. Threapleton DE, Evans CE, et al. Association between sugar sweet-ened and artificially sweetened soft drinks and Type-2 diabetes: systemic review and dose-response meta-analysis of prospective studies. *Br J Nutr.* 2014 Sep 14;112 (5):725–34.

153. Wjarnpreecha K, Thongprayoon C, Edmonds PJ, Cheungpasitporn W. Associations of sugar- and artificially sweetened soda with nonalcoholic fatty liver disease: a systemic review and dose-response meta-analysis of prospective studies. *Br J Nutr.* 2014 Sep 12;112 (5):725–34.

154. Malik VS. Sugar sweetened beverages and cardiometabolic health. *Curr Opin Cardinol.* 2017 Sep;32 (5):572–79.

155. Shomar, B. (2012). Zamzam water: Concentration of trace elements and other char-acteristics. *Chemosphere,* 86(6), 600–605. https://doi.org/10.1016/j.chemosphere.2011.10.025

156. Keramati Yazdi, F., Shabestani Monfared, A., Tashakkorian, H., Mahmoudzadeh, A., & Borzoueisileh, S. (2017). Radioprotective effect of Zamzam (alkaline) water: A cyto-genetic study. *Journal of Environmental Radioactivity,* 167, 166–169. https://doi.org/10.1016/j.jenvrad.2016.10.019

157. Bjarnadottir A. Science: coffee is the world's biggest source of antioxidants. https://authoritynutrition.com/coffee-world-biggest-source-of-antioxidants/. Retrieved February 25, 2020.

158. Ding M Satija A, Bhupathiraju SN, et al. Association of coffee consumption with total and cause-specific mortality in 3 large prospective cohorts. *Circulation.* 2015 November; 132:2305–15. Kennedy OJ, Roderick P, Buchanan R, Fallowfield JA, Hayes PC, Parkes J. Systematic review with meta-analysis: coffee consumption and the risk of cirrhosis. *Aliment Pharmacol Ther.* 2016 Mar; 43(5):562–74. O'Keefe JH, Bhatti SK, Patil HR, et al. Effects of habitual coffee consumption on cardiometabolic disease, cardiovascular health and all-cause mortality. *J Am Coll Cardiol.* 2013 Sep 17;62 (12):1043–51. Wu L, Sun D, He Y. Coffee intake and the incident risk of cognitive disorders: a dose response meta-analysis of nine prospective cohort studies. *Clin Nutr.* 2016 May 30. S0261-5614 (16)30111-X.

159. Van Dam RM, Pasman WJ, Verhoef P. Effects of coffee consumption of fasting blood sugar and insulin concentrations: randomized controlled trials in healthy volunteers. *Diabetes Care.* 2004 Dec; 27 (12): 2990–92.

160. Lovallo WR, Al'Absi M, Blick K, et al. Stress like adrenocorticotropin repsonses to caffeine in young men. *Pharmacol Biochem Behav.* 1996 Nov;55 (3):365–69.)

161. Brighenti, F., Castellani, G., Benini, L., Casiraghi, M. C., Leopardi, E., Crovetti, R., & Testolin, G. (1995). Effect of neutralized and native vinegar on blood glucose and acetate responses to a mixed meal in healthy subjects. European Journal of Clinical Nutrition, 49(4), 242–247.

162. Ostman, E., Granfeldt, Y., Persson, L., & Björck, I. (2005). Vinegar supplementation lowers glucose and insulin responses and increases satiety after a bread meal in healthy subjects. European *Journal of Clinical Nutrition*, 59(9), 983–988. https://doi.org/10.1038/sj.ejcn.1602197

163. Entani, E., Asai, M., Tsujihata, S., Tsukamoto, Y., & Ohta, M. (1998). Antibacterial action of vinegar against food-borne pathogenic bacteria including Escherichia coli O157:H7 *Journal of Food Protection*, 61(8), 953–959. https://doi.org/10.4315/0362-028x-61.8.953

164. Shishehbor, F., Mansoori, A., Sarkaki, A. R., Jalali, M. T., & Latifi, S. M. (2008). Apple cider vinegar attenuates lipid profile in normal and diabetic rats. *Pakistan Journal of Biological Sciences: PJBS*, 11(23), 2634–2638. https://doi.org/10.3923/pjbs.2008.2634.2638

165. Choi, In Hwa, Jeong Sook Noh, Ji-Sook Han, Hyun Ju Kim, Eung-Soo Han, and Yeong Ok Song. "Kimchi, a Fermented Vegetable, Improves Serum Lipid Profiles in Healthy Young Adults: Randomized Clinical Trial." *Journal of Medicinal Food* 16, no. 3 (March 2013): 223–29. doi:10.1089/jmf.2012.2563.

166. Sun, P., J. Q. Wang, and H. T. Zhang. "Effects of Bacillus Subtilis Natto on Performance and Immune Function of Preweaning Calves." *Journal of Dairy Science* 93, no. 12 (December 2010): 5851–55. doi:10.3168/jds.2010-3263.

167. He FJ, Nowson CA, Lucas M, et al. Increased consumption of fruit and vegetables is related to a reduced risk of coronary heart disease: meta-analysis of cohort studies. *J Hum Hypertens*. 2007 Sep; 21(9):717–28.

168. He FJ, Nowson CA, MacGregor GA. Fruit and vegetable consumption and stroke: meta-analysis of cohort studies. *Lancet*. 2006 Jan 28;367 (9507):320–26.

169. Nooyens AC, Bueno-de-Mesquita HB, van Boxtel MP, et al. Fruit and vegetable intake and cognitive decline in middle-aged men and women: the Doetinchem Cohort Study. *Br J Nutr*. 2001 Sep;106(5):752–61.

170. (Meyer BJ, de Bruin EJ, Du Plessis DG, et al. Some biochemical effects of mainly fruit diet in man. *S Afr Med J*. 1971;45 (10):253–61.).

171. Ali, S. A., Parveen, N., & Ali, A. S. (2018). Links between the Prophet Muhammad (PBUH) recommended foods and disease management: A review in the light of modern superfoods. *International Journal of Health Sciences*, 12(2), 61–69.

172. Russo, F., Caporaso, N., Paduano, A., & Sacchi, R. (2014). Phenolic compounds in fresh and dried figs from Cilento (Italy), by considering breba crop and full crop, in comparison to Turkish and Greek dried figs. Journal of Food Science, 79(7), C1278–1284. https://doi.org/10.1111/1750-3841.12505, Ercisli, S., Tosun, M., Karlidag, H., Dzubur, A., Hadziabulic, S., & Aliman, Y. (2012). Colour and antioxidant characteristics of some fresh fig (Ficus carica L.) genotypes from northeastern Turkey. *Plant Foods for Human Nutrition* (Dordrecht, Netherlands), 67(3), 271–276. https://doi.org/10.1007/s11130-012-0292-2

173. Ammar, S., del Mar Contreras, M., Belguith-Hadrich, O., Segura-Carretero, A., & Bouaziz, M. (2015). Assessment of the distribution of phenolic compounds and contribution to the antioxidant activity in Tunisian fig leaves, fruits, skins and pulps using mass spectrometry-based analysis. *Food & Function*, 6(12), 3663–3677. https://doi.org /10.1039/c5fo00837a

174. Jing, L., Zhang, Y.-M., Luo, J.-G., & Kong, L.-Y. (2015). Tirucallane-type triterpenoids from the fruit of Ficus carica and their cytotoxic activity. *Chemical & Pharmaceutical Bulletin*, 63(3), 237–243. https://doi.org/10.1248/cpb.c14-00779

175. Badgujar, S. B., Patel, V. V., Bandivdekar, A. H., & Mahajan, R. T. (2014). Traditional uses, phytochemistry and pharmacology of Ficus carica: A review. *Pharmaceutical Biology*, 52(11), 1487–1503. https://doi.org/10.3109/13880209.2014.892515

176. Yang, X., Guo, J. L., Ye, J. Y., Zhang, Y. X., & Wang, W. (2015). The effects of Ficus carica polysaccharide on immune response and expression of some immune-related genes in grass carp, Ctenopharyngodon idella. *Fish & Shellfish Immunology*, 42(1), 132–137. https://doi.org/10.1016/j.fsi.2014.10.037

177. Soltana, H., Pinon, A., Limami, Y., Zaid, Y., Khalki, L., Zaid, N., Salah, D., Sabitaliyevich, U. Y., Simon, A., Liagre, B., & Hammami, M. (2019). Antitumoral activity of Ficus carica L. on colourectal cancer cell lines. *Cellular and Molecular Biology* (Noisy-Le-Grand, France), 65(6), 6–11.

178. IDOSI Journals Databases. (n.d.). Retrieved February 26, 2020, from https://idosi.org /dbases.htm

179. Slatnar, A., Klancar, U., Stampar, F., & Veberic, R. (2011). Effect of drying of figs (Ficus carica L.) on the contents of sugars, organic acids, and phenolic compounds. *Journal of Agricultural and Food Chemistry*, 59(21), 11696–11702. https://doi.org/10 .1021/jf202707y

180. Georgiev, V., Ananga, A., & Tsolova, V. (2014). Recent Advances and Uses of Grape Flavonoids as Nutraceuticals. *Nutrients*, 6(1), 391–415. https://doi.org/10.3390 /nu6010391

181. Yadav, D., Kumar, A., Kumar, P., & Mishra, D. (2015). Antimicrobial properties of black grape (Vitis vinifera L.) peel extracts against antibiotic-resistant pathogenic bacteria and toxin producing moulds. *Indian Journal of Pharmacology*, 47(6), 663–667. https://doi.org/10.4103/0253-7613.169591

182. Luan, Y.-Y., Liu, Z.-M., Zhong, J.-Y., Yao, R.-Y., & Yu, H.-S. (2015). Effect of grape seed proanthocyanidins on tumor vasculogenic mimicry in human triple-negative breast cancer cells. Asian *Pacific Journal of Cancer Prevention: APJCP*, 16(2), 531–535. https://doi.org/10.7314/apjcp.2015.16.2.531

183. Wang, L., Xu, M., Liu, C., Wang, J., Xi, H., Wu, B., Loescher, W., Duan, W., Fan, P., & Li, S. (2013). Resveratrols in Grape Berry Skins and Leaves in Vitis Germplasm. *PLoS ONE*, 8(4). https://doi.org/10.1371/journal.pone.0061642

184. Paiotti, A. P. R., Neto, R. A., Marchi, P., Silva, R. M., Pazine, V. L., Noguti, J., Pastrelo, M. M., Gollücke, A. P. B., Miszputen, S. J., & Ribeiro, D. A. (2013). The anti-inflammatory potential of phenolic compounds in grape juice concentrate (G8000TM) on 2,4,6-trinitrobenzene sulphonic acid-induced colitis. *The British Journal of Nutrition*, 110(6), 973–980. https://doi.org/10.1017/S000711451300007X

185. Zarfeshany, A., Asgary, S., & Javanmard, S. H. (2014). Potent health effects of pomegranate. *Advanced Biomedical Research*, 3. https://doi.org/10.4103/2277-9175.129371

186. Punicic acid is an omega-5 fatty acid capable of inhibiting breast cancer proliferation .Michael E. Grossmann, Nancy K. Mizuno, Todd Schuster, Margot P. Cleary *Int J Oncol*. 2010 Feb; 36(2): 421–426. Shirode, A. B., Kovvuru, P., Chittur, S. V., Henning, S. M., Heber, D., & Reliene, R. (2014). Antiproliferative effects of pomegranate extract in MCF-7 breast cancer cells are associated with reduced DNA repair gene expression and induction of double strand breaks. *Molecular Carcinogenesis*, 53(6), 458–470. https://doi.org/10.1002/mc.21995.

187. Shukla, Meenakshi, Kalpana Gupta, Zafar Rasheed, Khursheed A. Khan, and Tariq M. Haqqi. "Bioavailable Constituents/Metabolites of Pomegranate (Punica Granatum L) Preferentially Inhibit COX2 Activity ex Vivo and IL-1beta-induced PGE2 Production in Human

188. Asgary, S., Keshvari, M., Sahebkar, A., Hashemi, M., & Rafieian-Kopaei, M. (2013). Clinical investigation of the acute effects of pomegranate juice on blood pressure and endothelial function in hypertensive individuals. *ARYA atherosclerosis*, 9(6), 326–331.

189. M. Schneeberger et al., "Akkermansia Muciniphila Inversely Correlates with the Onset of Inflammation, Altered Adiposetissue Metabolism, and Metabolic Disorders during Obesity in Mice," *Science Reports* 5 (2015):16643.

190. Rashidkhani, B., Lindblad, P., & Wolk, A. (2005). Fruits, vegetables and risk of renal cell carcinoma: A prospective study of Swedish women. *International Journal of Cancer*, 113(3), 451–455. https://doi.org/10.1002/ijc.20577

191. Houston, M. C. (2011). The importance of potassium in managing hypertension. Current Hypertension Reports, 13(4), 309–317. https://doi.org/10.1007/s11906-011-0197-8

192. Rosique-Esteban, N., Guasch-Ferré, M., Hernández-Alonso, P., & Salas-Salvadó, J. (2018). Dietary Magnesium and Cardiovascular Disease: A Review with Emphasis in Epidemiological Studies. *Nutrients,* 10(2). https://doi.org/10.3390/nu10020168

193. Clark, M. J., & Slavin, J. L. (2013). The effect of fibre on satiety and food intake: A systematic review. *Journal of the American College of Nutrition*, 32(3), 200–211. https://doi.org/10.1080/07315724.2013.791194

194. Effects of Fresh Watermelon Consumption on the Acute Satiety Response and Cardiometabolic Risk Factors in Overweight and Obese Adults. (n.d.). Retrieved February 25, 2021, from https://www.ncbi.nlm.nih.gov/pmc/articles/PMC6470521/

195. Naz, A., Butt, M. S., Sultan, M. T., Qayyum, M. M. N., & Niaz, R. S. (2014). Watermelon lycopene and allied health claims. *EXCLI Journal*, 13, 650–660.

196. Bowers, L. W., Rossi, E. L., O'Flanagan, C. H., deGraffenried, L. A., & Hursting, S. D. (2015). The Role of the Insulin/IGF System in Cancer: Lessons Learned from Clinical Trials and the Energy Balance-Cancer Link. *Frontiers in Endocrinology*, 6, 77. https://doi.org/10.3389/fendo.2015.00077

197. Figueroa, A., Wong, A., Hooshmand, S., & Sanchez-Gonzalez, M. A. (2013). Effects of watermelon supplementation on arterial stiffness and wave reflection amplitude in postmenopausal women. *Menopause* (New York, N.Y.), 20(5), 573–577. https://doi.org/10.1097/GME.0b013e3182733794

198. Ellis, A. C., Dudenbostel, T., & Crowe-White, K. (2019). Watermelon Juice: A Novel Functional Food to Increase Circulating Lycopene in Older Adult Women. *Plant Foods for Human Nutrition* (Dordrecht, Netherlands), 74(2), 200–203. https://doi.org/10.1007/s11130-019-00719-9

199. Tarazona-Díaz, M. P., Alacid, F., Carrasco, M., Martínez, I., & Aguayo, E. (2013). Watermelon juice: Potential functional drink for sore muscle relief in athletes. *Journal of Agricultural and Food Chemistry*, 61(31), 7522–7528. https://doi.org/10.1021/jf400964r

200. Puertollano, M. A., Puertollano, E., de Cienfuegos, G. Á., & de Pablo, M. A. (2011). Dietary antioxidants: Immunity and host defense. Current Topics in Medicinal Chemistry, 11(14), 1752–1766. https://doi.org/10.2174/156802611796235107,Wintergerst, E. S., Maggini, S., & Hornig, D. H. (2006). Immune-enhancing role of vitamin C and zinc and effect on clinical conditions. *Annals of Nutrition & Metabolism*, 50(2), 85–94. https://doi.org/10.1159/000090495

201. Anti-inflammatory effect of essential oil and its constituents from fingered citron (Citrus medica L. var. Sarcodactylis) through blocking JNK, ERK... – PubMed – NCBI. (n.d.). Retrieved February 25, 2020, from https://www.ncbi.nlm.nih.gov/pubmed/23541436

202. Aune, D., Giovannucci, E., Boffetta, P., Fadnes, L. T., Keum, N., Norat, T., Greenwood, D. C., Riboli, E., Vatten, L. J., & Tonstad, S. (2017). Fruit and vegetable intake and the risk of cardiovascular disease, total cancer and all-cause mortality-a systematic review and dose-response meta-analysis of prospective studies. *International Journal of Epidemiology*, 46(3), 1029–1056. https://doi.org/10.1093/ije/dyw319

203. Wu, Z., Li, H., Tu, D., Yang, Y., & Zhan, Y. (2013). Extraction optimization, preliminary characterization, and in vitro antioxidant activities of crude polysaccharides from finger citron. Industrial Crops and Products, 44, 145–151. https://doi.org/10.1016/j.indcrop.2012.11.008

204. *Citrus fruit and cancer risk in a network of case-control studies. – PubMed – NCBI.* (n.d.). Retrieved February 25, 2020, from https://www.ncbi.nlm.nih.gov/pubmed/19856118, Cirmi, S., Ferlazzo, N., Lombardo, G. E., Maugeri, A., Calapai, G., Gangemi, S., & Navarra, M. (2016). Chemopreventive Agents and Inhibitors of Cancer Hallmarks:

May Citrus Offer New Perspectives? *Nutrients*, 8(11). https://doi.org/10.3390/nu8110698, *Citrus Fruit Intake and Breast Cancer Risk: A Quantitative Systematic Review*. (n.d.). Retrieved February 25, 2020, from https://www.ncbi.nlm.nih.gov/pmc/articles/PMC3625773/

205. Abdoul-Azize, S. (2016). Potential Benefits of Jujube (Zizyphus Lotus L.) Bioactive Compounds for Nutrition and Health. *Journal of Nutrition and Metabolism*, 2016. https://doi.org/10.1155/2016/2067470

206. Zhang, L., Liu, X., Wang, Y., Liu, G., Zhang, Z., Zhao, Z., & Cheng, H. (2017). In vitro antioxidative and immunological activities of polysaccharides from Zizyphus Jujuba cv. Muzao. *International Journal of Biological Macromolecules*, 95, 1119–1125. https://doi.org/10.1016/j.ijbiomac.2016.10.102

207. San, A. M. M., Thongpraditchote, S., Sithisarn, P., & Gritsanapan, W. (2013). Total Phenolics and Total Flavonoids Contents and Hypnotic Effect in Mice of Ziziphus mauritiana Lam. Seed Extract. *Evidence-Based Complementary and Alternative Medicine: ECAM*, 2013, 835854. https://doi.org/10.1155/2013/835854, Shi, G.-B., Wu, Q., Zhang, B., Sun, X.-H., Zong, W.-T., Zhao, X.-R., Xin, Y., Zhao, Q.-C., & Chen, Y.-F. (2013). Possible mechanism involved in the sedative activity of jujubasaponins I in mice. *CNS Neuroscience & Therapeutics*, 19(4), 282–284. https://doi.org/10.1111/cns.12070

208. Vahedi, F., Fathi Najafi, M., & Bozari, K. (2008). Evaluation of inhibitory effect and apoptosis induction of Zyzyphus Jujube on tumor cell lines, an in vitro preliminary study. *Cytotechnology*, 56(2), 105–111. https://doi.org/10.1007/s10616-008-9131-6

209. Yue, Y., Wu, S., Li, Z., Li, J., Li, X., Xiang, J., & Ding, H. (2015). Wild jujube polysaccharides protect against experimental inflammatory bowel disease by enabling enhanced intestinal barrier function. Food & Function, 6(8), 2568–2577. https://doi.org/10.1039/c5fo00378d, Effects of Water-Soluble Carbohydrate Concentrate from Chinese Jujube on Different Intestinal and Fecal Indices | *Journal of Agricultural and Food Chemistry*. (n.d.). Retrieved February 25, 2020, from https://pubs.acs.org/doi/abs/10.1021/jf072664z

210. Holscher, H. D. (2017). Dietary fibre and prebiotics and the gastrointestinal microbiota. *Gut Microbes*, 8(2), 172–184. https://doi.org/10.1080/19490976.2017.1290756

211. Peterson, J., Dwyer, J., Adlercreutz, H., Scalbert, A., Jacques, P., & McCullough, M. L. (2010). Dietary lignans: Physiology and potential for cardiovascular disease risk reduction. *Nutrition Reviews*, 68(10), 571–603. https://doi.org/10.1111/j.1753-4887.2010.00319.x

212. Johnson, S. A., & Arjmandi, B. H. (2013). Evidence for anti-cancer properties of blueberries: A mini-review. *Anti-Cancer Agents in Medicinal Chemistry*, 13(8), 1142–1148. https://doi.org/10.2174/18715206113139990137.

213. Rodriguez-Mateos A, Rendeiro C, Bergillos-Meca T, et al. Intake and time dependence of blueberry flavonoid-induced improvements in vascular function: a randomized, controlled, double blind, crossover intervention study with mechanistic insights into biological activity. *Am J Clin Nutr.* 2013 Nov;98 (5):1179–91.

214. Schroder, K. E. E. (2010). Effects of fruit consumption on body mass index and weight loss in a sample of overweight and obese dieters enrolled in a weight-loss intervention trial. *Nutrition* (Burbank, Los Angeles County, Calif.), 26(7–8), 727–734. https://doi .org/10.1016/j.nut.2009.08.009

215. Mijanur Rahman, M., Gan, S. H., & Khalil, M. I. (2014). Neurological effects of honey: Current and future prospects. *Evidence-Based Complementary and Alternative Medicine: ECAM*, 2014, 958721. https://doi.org/10.1155/2014/958721.

216. Legault, J., Girard-Lalancette, K., Grenon, C., Dussault, C., & Pichette, A. (2010). Antioxidant activity, inhibition of nitric oxide overproduction, and in vitro antiproliferative effect of maple sap and syrup from Acer saccharum. *Journal of Medicinal Food*, 13(2), 460–468. https://doi.org/10.1089/jmf.2009.0029 ; High-performance liquid chromatography characterization and identification of antioxidant polyphenols in maple syrup | Canadian Forest Service Publications | Natural Resources Canada. (n.d.). Retrieved February 28, 2020, from https://cfs.nrcan.gc.ca/publications?id=28297.

217. Nagai, N., Ito, Y., & Taga, A. (2013). Comparison of the enhancement of plasma glucose levels in Type-2 diabetes Otsuka Long-Evans Tokushima Fatty rats by oral administration of sucrose or maple syrup. *Journal of Oleo Science*, 62(9), 737–743. https://doi .org/10.5650/jos.62.737, 220Nagai, N., Yamamoto, T., Tanabe, W., Ito, Y., Kurabuchi, S., Mitamura, K., & Taga, A. (2015). Changes in plasma glucose in Otsuka Long-Evans Tokushima Fatty rats after oral administration of maple syrup. *Journal of Oleo Science*, 64(3), 331–335. https://doi.org/10.5650/jos.ess14075.

218. González-Sarrías, A., Li, L., & Seeram, N. P. (2012). Effects of maple (Acer) plant part extracts on proliferation, apoptosis and cell cycle arrest of human tumorigenic and non-tumorigenic colon cells. Phytotherapy Research: PTR, 26(7), 995–1002. https:// doi.org/10.1002/ptr.3677; González-Sarrías, A., Ma, H., Edmonds, M. E., & Seeram, N. P. (2013). Maple polyphenols, ginnalins A-C, induce S- and G2/M-cell cycle arrest in colon and breast cancer cells mediated by decreasing cyclins A and D1 levels. *Food Chemistry*, 136(2), 636–642. https://doi.org/10.1016/j.foodchem.2012.08.023. Moriyama, K. Mitamura, A. Taga. Yamamoto, T., Uemura, K., Moriyama, K., Mitamura, K., & Taga, A. (2015). Inhibitory effect of maple syrup on the cell growth and invasion of human colourectal cancer cells. *Oncology Reports*, 33(4), 1579–1584. https://doi.org/10 .3892/or.2015.3777.

219. Phillips, K. M., Carlsen, M. H., & Blomhoff, R. (2009). Total Antioxidant Content of Alternatives to Refined Sugar. *Journal of the American Dietetic Association*, 109(1), 64–71. https://doi.org/10.1016/j.jada.2008.10.014.

220. Adukwu, E. C., Allen, S. C. H., & Phillips, C. A. (2012). The anti-biofilm activity of lemongrass (Cymbopogon flexuosus) and grapefruit (Citrus paradisi) essential oils against five strains of Staphylococcus aureus. *Journal of Applied Microbiology*, 113(5), 1217–1227. https://doi.org/10.1111/j.1365-2672.2012.05418.x

221. Sforcin, J. M., Amaral, J. T., Fernandes, A., Sousa, J. P. B., & Bastos, J. K. (2009). Lemongrass effects on IL-1beta and IL-6 production by macrophages. *Natural Product Research*, 23(12), 1151–1159. https://doi.org/10.1080/14786410902000601

222. Boukhatem, M. N., Ferhat, M. A., Kameli, A., Saidi, F., & Kebir, H. T. (2014). Lemon grass (Cymbopogon citratus) essential oil as a potent anti-inflammatory and antifungal drugs. *The Libyan Journal of Medicine*, 9, 25431. https://doi.org/10.3402/ljm.v9.25431

223. Chaouki, W., Leger, D. Y., Liagre, B., Beneytout, J.-L., & Hmamouchi, M. (2009). Citral inhibits cell proliferation and induces apoptosis and cell cycle arrest in MCF-7 cells. *Fundamental & Clinical Pharmacology*, 23(5), 549–556. https://doi.org/10.1111/j.1472-8206.2009.00738.x

224. Costa, C. A. R. A., Bidinotto, L. T., Takahira, R. K., Salvadori, D. M. F., Barbisan, L. F., & Costa, M. (2011). Cholesterol reduction and lack of genotoxic or toxic effects in mice after repeated 21-day oral intake of lemongrass (Cymbopogon citratus) essential oil. *Food and Chemical Toxicology: An International Journal Published for the British Industrial Biological Research Association*, 49(9), 2268–2272. https://doi.org/10.1016/j.fct.2011.06.025

225. Shah, G., Shri, R., Panchal, V., Sharma, N., Singh, B., & Mann, A. S. (2011). Scientific basis for the therapeutic use of Cymbopogon citratus, stapf (Lemon grass). *Journal of Advanced Pharmaceutical Technology & Research*, 2(1), 3–8. https://doi.org/10.4103/2231-4040.79796

226. Antioxidant Activity of Basil. (n.d.). Retrieved February 25, 2020, from https://hort.purdue.edu/newcrop/ncnu02/v5-575.html

227. Ocimum sanctum L (Holy Basil or Tulsi) and its phytochemicals in the prevention and treatment of cancer. – PubMed – NCBI. (n.d.). Retrieved February 25, 2020, from https://www.ncbi.nlm.nih.gov/pubmed/23682780

228. Sienkiewicz, M., Łysakowska, M., Pastuszka, M., Bienias, W., & Kowalczyk, E. (2013). The potential of use basil and rosemary essential oils as effective antibacterial agents. *Molecules* (Basel, Switzerland), 18(8), 9334–9351. https://doi.org/10.3390/molecules18089334

229. Jyoti, S., Satendra, S., Sushma, S., Anjana, T., & Shashi, S. (2007). Antistressor activity of Ocimum sanctum (Tulsi) against experimentally induced oxidative stress in rabbits. *Methods and Findings in Experimental and Clinical Pharmacology*, 29(6), 411–416. https://doi.org/10.1358/mf.2007.29.6.1118135

230. Manikandan, P., Murugan, R. S., Abbas, H., Abraham, S. K., & Nagini, S. (2007). Ocimum sanctum Linn. (Holy Basil) ethanolic leaf extract protects against

7,12-dimethylbenz(a)anthracene-induced genotoxicity, oxidative stress, and imbalance in xenobiotic-metabolizing enzymes. *Journal of Medicinal Food*, 10(3), 495–502. https://doi.org/10.1089/jmf.2006.125

231. Agrawal, P., Rai, V., & Singh, R. B. (1996). Randomized placebo-controlled, single blind trial of holy basil leaves in patients with noninsulin-dependent diabetes mellitus. International Journal of Clinical Pharmacology and Therapeutics, 34(9), 406–409.

232. Sadlon, A. E., & Lamson, D. W. (2010). Immune-modifying and antimicrobial effects of Eucalyptus oil and simple inhalation devices. Alternative Medicine Review: *A Journal of Clinical Therapeutic*, 15(1), 33–47.,Schnitzler, P., Schön, K., & Reichling, J. (2001). Antiviral activity of Australian tea tree oil and eucalyptus oil against herpes simplex virus in cell culture. *Die Pharmazie*, 56(4), 343–347.

233. Effect of Eucalyptus Oil Inhalation on Pain and Inflammatory Responses after Total Knee Replacement: A Randomized Clinical Trial. (n.d.). Retrieved February 25, 2020, from https://www.ncbi.nlm.nih.gov/pmc/articles/PMC3703330/

234. Hannan, A., Saleem, S., Chaudhary, S., Barkaat, M., & Arshad, M. U. (2008). Anti bacterial activity of Nigella sativa against clinical isolates of methicillin resistant Staphylococcus aureus. Journal of *Ayūb Medical College, Abbottabad: JAMC*, 20(3), 72–74.

235. The antitumor activity of thymoquinone and thymohydroquinone in vitro and in vivo. – *PubMed – NCBI*. (n.d.). Retrieved February 26, 2020, from https://www.ncbi.nlm.nih.gov/pubmed/17080016, Salim, L. Z. A., Mohan, S., Othman, R., Abdelwahab, S. I., Kamalidehghan, B., Sheikh, B. Y., & Ibrahim, M. Y. (2013). Thymoquinone Induces Mitochondria-Mediated Apoptosis in Acute Lymphoblastic Leukaemia in Vitro. *Molecules*, 18(9), 11219–11240. https://doi.org/10.3390/molecules180911219, Rajput, S., Kumar, B. N. P., Dey, K. K., Pal, I., Parekh, A., & Mandal, M. (2013). Molecular targeting of Akt by thymoquinone promotes G(1) arrest through translation inhibition of cyclin D1 and induces apoptosis in breast cancer cells. *Life Sciences*, 93(21), 783–790. https://doi.org/10.1016/j.lfs.2013.09.009, Racoma, I. O., Meisen, W. H., Wang, Q.-E., Kaur, B., & Wani, A. A. (2013). Thymoquinone Inhibits Autophagy and Induces Cathepsin-Mediated, Caspase-Independent Cell Death in Glioblastoma Cells. *PLoS ONE*, 8(9). https://doi.org/10.1371/journal.pone.0072882

236. Mathur, M. L., Gaur, J., Sharma, R., & Haldiya, K. R. (2011). Antidiabetic Properties of a Spice Plant Nigella sativa. *Journal of Endocrinology and Metabolism*, 1(1), 1–8. https://doi.org/10.4021/jem.v1i1.15

237. Namazi, N., Larijani, B., Ayati, M. H., & Abdollahi, M. (2018). The effects of Nigella sativa L. on obesity: A systematic review and meta-analysis. *Journal of Ethnopharmacology*, 219, 173–181. https://doi.org/10.1016/j.jep.2018.03.001

238. Comparison of therapeutic effect of topical Nigella with Betamethasone and Eucerin in hand eczema. – PubMed – NCBI. (n.d.). Retrieved February 26, 2020, from https://www.ncbi.nlm.nih.gov/pubmed/23198836

239. Hamed, M. A., El-Rigal, N. S., & Ali, S. A. (2013). Effects of black seed oil on resolution of hepato-renal toxicity induced bybromobenzene in rats. *European Review for Medical and Pharmacological Sciences*, 17(5), 569–581.

240. Mashhadi, N. S., Ghiasvand, R., Askari, G., Hariri, M., Darvishi, L., & Mofid, M. R. (2013). Anti-Oxidative and Anti-Inflammatory Effects of Ginger in Health and Physical Activity: Review of Current Evidence. *International Journal of Preventive Medicine*, 4(Suppl 1), S36–S42.

241. Aghazadeh, M., Zahedi Bialvaei, A., Aghazadeh, M., Kabiri, F., Saliani, N., Yousefi, M., Eslami, H., & Samadi Kafil, H. (2016). Survey of the Antibiofilm and Antimicrobial Effects of Zingiber officinale (in Vitro Study). *Jundishapur Journal of Microbiology*, 9(2), e30167. https://doi.org/10.5812/jjm.30167

242. Rhode, J., Fogoros, S., Zick, S., Wahl, H., Griffith, K. A., Huang, J., & Liu, J. R. (2007). Ginger inhibits cell growth and modulates angiogenic factors in ovarian cancer cells. *BMC Complementary and Alternative Medicine*, 7, 44. https://doi.org/10.1186/1472-6882-7-44

243. Khandouzi, N., Shidfar, F., Rajab, A., Rahideh, T., Hosseini, P., & Mir Taheri, M. (2015). The Effects of Ginger on Fasting Blood Sugar, Hemoglobin A1c, Apolipoprotein B, Apolipoprotein A-I and Malondialdehyde in Type-2 Diabetic Patients. *Iranian Journal of Pharmaceutical Research: IJPR*, 14(1), 131–140.

244. Alizadeh-Navaei, R., Roozbeh, F., Saravi, M., Pouramir, M., Jalali, F., & Moghadamnia, A. A. (2008). Investigation of the effect of ginger on the lipid levels. A double blind controlled clinical trial. *Saudi Medical Journal*, 29(9), 1280–1284.

245. Hu, M.-L., Rayner, C. K., Wu, K.-L., Chuah, S.-K., Tai, W.-C., Chou, Y.-P., Chiu, Y.-C., Chiu, K.-W., & Hu, T.-H. (2011). Effect of ginger on gastric motility and symptoms of functional dyspepsia. *World Journal of Gastroenterology: WJG*, 17(1), 105–110. https://doi.org/10.3748/wjg.v17.i1.105

246. McMaster University. (2018, August 9). Pass the salt: Study finds average consumption safe for heart health: Public health strategies should be based on best evidence. ScienceDaily. Retrieved April 11, 2021 from www.sciencedaily.com/releases/2018/08/180809202057.htm.

247. Organic Foods vs Supermarket Foods: Element Levels. (n.d.). Retrieved February 27, 2020, from http://journeytoforever.org/farm_library/bobsmith.html.

248. Environmental Working Group. 2017 shopper's guide to pesticides in produce. http://www.ewg.org/foodnews/summary.php.

249. Bassil KL, Vakil C, Sanborn M, et al. Cancer health effects of pesticides: systemic review. *Can Fam Physician*. 2007 Oct;53 (10):1704–11.

250. Priyadarshi A, Khuder SA, Schaub EA, et al. A meta-analysis of Parkinson's disease and exposure to pesticides. *Neurotoxicology*. 2000 Aug;21(4):435–40.

251. Beard JD, Umback DM, Hoppin JA, et al. Pesticide exposure and depression among male private pesticide applicators in the agricultural health study. *Environ Health Perspect*. 2014 Sept;122 (9):984–91.

252. B. Smith, "Organic Foods vs Supermarket Foods: Element Levels," *Journal of Applied Nutrition* (1993).

253. Curl CL, Beresford SAA, Fenske RA, et al. Estimating pesticide exposure from (MESA). *Environ Health Perspect.* 2015 May;123 (5):475–83.

254. Heyman MB. Lactose intolerance in infants, children and adolescents. *Pediatrics.* 2006 Sep; 118 (3):1279–86.

255. Danby FW. Acne, dairy and cancer: the 5alpha-P link. *Dermatoendocrinol.* 2009 Jan; 1(1):12–16.

256. Hochwallner H, Schulmeister U, Swoboda I, et al. Microarray and allergenic activity assessment of milk allergens. *Clin Exp Allergy.* 2010 Dec; 40 (12)1809–18.

257. Azzouz, Abdelmonaim, Beatriz Jurado-Sánchez, Badredine Souhail, and Evaristo Ballesteros. "Simultaneous Determination of 20 Pharmacologically Active Substances in Cow's Milk, Goat's Milk, and Human Breast Milk by Gas Chromatography–Mass Spectrometry." *Journal of Agricultural and Food Chemistry* 59, no. 9 (May 2011): 5125–32. doi:10.1021/jf200364w.

258. Carroccio A, Brusca I, Mansueto P, et al. Fecal assays detect hypersensitivity to cow's milk protein and gluten in adults with irritable bowel syndrome. *Clin Gastroenterol Hapatol.* 2011 Nov;9 (11):965–71.

259. Aune D, Navarro Rosenblatt DA, Chan DS, et al. Dairy products, calcium, and prostate cancer: a systemic review and meta-analysis of cohort studies. *Am J Clin Nutr.* 2015 Jan;101 (1): 87–117.

260. Katta R, Schlickte M. Diet and dermatitis: food triggers. *J Clin Aesthet Dermatol.* 2014 Mar; 7(3):30–36

261. Howchwallner H, Schulmeister U, Swoboda I, et al. Cow's milk allergy: from allergens to new forms of diagnosis, therapy and prevention. *Methods.* 2014 Mar;66 (1):2–33.

262. Lill C, Loader B, Seemann R, et al. Milk allergy is frequent in patients with chronic sinusitis and nasal polyposis. *Am J Rhinol Allergy.* 2011 Nov-Dec; 25 (6):e221–e224.

263. You're Drinking the Wrong Kind of Milk – Mother Jones. (n.d.). Retrieved February 27, 2020, from https://www.motherjones.com/environment/2014/03/a1-milk-a2 -milk-america/.

264. Deth R, Clarke A, Ni J, Trivedi M. Clinical evaluation of glutathione concentration after consumption of milk containing different subtypes of B-casein: results from randomized, cross-over clinical trial. *Nutr J. 2016* Sep 29; 15(1):82.

265. Elliott RB, Harris DP, Hill JP, Bibby NJ, Wasmuth HE. Type-1 (insulin dependent) diabetes mellitus and cow milk: casein variant consumption. *Diabetologia.* 1999 Mar; 42 (3): 292–96.

266. Eat Wild – Super Natural. (n.d.). Retrieved February 27, 2020, from http://www .eatwild.com/articles/superhealthy.html.

267. Centre for Disease Control and Prevention, "Trends in Intake of Energy and Macronutrients in Adults from 1999–2000 through 2007–2008, *NCHS Data Brief* no. 49, November 2010.

268. Nutrients | Free Full-Text | The Dietary Intake of Wheat and other Cereal Grains and Their Role in Inflammation. (n.d.). Retrieved February 27, 2020, from https://www .mdpi.com/2072-6643/5/3/771.

269. Articles – Food and Nutrition Sciences – SCIRP. (n.d.). Retrieved February 27, 2020, from https://www.scirp.org/journal/allarticle.aspx?journalid=208.

270. Ludvigsson, Jonas F., Johan Reutfors, Urban Ösby, Anders Ekbom, and Scott M. Montgomery. "Coeliac Disease and Risk of Mood Disorders – A General Population-Based Cohort Study." *Journal of Affective Disorders* 99, no. 1–3 (April 2007): 117–26. doi:10.1016/j.jad.2006.08.032.

271. Millward, C., M. Ferriter, S. Calver, and G. Connell-Jones. "Gluten- and Casein-free Diets for Autistic Spectrum Disorder." Cochrane Database of Systematic Reviews, April 2004. doi:10.1002/14651858.cd003498.pub2.

272. Hu, W. T., Murray, J. A., Greenaway, M. C., Parisi, J. E., & Josephs, K. A. (2006). Cognitive Impairment and Celiac Disease. *Archives of Neurology*, 63(10), 1440–1446. https://doi.org/10.1001/archneur.63.10.1440.

273. Ludvigsson, Jonas F. "Small-Intestinal Histopathology and Mortality Risk in Celiac Disease." *JAMA* 302, no. 11 (September 2009): 1171. doi:10.1001/jama.2009.1320

274. Byrnes SE, Miller JC, Denyer GS. Amylopectin starch promotes the development of insulin resistance in rats. *J Nutr.* 1995 Jun;125 (6):1430–37.)

275. Punzi, John S., Martha Lamont, Diana Haynes, and Robert L. Epstein. "USDA Pesticide Data Program: Pesticide Residues on Fresh and Processed Fruit and Vegetables, Grains, Meats, Milk, and Drinking Water." *Outlooks on Pest Management* 16, no. 3 (June 2005): 131–37. doi:10.1564/16jun12.

276. Wang, Wen Le. "Zonula Occludin Toxin, a Microtubule Binding Protein." World Journal of Gastroenterology 6, no. 3 (2000): 330. doi:10.3748/wjg.v6.i3.330. Fasano, A. "Zonulin and Its Regulation of Intestinal Barrier Function: The Biological Door to Inflammation, Autoimmunity, and Cancer." *Physiological Reviews* 91, no. 1 (January 2011): 151–75. doi:10.1152/physrev.00003.2008.

277. Fasano, Alessio. "Intestinal Permeability and Its Regulation by Zonulin: Diagnostic and Therapeutic Implications." *Clinical Gastroenterology and Hepatology* 10, no. 10 (October 2012): 1096–100. doi:10.1016/j.cgh.2012.08.012.

278. Bernardo, D., J. A. Garrote, L. Fernandez-Salazar, S. Riestra, and E. Arranz. "Is Gliadin Really Safe for Non-Coeliac Individuals? Production of Interleukin 15 in Biopsy Culture from Non-Coeliac Individuals Challenged with Gliadin Peptides." *Gut* 56, no. 6 (June 2007): 889–90. doi:10.1136/gut.2006.118265.

279. Behall, K. M., Scholfield, D. J., Yuhaniak, I., & Canary, J. (1989). Diets containing high amylose vs amylopectin starch: Effects on metabolic variables in human subjects.

The American Journal of Clinical Nutrition, 49(2), 337–344. https://doi.org/10.1093 /ajcn/49.2.337.

280. Koehler, Peter, Georg Hartmann, Herbert Wieser, and Michael Rychlik. "Changes of Folates, Dietary Fibre, and Proteins in Wheat As Affected by Germination." *Journal of Agricultural and Food Chemistry* 55, no. 12 (June 2007): 4678–83. doi:10.1021/ jf0633037.

281. De Punder, K., & Pruimboom, L. (2013). The Dietary Intake of Wheat and other Cereal Grains and Their Role in Inflammation. *Nutrients*, 5(3), 771–787. https://doi .org/10.3390/nu5030771.

282. US Department of Agriculture. Adoption of genetically engineered crops in the U. S.: recent trends in GE adoption. November 3, 2016.

283. Sun Q, Spiegelman D, van Dam RM, et al. White rice, brown rice, and risk of Type-2 diabetes in US men and women. *Arch Intern Med.* 2010 June 14:170 (11):961–69. If you are going to have rice, make sure to eat traditional coloured varieties of rice, as it continues more antioxidants, and antiallergic protection. Deng GF, Xu XR, Zhang Y, et al. Phenolic compounds and bioactivites of pigmented rice. *Crit Rev Food Sci Nutr.* 2013; 53 (3):296–306.

284. Consumer Reports. Arsenic-in-your-food/index.htm. November 2012. Consumer Reports. How much arsenic is in your rice? http://www.consumerreports.org/cro /magazine/205/01/how-much-arsenic-is-in-your-rice/index.htm. January 2015.

285. Ebbeling CB, Swain JF, Feldman HA, et al. Effects of dietary composition on energy expenditure during weight- loss maintenance. *JAMA.* 2012 Jun 27;307 (24):2627–34.) (Ludwig DS, Majzoub JA, Al-Zahrani A, Dallal GE, Blanco I, Roberts SB. High gly-caemic index foods, overeating and obesity. *Pediatrics.* 1999 Mar;103 (3):E26.

286. Ravnskov U, Diamond DM, Hama R, et al. Lack of an association or an inverse asso-ciation between low density-lipoprotein cholesterol and mortality in the elderly: a sys-temic review, *BMJ Open.* 2016 Jun 12;6 (6):e010401.

287. Nutrition for Optimal Health Association. "Review of: Excitotoxins: The Taste that Kills." Nutrition Digest 38, No. 2 (1995). http://americannutritionassociation.org /newsletter/review-excitotoxins-taste-kills.

288. Kobylewski and Jacobson, "Food Dyes: A Rainbow of Risks."

289. Ibid.

290. International Agency for Research on Cancer, "Agents Classified by the IARC Monographs, Volumes 1–121."

291. Walsh, Bryan. "Do the Chemicals That Turn Soda Brown Also Cause Cancer?" *Time,* February 17, 2011. http://healthland.time.com/2011/02/17/do-the-chemicals-that-t urn-soda-brown-also-cause-cancer/; *Centre for Science in the Public Interest.* "Petition to bar the use of caramel colourings produced with ammonia and containing certain carcinogens." February 16, 2011. http://cspinet.org/resource/petition-bar-use-carmel -colourings-produced-ammonia-and-containing-certain-carcinogens.

292. Jing Ye et al. " Assessment of the Dermination of Azodicarbonamide and Its Decomposition Poduct Semicarbazide: Investigation of Variation in Flour and Flour Products." *Journal of Agricultural and Food Chemistry* 59, no. 17 (2011): 9313–18. https://www.ncbi.nlm.nih.gov/pubmed/21786817, Lefferts, Lisa. "FDA Should Ban Azodicarbonamide, Says CSPI," *Centre for Science in the Public Interest*, February 4, 2014. https://cspinet.org/new/201402041.html.

293. Henriques, Martha. "Additive in breakfast cereals could make the brain 'forget' to stop eating." International Business Times, August 10, 2017. http://www.ibtimes.co.uk /additive-breakfast-cereals-could-make-brain-forget-stop-eating-1634413.,

294. Environmental Working Group. "EWG's Dirty Dozen Guide to Food Additives." https://www.ewg.org/research/ewg-s-dirty-dozen-guide-food-additives/generally -recognized-as-safe-but-is-it#.W4hygpNKiRs.

295. Dengate, S. and A. Ruben. "Controlled trial of cumulative behavioural effects of a common bread preservative." *Journal of Paediatrics and Child Health* 38 (202):373–76. https://www.nch.lm.hih.gov/pubmed/12173999.

296. Esmaillzadeh, A., & Azadbakht, L. (2008). Home use of vegetable oils, markers of systemic inflammation, and endothelial dysfunction among women. *The American Journal of Clinical Nutrition*, 88(4), 913–921. https://doi.org/10.1093/ajcn/88.4.913 ., Charlton, K. M. et al. "Cardiac Lesons in Rats Fed Rapeseed Oils." *Canadian Journal of Comparative Medicine* 39, no.3 (1975):261–69. https://www.ncbi.nlm.nih.gov/pmc /articles/PMC1277456/.

297. Lerner, Aaron, and Torsten Matthias. "Changes in Intestinal Tight Junction Permeability Associated with Industrial Food Additives Explain the Rising Incidence of Autoimmune Disease." *Autoimmunity Reviews* 14, no. 6 (June 2015):479–89. doi:10.1016/j.autrev.2015 .01.009.

298. Gupta, Raj Kishor, Shivraj Singh Gangoliya, and Nand Kumar Singh. "Reduction of Phytic Acid and Enhancement of Bioavailable Micronutrients in Food Grains." *Journal of Food Science and Technology* 52.2 (2015):676–84. https://www.ncbi.nlm.nih.gov /pmc/articles/PMC4325021/.

299. Kelley, Geri and Sarina Gleason."Common Additive May Be Why You Have Food Allergies." Michigan State University, July 11, 2016. http://msutoday.msu.edu/news /2016/common-additives-may-be-why-you-have-food-allergies/.

300. Santarelli, Raphaëlle, Fabrice Pierre, and Denis Corpet. "Processed Meat and Colourectal Cancer: A Review of Epidemiologic and Experimental Evidence." *Nutrition and Cancer* 60, no. 2 (March 2008): 131–44. doi:10.1080/01635580701684872.

301. Environmental Working Group, "Synthetic Ingredients in Natural Flavors and Natural Flavors in Artificial Flavors."

302. Charles, A. K. and P.D. Darbre. "Combinations of parabens at concentrations measure in human breast tissue can increase proliferation of MCF-7 human breast cancer cells." Journal of Applied *Toxicology* 33 (2013): 390–98. https://onlinelibrary.wiley.com/doi

/abs/10.1002/jat.2850; Khanna S., P. R. Dash, and P. D. Darbre. "Exposure to para-bens at the concentration of maximal proliferative response increases migratory and invasive activity of human breast cancer cells in vitro." *J. Appl. Toxicol.* 34 (2014):1051–59. https://onlinelibrary.wiley.com/doi/abs/10.1002/jat.3003.

303. Environmental Working Group, "EWG's Dirty Dozen Guide to Food Additives."

304. Ramsden, C. E., D. Zamora, B. Leelarthaepin, S. F. Majchrzak-Hong, K. R. Faurot, C. M. Suchindran, A. Ringel, J. M. Davis, and J. R. Hibbeln. "Use of Dietary Linoleic Acid for Secondary Prevention of Coronary Heart Disease and Death: Evaluation of Recovered Data from the Sydney Diet Heart Study and Updated Metaanalysis." *BMJ* 346, no. 3 (February 2013). doi:10.1136/bmj.e8707

305. Simopoulos, A. P. "Importance of the Ratio of Omega-6/Omega-3 Essential Fatty Acids: Evolutionary Aspects." World Review of Nutrition and Dietetics Omega-6/Omega-3 Essential Fatty Acid Ratio: The Scientific Evidence, 2003, 1–22. doi:10.1159/0000 73788.

306. Trans Fat Leads To Weight Gain Even on Same Total Calories, Animal Study Shows. (n.d.). Retrieved February 27, 2020, from https://www1.wakehealth.edu/News-Releases/2006/Trans_Fat_Leads_To_Weight_Gain_Even_on_Same_Total_Calories,_Animal_Study_Shows.htm.

307. Shining the Spotlight on Trans Fats | The Nutrition Source | Harvard T.H. Chan School of Public Health. (n.d.). Retrieved February 27, 2020, from https://www.hsph.harvard.edu/nutritionsource/what-should-you-eat/fats-and-cholesterol/types-of-fat/transfats/.

308. Slattery, M. L., Benson, J., Ma, K.-N., Schaffer, D., & Potter, J. D. (2001). Trans-Fatty Acids and Colon Cancer. Nutrition and Cancer, 39(2), 170–175. https://doi.org/10.1207/S15327914nc392_2. Chajès, Véronique, Anne C. M. Thiébaut, Maxime Rotival, Estelle Gauthier, Virginie Maillard, Marie-Christine Boutron-Ruault, Virginie Joulin, Gilbert M. Lenoir, and Françoise Clavel-Chapelon, (PDF) Association between Serum trans-Monounsaturated Fatty Acids and Breast Cancer Risk in the E3N-EPIC Study. (n.d.). Retrieved February 27, 2020, from https://www.researchgate.net/publication/5461399_Association_between_Serum_trans-Monounsaturated_Fatty_Acids_and_Breast_Cancer_Risk_in_the_E3N-EPIC_Study.

309. Wang Q P, Lin YQ, Zhang L, et al. Sucralose promotes food intake through NPY and a neuronal fasting response. Cell Metab. 2016 Jul 12;24 (1):75–90. Swithers SE, Davidson TL. A role of sweet taste: calorie predictive relations in energy regulation by rats. *Behav Neurosci.* 2008 Feb; 122 (1):161–73.

310. Maher TJ, Wurtman RJ. Possible neurologic effects of aspartame, a widely used food additive. *Environ Health Perspect.* 1987 Nov;75:53–57.

311. Suez J, Korem T, Zeevi D, et al. Artificial sweeteners induce glucose intolerance by altering the gut microbiota. *Nature.* 2014;514 (7521):181–86.

312. Ruiz-Ojeda, F. J., Plaza-Díaz, J., Sáez-Lara, M. J., & Gil, A. (2019). Effects of Sweeteners on the Gut Microbiota: A Review of Experimental Studies and Clinical Trials. *Advances*

in nutrition (Bethesda, Md.), 10(suppl_1), S31–S48. https://doi.org/10.1093/advances/nmy037

313. Soffritti M, Belpoggi (F, Manservigi M, et al. Aspartame administered in feed, beginning prenatally through life span, induces cancer of the liver and lung in male Swill mice. *Am J Ind Med.* 2010 Dec;53 (53 (12):1197–1206.

314. Schiffman, Susan S., and Kristina I. Rother. "Sucralose, A Synthetic Organochlorine Sweetener. Overview of Biological Issues." *Journal of Toxicology and Environmental Health*, Part B 16, no. 7 (October 2013): 399–451. doi:10.1080/10937404.2013.842523

315. Abou-Donia, Mohamed B., Eman M. El-Masry, Ali A. Abdel-Rahman, Roger E. Mclendon, and Susan S. Schiffman. "Splenda Alters Gut Microflora and Increases Intestinal P-Glycoprotein and Cytochrome P-450 in Male Rats." *Journal of Toxicology and Environmental Health*, Part A 71, no. 21 (September 2008): 1415–29. doi:10.1080/15287390802328630.

316. Nettleton, J. A., P. L. Lutsey, Y. Wang, J. A. Lima, E. D. Michos, and D. R. Jacobs. "Diet Soda Intake and Risk of Incident Metabolic Syndrome and Type-2 Diabetes in the Multi-Ethnic Study of Atherosclerosis (MESA)." *Diabetes Care* 32, no. 4 (January 2009): 688–94. doi:10.2337/dc08-1799.

317. Suez, Jotham, Tal Korem, David Zeevi, Gili Zilberman-Schapira, Christoph A. Thaiss, Ori Maza, David Israeli, Niv Zmora, Shlomit Gilad, Adina Weinberger, Yael Kuperman, Alon Harmelin, Ilana Kolodkin-Gal, Hagit Shapiro, Zamir Halpern, Eran Segal, and Eran Elinav. "Artificial Sweeteners Induce Glucose Intolerance by Altering the Gut Microbiota." *Obstetrical & Gynecological Survey* 70, no. 1 (January 2015): 31–32. doi:10.1097/01.ogx.0000460711.58331.94.

318. Yang Q. Gain weight by "going diet"? Artificial sweeteners and neurobiology of sugar cravings: Neuroscience 2010. *Yale Journal of Biology and Medicine.* 2010: 83 (2): 101–8.

319. https://www.nongmoproject.org/gmo-facts/.

320. "The Microbiome for Gastroenterologists." Gastroenterology & Endoscopy News. 2015; 66: 4.

321. Samsel A, Seneff S. Glyphosate, pathways to modern diseases II: celiac sprue and gluten intolerance. Interdisciplinary Toxicology. 2013; 6(4): 159–84. Samsel A, Seneff S. Glyphosate's suppression of cytcochrome P450 enzymes and amino acid biosynthesis by the gut microbiome: pathways to modern disease. *Entropy.* 2013; 15: 1416–63.

322. Stephen R. Padgette et al, "The Composition of Glyphosate-Tolerant Soybean Seeds Is Equivalent to That of Conventional Soybeans," *The Journal of Nutrition* 126, no. 4, (April 1996)

323. Soy disrupts the endocrine system, especially dysregulating thyroid and oestrogen, and interferes with leptin, leading to leptin resistance, making you overeat, leading to leaky gut syndrome (when remains undigested) as it stimulates the immune system to produce antibodies, food sensitivities, and inflammation. Glyphosate, pathways to modern

diseases II: Celiac sprue and gluten intolerance in: Interdisciplinary Toxicology Volume 6 Issue 4 (). (n.d.). Retrieved February 27, 2021, from https://content.sciendo.com /configurable/contentpage/journals$002fintox$002f6$002f4$002farticle-p159.xml.

324. Lenoir M, Serre F, Cantin L, Ahmed SH. Intense sweetness surpasses cocaine reward. *PLoS One* 2007 Aug 1;2 (8):e698.

325. Neuroreport, November 16, 2001; 12(16): 3549–52. Sugar stimulates the brain reward centres via the neurotransmitter dopamine like other addictive drugs.

326. Mastrocola R, Nigro D, Cento AS, et al. High-fructose intake as risk factor for neurogeneration:key role for carboxy methyllysine accumulation in mice hippocampal neurons. *Neurobiol Dis.* 2016 May;89:65–75.

327. Te Morenga LA, Howatson AJ, Jones RM, et al. Dietary sugars and cardiomtabolic effects on blood pressure and lipids. Am J Clin Nutr. 2014 Jul;100 (1): 65–79. Ruff RR. Sugar-sweetended beferage consumption is linked to global adult morbidity and mortality through diabetes mellitus, cardiovascular disease and adiposity-related cancers. *Evid Based Med.* 2015 Dec;20 (6):223–24.

328. Stephan BC, Wells JC, Brayne C, et al. Increased fructose intake as a risk factor for dementia. *J Gerontol A Biol Sci Med Sci.* 2010 Aug;65 (8): 809–14.

329. Felix DR, Costenaro F, Gottschall CB, et al. Non-alcoholic fatty liver disease 2016 Nov 15;16 (1): 187. Kavanagh K, Wylie AT, Tucker KL, et al. Dietary fructose induces endotoxemia and hepatic injury in calorically controlled primates. *Am J Clin Nutr.* 2013 Aug;98 (2):349–57.

330. Yang, Q., Zhang, Z., Gregg, E. W., Flanders, W. D., Merritt, R., & Hu, F. B. (2014). Added Sugar Intake and Cardiovascular Diseases Mortality Among US Adults. JAMA Internal Medicine, 174(4), 516–524. https://doi.org/10.1001/jamainternmed.2013 .13563.

331. Hootman KC, Trezzi JP, Kraemer L, et al. Erythritol is a pentose- phosphate pathway metabolite and associated with adiposity gain in young adults. Proc Natl Acad Sci US A. 2017 May 23;114 (21): E4233-E4240. doi:10.1073/pnas. 1620079114.

332. Purohit, Vishnudutt, J. Christian Bode, Christiane Bode, David A. Brenner, Mashkoor A. Choudhry, Frank Hamilton, Y. James Kang, Ali Keshavarzian, Radhakrishna Rao, R. Balfour Sartor, Christine Swanson, and Jerrold R. Turner, Alcohol, intestinal bacterial growth, intestinal permeability to endotoxin, and medical consequences: Summary of a symposium – ScienceDirect. (n.d.). Retrieved February 27, 2021, from https://www .sciencedirect.com/science/article/abs/pii/S0741832908002036?viapercent3Dihub.

Fasting

1. Tinsley, G. M., & La Bounty, P. M. (2015). Effects of intermittent fasting on body composition and clinical health markers in humans. Nutrition Reviews, 73(10), 661–674. https://doi.org/10.1093/nutrit/nuv041

Boston, 677 Huntington Avenue, & Ma 02115 +1495-1000. (2018, January 16). Diet Review: Intermittent Fasting for Weight Loss. *The Nutrition Source.* https://www.hsph .harvard.edu/nutritionsource/healthy-weight/diet-reviews/intermittent-fasting/

2. Arnason, T. G., Bowen, M. W., & Mansell, K. D. (2017). Effects of intermittent fasting on health markers in those with Type-2 diabetes: A pilot study. World Journal of Diabetes, 8(4), 154–164. https://doi.org/10.4239/wjd.v8.i4.154, Barnosky, A. R., Hoddy, K. K., Unterman, T. G., & Varady, K. A. (2014). Intermittent fasting vs daily caloric restriction for Type-2 diabetes prevention: A review of human findings. Translational Research, 164(4), 302–311. https://doi.org/10.1016/j.trsl.2014.05.013, Fasting-mimicking diet and markers/risk factors for aging, diabetes, cancer, and cardiovascular disease | Science Translational Medicine. (n.d.). Retrieved February 25, 2020, from https:// stm .sciencemag.org/content/9/377/eaai8700

3. Varady, K. A., Bhutani, S., Church, E. C., & Klempel, M. C. (2009). Short-term modi- fied alternate-day fasting: A novel dietary strategy for weight loss and cardioprotection in obese adults. *The American Journal of Clinical Nutrition,* 90(5), 1138–1143. https://doi .org/10.3945/ajcn.2009.28380

4. Carlson, A. J., & Hoelzel, F. (1946). Apparent prolongation of the life span of rats by intermittent fasting. *The Journal of Nutrition,* 31, 363–375. https://doi.org/10.1093/jn /31.3.363
    Sogawa, H., & Kubo, C. (2000). Influence of short-term repeated fasting on the lon- gevity of female (NZB×NZW)F1 mice. *Mechanisms of Ageing and Development,* 115(1), 61–71. https://doi.org/10.1016/S0047-6374(00)00109-3

5. S. Periyasamy-Thandavan et al., "Caloric Restriction and the Adipokine Leptin Alter the SDF-1 Signaling Axis in Bone Marrow and in Bone Marrow Derived Mesenchymal Stem Cells," Molecular and *Cellular Endocrinology* 410 (2015):64–72.

Detoxing Your Body with a *Ṭayyib* Environment

1. Bitto, Alessandra, Gabriele Pizzino, Natasha Irrera, Federica Galfo, and Francesco Squadrito. "Epigenetic Modifications Due to Heavy Metals Exposure in Children Living in Polluted Areas." Current Genomics. December 2014. Accessed February 25, 2020. http://www.ncbi.nlm.nih.gov/pmc/articles/PMC4311390/.

2. Shanna H. Swan, "Environmental phthalate exposure in relation to reproductive out- comes and other health endpoints in humans." *Environmental Research,* 108 (2), 2008 Oct:177–84, doi:10.1016/j.envres. 2008.08.007. Rishikesh Mankidy, et al., "Biological impact of phthalates." Toxicology Letters, 217, (2013): 50–58 http://www.usask.ca /toxicology/jgiesy/pdf/publications/JA-712.pdf.

3. Toxic effects of the easily avoidable phthalates and parabens. Walter J. Crinnion, *Altern Med Rev.* 2010 Sep; 15(3): 190–196.

4. Kim, S. A., Moon, H., Lee, K., & Rhee, M. S. (2015). Bactericidal effects of triclosan in soap both in vitro and in vivo. *Journal of Antimicrobial Chemotherapy*, 70(12), 3345–3352. https://doi.org/10.1093/jac/dkv275.

5. CFR – Code of Federal Regulations Title 21. (n.d.). Retrieved February 27, 2020, from https://www.accessdata.fda.gov/scripts/cdrh/cfdocs/cfcfr/cfrsearch.cfm.

6. Hellwig, E., & Lennon, Á. M. (2004). Systemic versus Topical Fluoride. *Caries Research*, 38(3), 258–262. https://doi.org/10.1159/000077764.

7. Neurobehavioural effects of developmental toxicity – The Lancet Neurology. (n.d.). Retrieved February 27, 2020, from https://www.thelancet.com/journals/laneur/article/PIIS1474-4422(13)70278-3/fulltext.

8. Beltrán-Aguilar ED, Barker L, Dye BA.Prevalence and severity of dental fluorosis in the United States, 1999–2004. NCHS data brief, no 53. Hyattsville, MD: National Centre for Health Statistics. 2010. Retrieved February 27, 2020, from. https://www.cdc.gov/nchs/data/databriefs/db53.pdf.

9. Konieczna, A., Rutkowska, A., & Rachoń, D. (2015). Health risk of exposure to Bisphenol A (BPA). Undefined. /paper/Health-risk-of-exposure-to-Bisphenol-A-(BPA).-Konieczna-Rutkowska/42fbd0f59c0e6935c65a24352e4ab0ecbb3086d6.

10. Rice, K. M., Walker, E. M., Wu, M., Gillette, C., & Blough, E. R. (2014). Environmental Mercury and Its Toxic Effects. *Journal of Preventive Medicine and Public Health*, 47(2), 74–83. https://doi.org/10.3961/jpmph.2014.47.2.74.

11. Hong, Y.-S., Song, K.-H., & Chung, J.-Y. (2014). Health Effects of Chronic Arsenic Exposure. *Journal of Preventive Medicine and Public Health*, 47(5), 245–252. https://doi.org/10.3961/jpmph.14.035

12. Dahiya, P., Kamal, R., Luthra, R. P., Mishra, R., & Saini, G. (2012). Miswak: A periodontist's perspective. *Journal of Ayurveda and Integrative Medicine*, 3(4), 184–187. https://doi.org/10.4103/0975-9476.104431

13. Bandara, Priyanka, et al., "Planetary Electromegnetic Pollution: It is Time to Assess Its Impact," Lancet Planetary Health 2, no.12 (December 2018): e512-14. doi:10.1016/S2542-5196(18)30221-3.

Part 2: Chapter 4

Stress

1. M. K. Hhasin et al., "Relaxation Response induces Temporal Transcriptome Changes in Energy Metabolism, Insulin Secretion and Inflammatory Pathways," *PLoS One 8*, no.5 (May2013): e 62817.

2. J. A. Rosenkranz, E.R. Venheim, and M. Padival, "Chronic Stress Causes Amygdala Hyperexcitability in Rodents," *Biol. Psychiatry* 67, no. 12 (June 2010):1128–36.

3. Kivimaki, M., D. A. Lawlor, A. Singh-Manoux, G. D. Batty, J. E. Ferrie, M. J. Shipley, H. Nabi, S. Sabia, M. G. Marmot, and M. Jokela. "Common Mental Disorder and Obesity: Insight from Four Repeat Measures over 19 Years: Prospective Whitehall II Cohort Study." *Bmj* 339, no. 2 (October 6, 2009). doi:10.1136/bmj.b3765.

4. Eriksson, A.-K., A. Ekbom, F. Granath, A. Hilding, S. Efendic, and C.-G. Stenson. "Psychological Distress and Risk of Pre-diabetes and Type2 Diabetes in a Prospective Study of Swedish Middle aged Men and Women." *Diabetic Medicine* 25, no. 7 (July 2008): 834–42. doi:10.1111/j.1464-5491.2008.02463.x.

5. Vogelzangs, Nicole, Aartjan T. F. Beekman, Yuri Milaneschi, Stefania Bandinelli, Luigi Ferrucci, and Brenda W. J. H. Penninx. "Urinary Cortisol and Six-Year Risk of All-Cause and Cardiovascular Mortality." *The Journal of Clinical Endocrinology & Metabolism* 95, no. 11 (November 2010): 4959–64. doi:10.1210/jc.2010-0192.

6. Johansson, L., X. Guo, M. Waern, S. Ostling, D. Gustafson, C. Bengtsson, and I. Skoog. "Midlife Psychological Stress and Risk of Dementia: A 35-Year Longitudinal Population Study." *Brain* 133, no. 8 (May 2010): 2217–24. doi:10.1093/brain/awq116.

7. Kuper, Hannah, Ling Yang, Tores Theorell, and Elisabete Weiderpass. "Job Strain and Risk of Breast Cancer." *Epidemiology* 18, no. 6 (November 2007): 764–68. doi:10.1097/ede.0b013e318142c534.

8. Rai, Dheeraj, Kyriaki Kosidou, Michael Lundberg, Ricardo Araya, Glyn Lewis, and Cecilia Magnusson. "Psychological Distress and Risk of Long-Term Disability: Population-based Longitudinal Study." *Journal of Epidemiology and Community Health* 66, no. 7 (March 2011):586–92. doi:10.1136/jech.2010.119644.

9. Aboa-Éboulé, Corine, Chantal Brisson, Elizabeth Maunsell, Benoît Mâsse, Renée Bourbonnais, Michel Vézina, Alain Milot, Pierre Théroux, and Gilles R. Dagenais. "Job Strain and Risk of Acute Recurrent Coronary Heart Disease Events." *JAMA* 298, no. 14 (October 2007): 1652. doi:10.1001/jama.298.14.1652.

10. Campos-Rodríguez, R. P., Godínez-Victoria, M. P., Abarca-Rojano, E. P., Pacheco-Yepez, J. P., Reyna-Garfias, H. M., Barbosa-Cabrera, R. E. P., & Drago-Serrano, M. E. (2013). Stress modulates intestinal secretory immunoglobulin A. *Frontiers in Integrative Neuroscience,* 7. https://doi.org/10.3389/fnint.2013.00086.

11. Vanuytsel, Tim, Sander Van Wanrooy, Hanne Vanheel, Christophe Vanormelingen, Sofie Verschueren, Els Houben, Shadea Salim Rasoel, Joran Tóth, Lieselot Holvoet, Ricard Farré, Lukas Van Oudenhove, Guy Boeckxstaens, Kristin Verbeke, and Jan Tack. "Psychological Stress and Corticotropin-Releasing Hormone Increase Intestinal Permeability in Humans by a Mast Cell-Dependent Mechanism." *Gut* 63, no. 8 (October 2013): 1293–99. doi:10.1136/gutjnl-2013-305690.

12. Vanuytsel, Tim, Sander Van Wanrooy, Hanne Vanheel, Christophe Vanormelingen, Sofie Verschueren, Els Houben, Shadea Salim Rasoel, Joran Tóth, Lieselot Holvoet, Ricard Farré, Lukas Van Oudenhove, Guy Boeckxstaens, Kristin Verbeke, and Jan Tack. "Psychological Stress and Corticotropin-Releasing Hormone Increase Intestinal

Permeability in Humans by a Mast Cell-Dependent Mechanism." *Gut* 63, no. 8 (October 2013): 1293–99. doi:10.1136/gutjnl-2013-305690.

13. Alcock, Joe, Carlo C. Maley, and C. Athena Aktipis. "Is Eating behaviour Manipulated by the Gastrointestinal Microbiota? Evolutionary Pressures and Potential Mechanisms." *BioEssays* 36, no. 10 (August 2014): 940–49. doi:10.1002/bies.201400071.

14. Kelly, John R., Paul J. Kennedy, John F. Cryan, Timothy G. Dinan, Gerard Clarke, and Niall P. Hyland. "Breaking Down the Barriers: The Gut Microbiome, Intestinal Permeability and Stress-Related Psychiatric Disorders." *Frontiers in Cellular Neuroscience* 9 (October 2015). doi:10.3389/fncel.2015.00392.

15. Mindfulness Matters | NIH News in Health. (n.d.). Retrieved February 27, 2020, from https://newsinhealth.nih.gov/2012/01/mindfulness-matters.

16. Bested, Alison C., Alan C. Logan, and Eva M. Selhub. "Intestinal Microbiota, Probiotics and Mental Health: From Metchnikoff to Modern Advances: Part II – Contemporary Contextual Research." *Gut Pathogens* 5, no. 1 (2013): 3. doi:10.1186/1757-4749-5-3

17. Bercik, P., A. J. Park, D. Sinclair, A. Khoshdel, J. Lu, X. Huang, Y. Deng, P. A. Blennerhassett, M. Fahnestock, D. Moine, B. Berger, J. D. Huizinga, W. Kunze, P. G. Mclean, G. E. Bergonzelli, S. M. Collins, and E. F. Verdu. "The Anxiolytic Effect of Bifidobacterium Longum NCC3001 Involves Vagal Pathways for Gut-Brain Communication." *Neurogastroenterology & Motility* 23, no. 12 (October 2011): 1132–39. doi:10.1111/j.1365-2982.2011.01796.x.

18. Bravo, J. A., Forsythe, P., Chew, M. V., Escaravage, E., Savignac, H. M., Dinan, T. G., Bienenstock, J., & Cryan, J. F. (2011). Ingestion of Lactobacillus strain regulates emotional behaviour and central GABA receptor expression in a mouse via the vagus nerve. Proceedings of the National Academy of Sciences, 108(38), 16050–16055. https://doi.org/10.1073/pnas.1102999108.

19. Schmidt, K., P. Cowen, C. J. Harmer, G. Tzortzis, and P. W. J. Burnet. "P.1.e.003 Prebiotic Intake Reduces the Waking Cortisol Response and Alters Emotional Bias in Healthy Volunteers." *European Neuropsychopharmacology* 24 (October 2014). doi:10.1016/s0924-977x(14)70294-9.

20. Li, L., Li, X., Zhou, W., & Messina, J. L. (2013). Acute psychological stress results in the rapid development of insulin resistance. *Journal of Endocrinology*, 217(2), 175–184. https://doi.org/10.1530/JOE-12-0559.

21. Harding, J. L., Backholer, K., Williams, E. D., Peeters, A., Cameron, A. J., Hare, M. J., Shaw, J. E., & Magliano, D. J. (2014). Psychosocial stress is positively associated with body mass index gain over 5 years: Evidence from the longitudinal AusDiab study. *Obesity*, 22(1), 277–286. https://doi.org/10.1002/oby.20423.

22. Wellen, K. E., & Hotamisligil, G. S. (2005). Inflammation, stress, and diabetes. *The Journal of Clinical Investigation*, 115(5), 1111–1119. https://doi.org/10.1172/JCI25102.

23. Hanson, Rick. "Relaxed and Contented: Activating the Parasympathetic Wave of Your Nervous System," Retrieved February 27, 2020, from https://www.wisebrain.org /ParasympatheticNS.pdf.

24. Koopman, F. A., Stoof, S. P., Straub, R. H., Maanen, M. A. van, Vervoordeldonk, M. J., & Tak, P. P. (2011). Restoring the Balance of the Autonomic Nervous System as an Innovative Approach to the Treatment of Rheumatoid Arthritis. Molecular Medicine, 17(9), 937 948. httpoi//doi.org/10.2119/molmed.2011.00065.

25. Wayne C. Zipperer and Steward T. A. Pickett, "Urban Ecology: Patterns of Population Growth and Ecological Effects," in *Encyclopedia of Life Sciences* (Chichester, UK: John Wiley & Sons, 2012), 1–8.

26. Numerous papers have covered the relationship between exposure to nature and human health. For a recent basic review, see M. A. Repke st al., "How Does Nature Exposure Make People Healthier?: Evidence for the Role of Impulsivity and Expanded Space Perception," *PLoS One* 13, no.8 (August 2018):e0202246.

27. Q. Li et al., "A Forest Bathing Trip Increases Human Natural Killer Activity and Expression of Anti-Cancer Proteins in Female Subjects," *J. Biol, Regul. Homeost.* Agents 22, no. 1 (January-March 2008):45–55.) and cognition (K. Sowndhararanjan and S. Kim, "Influence of Fragrances on Human Psychophysiological Activity: With Special Reference to Human Electroencephalographic Response," *Sci. Pharm.* 84, no.4 (November 2016):724–52.

28. L. Hilton et al., "Mindfulness Meditation for Chronic Pain: Systemic Review and Meta-Analysis," *Ann. Behav. Med.* 51, no.2 (April 2017): 199–213.

29. Tang, Y.-Y., Lu, Q., Feng, H., Tang, R., & Posner, M. I. (2015). Short-term meditation increases blood flow in anterior cingulate cortex and insula. *Frontiers in Psychology*, 6. https://doi.org/10.3389/fpsyg.2015.00212.

30. Marchiori, M. de F. R., Kozasa, E. H., Miranda, R. D., Andrade, A. L. M., Perrotti, T. C., & Leite, J. R. (2015). Decrease in blood pressure and improved psychological aspects through meditation training in hypertensive older adults: A randomized control study. *Geriatrics & Gerontology International*, 15(10), 1158–1164. https://doi.org/10.1111/ggi.12414.

31. Meditation: In Depth | NCCIH. (n.d.). Retrieved February 27, 2020, from https://nccih .nih.gov/health/meditation/overview.htm.

32. A. A. Taren, J. D. Creswell, and P. J. Gianaros, "Dispositional Mindfulness Co-Varies with Smaller Amygdala and Caudate Volumes in Community Adults," *PLoS One* 8, no.5 (May 2013):e64574.

33. Alcock, Joe, Carlo C. Maley, and C. Athena Aktipis. "Is Eating behaviour Manipulated by the Gastrointestinal Microbiota? Evolutionary Pressures and Potential Mechanisms." *BioEssays* 36, no. 10 (August 2014): 940–49. doi:10.1002/bies.201400071

34. Saatcioglu, F. (2013). Regulation of gene expression by yoga, meditation and related practices: A review of recent studies. *Asian Journal of Psychiatry*, 6(1), 74–77. https://doi .org/10.1016/j.ajp.2012.10.002.

35. D.S. Black and G. M. Slavich, "Mindfulness Meditation and the Immune System: A Systemic Review of Randomized Controlled Trials," *Ann. N. Y. Acad. Sci* 1373, no. 1 (June 2016): 13–24.

36. Y-Y. Tang, B. K. Holzel, and M. I. Posner, "The Neuroscience of Mindfulness Meditation," *Nat. Rev. Neurosci.* 16, no.4 (April 2015): 213–25.

37. Doufesh, H., Ibrahim, F., Ismail, N. A., & Wan Ahmad, W. A. (2014). Effect of Muslim Prayer (Salat) on α Electroencephalography and Its Relationship with Autonomic Nervous System Activity. Journal of Alternative and Complementary Medicine, 20(7), 558–562. https://doi.org/10.1089/acm.2013.0426

38. Saniotis, A. (2018). Understanding Mind/Body Medicine from Muslim Religious Practices of Salat and Dhikr. *Journal of Religion and Health*, 57(3), 849–857. https://doi .org/10.1007/s10943-014-9992-2

39. Al-Tuwayjirī, Muḥammad ibn Ibrāhīm. *Mawsū'at Fiqh Al-Qulūb*. (Ammān: Bayt al-Afkār al-Dawlīyah, 2006), 2:1997

40. Doufesh, H., Ibrahim, F., Ismail, N. A., & Wan Ahmad, W. A. (2014). Effect of Muslim Prayer (Salat) on α Electroencephalography and Its Relationship with Autonomic Nervous System Activity. Journal of Alternative and Complementary Medicine, 20(7), 558–562. https://doi.org/10.1089/acm.2013.0426

41. Doufesh, H., Ibrahim, F., & Safari, M. (2016). Effects of Muslims praying (Salat) on EEG gamma activity. Complementary Therapies in Clinical Practice, 24, 6–10. https:// doi.org/10.1016/j.ctcp.2016.04.004

42. Osama, M., & Malik, R. J. (2019). Salat (Muslim prayer) as a therapeutic exercise. JPMA. The Journal of the Pakistan Medical Association, 69(3), 399–404.

43. Hosseini, L., Lotfi Kashani, F., Akbari, S., Akbari, M. E., & Sarafraz Mehr, S. (2016). The Islamic Perspective of Spiritual Intervention Effectiveness on Bio-Psychological Health Displayed by Gene Expression in Breast Cancer Patients. *Iranian Journal of Cancer Prevention*, 9(2). https://doi.org/10.17795/ijcp-6360

44. D. Aune et al., "Physical Activity and the risk of Type-2 Diabetes: ASystemic Review and Dose-Respone Met-Analysis," *Eur. J. Epidemiol.* 30, no. 7 (July 2015): 529–42.

45. E. E. Hill et al., "Exercise and Circulating Cortisol Levles: The Intesity Threshold Effet," *J. Endol crinol.* Invest. 31, no. 7 (July 2008):587–91.

46. G. M. Cooney et al., "Exercise for Depression," *Cochrane Database Syst. Rev.* (September 2013): CD004366.

47. Vina, J., Sanchis-Gomar, F., Martinez-Bello, V., & Gomez-Cabrera, M. (2012). Exercise acts as a drug; the pharmacological benefits of exercise: Exercise acts as a drug. *British Journal of Pharmacology*, 167(1), 1–12. https://doi.org/10.1111/j.1476-5381.2012.01970.x.

48. Bartholomae E, Johnson Z, Moore J, Ward K, Kressler J. Reducing Glycaemic Indicators with Moderate Intensity Stepping of Varied, Short Durations in People with Pre-Diabetes. *J Sports Sci Med*. 2018;17(4):680-685. Published 2018 Nov 20.)

Sleep

1. Centres for Disease Control and Prevention, "Short Sleep Duration Amonth U.S. Adults", https://www.cdc.gov/sleep/data_statistics.hlml.

2. For access to a library of resources and data about sleep, see the National Sleep Foundation's website at SleepFoundation.org.

3. C. S. Moller-Level et al., "Effects of Insufficient Sleep on Circadioan Rhythmicity and Expression Amplitude of The Humin Blood Transcriptome," Proc. Natl. Acad. Sci. USA 110, no. 12 (March 2013):E1132–41.

4. Jackson, Melinda L., Ewa M. Sztendur, Neil T. Diamond, Julie E. Byles, and Dorothy Bruck. "Sleep Difficulties and the Development of Depression and Anxiety: A Longitudinal Study of Young Australian Women." *Archives of Women's Mental Health* 17, no. 3 (March 2014): 189–98. doi:10.1007/s00737-014-0417

5. T. B. Meier et al., "Relationship Between Neruotoxic Kynurenine Metabolites and Reduction in Right Medial Prefrontal Cortical Thickness in Major Depressive Disorder," *Brain Behav. Immun.* 53 (March 2016):39–48.

6. Sleep deprivation doubles risks of obesity in both children and adults. (n.d.). Retrieved February 27, 2020, from https://warwick.ac.uk/newsandevents/pressreleases /ne100000021440/.

7. J. S. Rihm et al., "Sleep Deprivation Selectively Upgrades an Amygdala-Hypothalamic Circuit Involved in Food Reward," *J. Neurosci.* 39, no. 5 (January 2019:888–99)

8. Patel, S. R., A. Malhotra, D. P. White, D. J. Gottlieb, and F. B. Hu. "Association between Reduced Sleep and Weight Gain in Women." *American Journal of Epidemiology* 164, no. 10 (September 2006): 947–54. doi:10.1093/aje/kwj280

9. M.R. Irwin, R. Olmstead, and J. E. Carroll, "Sleep Disturbance, Sleep Duration, and Inflammation: A Systemic Review and Meta-Analysis of Cohort Studies and Experimental Sleep Deprivation," Bio. Psychiatry 80, no. 1 (July 2016):40.

10. Sleep your way to a slimmer body | New Scientist. (n.d.). Retrieved February 27, 2020, from https://www.newscientist.com/article/mg19025535-600-sleep-your-way-to-a-slimmer -body/.

11. Känel, Roland Von, José S. Loredo, Sonia Ancoli-Israel, Paul J. Mills, Loki Natarajan, and Joel E. Dimsdale. "Association between Polysomnographic Measures of Disrupted Sleep and Prothrombotic Factors." *Chest* 131, no. 3 (March 2007): 733–39. doi:10.1378/ chest.06-2006.

12. J.J. Iliff et al.," A Parvascular Pathway Facilitates CSF Flow Through The Brain Parenchyma and the Clearance of Interstitial Solutes, Including Amyloid B, " *Sci. Transl. Med.* 4, no. 147 (August 2012):147ra111.

13. L, K. Barger et at., "Short Sleep Duration, Obstructive Sleep Apnea, Shiftwork, and the Risk of Adverse Cardiovascular Events in Patients After an Acute Coronary Syndrome,"*J. Am. Heart Associ.* 6, no.10 (October 2017):e006959.

14. C. W. Kim et., "Sleep Duration and Progression to Diabetes in People with Prediabetes Defined by HbA1c Concentration," *Diabet. Med.* 34, no.11 (November 2017): 1591–98.

15. P. James et al., "Outdoor Light at Night and Breast Cancer Incidence in the Nurses' Health Study II," *Environ. Health Perspec.* 125, no. 8 (August 2017): 087010.

16. Miles, A. (2011). PubMed Health. *Journal of the Medical Library Association: JMLA,* 99(3), 265–266. https://doi.org/10.3163/1536-5050.99.3.018

17. BaHammam, A. S. (2011). Sleep from an Islamic perspective. *Annals of Thoracic Medicine,* 6(4), 187–192. https://doi.org/10.4103/1817-1737.84771

Social Support

1. Kearns, A., Whitley, E., Tannahill, C., & Ellaway, A. (2015). Loneliness, Social Relations and Health and Well-being in Deprived Communities. *Psychology, Health & Medicine,* 20(3), 332–344. https://doi.org/10.1080/13548506.2014.940354

2. Engeland, C. G., Hugo, F. N., Hilgert, J. B., Nascimento, G. G., Junges, R., Lim, H.-J., Marucha, P. T., & Bosch, J. A. (2016). Psychological distress and salivary secretory immunity. Brain, behaviour, and Immunity, 52, 11–17. https://doi.org/10.1016/j.bbi.2015.08.017.

3. Uchino BN, Trettevik R, Kent de Grey RG, Cronan S, Hogan J, Baucom BRW. Social support, social integration, and inflammatory cytokines: A meta-analysis. Health Psychol. 2018 May;37(5):462-471. doi:10.1037/hea0000594. Epub 2018 Mar 22. PMID: 29565600.

4. Ford J, Anderson C, Gillespie S, Giurgescu C, Nolan T, Nowak A, Williams KP. Social Integration and Quality of Social Relationships as Protective Factors for Inflammation in a Nationally Representative Sample of Black Women. J Urban Health. 2019 Mar;96(Suppl 1):35-43. doi:10.1007/s11524-018-00337-x. PMID: 30617636; PMCID: PMC6430279.

5. Yeung, J. W. K., Zhang, Z., & Kim, T. Y. (2017). Volunteering and health benefits in general adults: Cumulative effects and forms. *BMC Public Health,* 18. https://doi.org/10.1186/s12889-017-4561-8

Spiritual Support

1. In praise of gratitude – Harvard Health Blog – Harvard Health Publishing. (n.d.). Retrieved February 27, 2020, from https://www.health.harvard.edu/blog/in-praise-of-gratitude-201211215561.

2. Mills, P. J., Redwine, L., Wilson, K., Pung, M. A., Chinh, K., Greenberg, B. H., Lunde, O., Maisel, A., Raisinghani, A., Wood, A., & Chopra, D. (2015). The role of gratitude in spiritual well-being in asymptomatic heart failure patients. *Spirituality in Clinical Practice,* 2(1), 5–17. https://doi.org/10.1037/scp0000050.

3. Fadardi, J. S., & Azadi, Z. (2017). The Relationship Between Trust-in-God, Positive and Negative Affect, and Hope. *Journal of Religion and Health*, 56(3), 796–806. https://doi.org/10.1007/s10943-015-0134-2.

4. Koenig, H. G. (2012). Religion, Spirituality, and Health: The Research and Clinical Implications. *ISRN Psychiatry*, 2012. https://doi.org/10.5402/2012/278730

5. Ghiasi, A., & Keramat, A. (2018). The Effect of Listening to Holy Qur'an Recitation on Anxiety: A Systematic Review. *Iranian Journal of Nursing and Midwifery Research*, 23(6), 411–420. https://doi.org/10.4103/ijnmr.IJNMR_173_17

6. Frih, B., Mkacher, W., Bouzguenda, A., Jaafar, H., ALkandari, S. A., Ben Salah, Z., Sas, B., Hammami, M., & Frih, A. (2017). Effects of listening to Holy Qur'an recitation and physical training on dialysis efficacy, functional capacity, and psychosocial outcomes in elderly patients undergoing haemodialysis. *The Libyan Journal of Medicine*, 12(1). https://doi.org/10.1080/19932820.2017.1372032

7. Saged, A. A. G., Mohd Yusoff, M. Y. Z., Abdul Latif, F., Hilmi, S. M., Al-Rahmi, W. M., Al-Samman, A., Alias, N., & Zeki, A. M. (2018). Impact of Qur'an in Treatment of the Psychological Disorder and Spiritual Illness. *Journal of Religion and Health*. https://doi.org/10.1007/s10943-018-0572-8

Part 3: Using Qur'an for Healing

1. Cortés-Giraldo, Isabel, Julio Girón-Calle, Manuel Alaiz, Javier Vioque, and Cristina Megías. "Hemagglutinating Activity of Polyphenols Extracts from Six Grain Legumes." *Food and Chemical* Toxicology 50, no. 6 (June 2012): 1951–54. doi:10.1016/j.fct.2012.03.071.

2. Sandberg, Ann-Sofie. "Bioavailability of Minerals in Legumes." *British Journal of Nutrition* 88, no. S3 (December 2002): 281. doi:10.1079/bjn/2002718

3. Greer F, Pusztai A. Toxicity of kidney bean (Phaseolus vulgaris)in rates: changes in intestinal permeability. *Digestion*. 1985;32 (1):42–46

4. Frauenknecht V, Theil S, Storm L, et al. Plasma levels of manna-binding lectin (MBL)-associated serine proteases (MASPs) and MBL-associated protein in cardio and cerebrovascular disease. *Clin Exp Immunolo*. 2013 Jul;173(1):112–20.)

5. Freed DLJ. Do dietary lectins cause disease? *BMJ*. 1999 Apr 17;318 (7190):1023–24.).

6. Nachbar MS, Oppenheim JD. Lectins in the United States diet: a survey of lectins in commonly consumed foods and a review of the literature. *Am J Clin Nutr*. 1980 Nov:33 (11):2338–45.)

7. Sisson M. The lowdown on lectins. Mark's Daily Apple. June 4, 2010.

8. Macfarlane BJ, Bezwoda WR, Bothwell TH, et al. Inhibitory effect of nuts on iron absoption. *AM J Clin Nutr*. 1988 Feb;47 (2): 270–74.

9. Prudden, John F., and Leslie L. Balassa. "The Biological Activity of Bovine Cartilage Preparations." Seminars in Arthritis and Rheumatism 3, no. 4 (June 1974): 287–321.

doi:10.1016/0049-0172(74)90003-1. Samonina, G., L. Lyapina, G. Kopylova, V. Pastorova, Z. Bakaeva, N. Jeliaznik, S. Zuykova, and I. Ashmarin. "Protection of Gastric Mucosal Integrity by Gelatin and Simple Proline-Containing Peptides." *Pathophysiology* 7, no. 1 (April 2000): 69–73. doi:10.1016/s0928-4680(00)00045-6

10. Mandel, David R., Katy Eichas, and Judith Holmes. "Bacillus Coagulans: A Viable Adjunct Therapy for Relieving Symptoms of Rheumatoid Arthritis according to a Randomized, Controlled Trial." *BMC Complementary and Alternative Medicine* 10, no. 1 (January 2010). doi:10.1186/1472-6882-10-1.

11. Hertzler, Steven R., and Shannon M. Clancy. "Kefir Improves Lactose Digestion and Tolerance in Adults with Lactose Maldigestion." *Journal of the American Dietetic Association* 103, no. 5 (May 2003): 582–87. doi:10.1053/jada.2003.50111

12. Guslandi, Mario, Patrizia Giollo, and Pier Alberto Testoni. "A Pilot Trial of Saccharomyces Boulardii in Ulcerative Colitis." *European Journal of Gastroenterology & Hepatology* 15, no. 6 (June 2003): 697–98. doi:10.1097/00042737-200306000-00017. Castagliuolo, I., L. Valenick, M. Riegler, Jt Lamont, and C. Pothoulakis. "Saccharomyces Boulardii Protease Inhibits Clostridium Difficile Toxin a and B-induced Effects in Human Colonic Mucosa." *Gastroenterology* 114 (April 1998). doi:10.1016/s0016-5085(98)83862-6. Buts, Jean-Paul, Nadine De Keyser, and Laurence De Raedemaeker. "Saccharomyces Boulardii Enhances Rat Intestinal Enzyme Expression by Endoluminal Release of Polyamines." *Pediatric Research* 36, no. 4 (October 1994): 522–27. doi:10.1203/00006450-199410000-00019.

13. Recent developments in prebiotics to selectively impact beneficial microbes and promote intestinal health. – PubMed – NCBI. (n.d.). Retrieved February 27, 2020, from https://www.ncbi.nlm.nih.gov/pubmed/25448231.

14. Katz, Uriel, Yehuda Shoenfeld, Varda Zakin, Yaniv Sherer, and Shaul Sukenik. "Scientific Evidence of the Therapeutic Effects of Dead Sea Treatments: A Systematic Review." *Seminars in Arthritis and Rheumatism* 42, no. 2 (October 2012): 186–200. doi:10.1016/j.semarthrit.2012.02.006.

15. Wegienka, G., C. C. Johnson, S. Havstad, D. R. Ownby, C. Nicholas, and E. M. Zoratti. "Lifetime Dog and Cat Exposure and Dog- and Cat-Specific Sensitization at Age 18 Years." *Clinical & Experimental Allergy* 41, no. 7 (June 2011): 979–86. doi:10.1111/j.1365-2222.2011.03747.x.

16. The implication of vitamin D and autoimmunity: A comprehensive review. – PubMed – NCBI. (n.d.). Retrieved February 27, 2020, from https://www.ncbi.nlm.nih.gov/pubmed/23359064.

17. Magnesium in disease. (n.d.). Retrieved February 27, 2020, from https://www.ncbi.nlm.nih.gov/pmc/articles/PMC4455821/.

18. Suboptimal magnesium status in the United States: Are the health consequences underestimated? – PubMed – NCBI. (n.d.). Retrieved February 27, 2020, from https://www.ncbi.nlm.nih.gov/pubmed/22364157.

19. The multifaceted and widespread pathology of magnesium deficiency. – PubMed – NCBI. (n.d.). Retrieved February 27, 2020, from https://www.ncbi.nlm.nih.gov /pubmed/11425281.

20. Hypomagnesemia and cardiovascular system. (n.d.). Retrieved February 27, 2020, from https://www.ncbi.nlm.nih.gov/pmc/articles/PMC2464251/.

21. The multifaceted and widespread pathology of magnesium deficiency. – PubMed – NCBI. (n d). Retrieved February 27, 2020, from https://www.ncbi.nlm.nih.gov /pubmed/11425281.

22. Surette, M. E., J. Whelan, K. S. Broughton, and J. E. Kinsella. "Evidence for Mechanisms of the Hypotriglyceridemic Effect of N – 3 Polyunsaturated Fatty Acids." Biochimica Et Biophysica Acta (*BBA – Lipids and Lipid Metabolism*) 1126, no. 2 (June 1992): 199–205. doi:10.1016/0005-2760(92)90291-3.

23. Omega-3 Fatty Acids and Our Health – Wake Internal Medicine. (n.d.). Retrieved February 27, 2020, from https://wakeinternalmedicine.com/omega-3-fatty-acids -health/.

24. *Nutr Cancer* (2010) 62:284–96; *Cancer Prev Res.* (2011) 2062–71; *Cancer* (2011); 117: 3774–80.

25. Yurko-Mauro K, Kralovec J, Bailey-Hall E, et al.Similar eicosapentaenoic acid and docosakexaenoic acid plasma level achieved with fish oil or krill oil in a randomized double-blind four-week bioavailbility study. *Lipids Health Dis.* 2015 Sep 2;14–99.

About the Author

Madiha Saeed, MD, also known as HolisticMom, MD on social media, is a practising board-certified family physician in the USA, a health influencer, international speaker, and best-selling author. Her best-selling books include: *The Holistic Rx: Your Guide to Healing Chronic Inflammation and Disease*, a best-selling functional medicine children's book series, *Adam's Healing Adventures Series* (one of Dr. Mark Hyman's favourite pics), *The Pandemic Prescription: Restoring Hope from the Qur'an, Sunnah and Science,* and *The Holistic Rx for Kids: Parenting Healthy Brains and Bodies in a Changing World.*

Dr Saeed is the current president of Nagamia Institute of Islamic Medicine and Sciences, director of education of Documenting Hope and KnoWEwell and on sits other medical advisory boards including Wellness Mama. Dr Saeed and her children speak internationally at the most prestigious holistic conferences, summits, radio, newspapers, and TV (ABC, NBC and CBS), and podcasts (including Mind Body Green). She is a regular on the international Emmy-winning medical talk show, The Dr. Nandi Show.

Dr Saeed's children host "The Holistic Kids' Show" podcast, interviewing the biggest names in the functional, holistic, and integrative medicine world, helping kids empower and educate other kids. She started a channel with her mother-in-law Tahira Mumtaz called Holistic Urdu, MD together impacting millions of lives. She and her family speak internationally, igniting the world with their energy and passion to ignite a healing revolution to save our children.

Index

worries, 132, 141–142, 158, 184–186, 189

worship, 26–29, 32–33, 39, 53, 141, 143–146, 162–163, 185–186, 194–195, 229

X

xenoestrogens, 115

Y

yeast, 48, 50, 200, 202, 204, 214, 222
yoga, 147, 154
yoghurt, 94, 203, 234, 236–237
youth, 170–171

Z

Zakāt, 167–168
zinc, 72–73, 88, 93, 97, 107, 204, 209, 220, 246
zucchini, 63, 106, 129, 255–256